ADDITIONAL PRAISE

D0362491

DISCARD

"The worldwide trend toward delayed m_____ r women. But does having children later in life really give more life choices and freedoms for women worldwide? Using her creative insights and keen intellect, Selvaratnam tells her personal story. Read this book and reflect on her unique Asian American journey."

—Soon-Young Yoon,
United Nations representative
for the International Alliance of Women

"Through detailed research and personal insights, Selvaratnam sheds light on one of the most important issues facing women in today's society—that is, infertility. [She] bravely shares her story so that we can all reexamine our notions of how a family is built. This book not only arms us with the information, guidance, and support to face infertility but also provides the honesty, vulnerability, and hope to comfort us."

—Mindy Berkson, infertility consultant, Lotus Blossom Consulting

"Forty may be the new thirty, and women are looking and feeling younger than their years—but try telling that to your ovaries! There is a disconnect between what women see in the mirror and what's happening to their reproductive organs. Selvaratnam's book will help women better understand their biological age and fertility health. It will also educate on the incredible advances being made in fertility treatment so that women are informed about their fertility options and choices."

—Carole Kowalczyk, MD,
board-certified reproductive endocrinologist;
director, Michigan Center for Fertility and Women's Health

"This book will be a wake-up call for the many women who are (voluntarily or involuntarily) postponing reproduction. I applaud the desire of Selvaratnam to dispel myths and tell the truth about the 'biological clock.' We cannot 'rewind' it, but today we can stop it with egg freezing. This technology is powerful, revolutionary, and will change the lives of women in the twenty-first century."

—Pasquale Patrizio, MD, MBE, professor,
reproductive bioethicist, and director, Yale Fertility Center

THE BIG LIE

THE BIG LIE

MOTHERHOOD, FEMINISM, AND THE REALITY OF THE BIOLOGICAL CLOCK

Tanya Selvaratnam

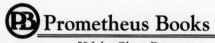 **Prometheus Books**

59 John Glenn Drive
Amherst, New York 14228

Published 2014 by Prometheus Books

Prometheus Books recognizes the following registered trademarks, trademarks, and service marks mentioned within the text: BabyCenter®, Clomid®, Colace®, Dave Thomas Foundation for Adoption®, Dilaudid®, Eggsurance™, Extend Fertility®, Facebook®, *Fertility and Sterility*®, Forever 21®, iPeriod®, Girls Inc.® , Gonal-F®, Google®, Growing Generations®, Life Raft Group®, Lehman Brothers®, Live**Strong**®, Lupron®, MAKERS®, McDonalds®, Menopur®, MoveOn.org®, My Mobile Fertility®, National Infertility Awareness Week 2012®, Oleg Cassini®, OvaScience®, Patients beyond Borders®, Planned Parenthood®, Race for the Family®, RESOLVE®, Schering-Plough®, Skype®, SpermCheck Fertility®, Sprout™, Vicodin®, Vivelle®, Whole Foods®, *Wikipedia*®, Yaddo®, Yahoo!®.

Cover image © Tony Cordoza/Media Bakery
Cover design by Jacqueline Nasso Cooke

Inquiries should be addressed to
Prometheus Books
59 John Glenn Drive • Amherst, New York 14228
VOICE: 716–691–0133 • FAX: 716–691–0137
WWW.PROMETHEUSBOOKS.COM

18 17 16 15 14   5 4 3 2 1

Library of Congress Cataloging-in-Publication Data

Selvaratnam, Tanya.
    The big lie : motherhood, feminism, and the reality of the biological clock / Tanya Selvaratnam.
        pages cm
    Includes bibliographical references and index.
    ISBN 978-1-61614-845-4 (pbk.) • ISBN 978-1-61614-846-1 (ebook)
    1. Miscarriage—Personal narratives. 2. Motherhood—Age factors. 3. Generative organs, Female—Aging. 4. Feminism. I. Title.

RG648.S438 2014
618.3'9—dc23

2013031767

Printed in the United States of America

for my mother

how can I give you
        all your due
               take courage from your courage

                  —from "Heroines" by Adrienne Rich,
                  Later Poems: Selected and New, 1971–2012

Some names have been omitted to protect the privacy of the individuals involved.

CONTENTS

INTRODUCTION

For all the news stories about age and infertility, egg freezing, sperm donation, in vitro fertilization (IVF), and the like, many women believe in the fantasy that they can become mothers on their own timetables. Thinking you can have kids when you are ready is a flawed belief with devastating consequences. I am one of millions who made that mistake.

There are excellent books by authors such as Amy Richards and Peggy Orenstein that address the interplay of feminism and the biological clock. What I've tried to do in this book is draw from earlier writings, update the research, present different points of view, and offer my personal experience.

This is a story of heartbreak and self-discovery for which no class or book could have prepared me. I work in the arts, as a performer and producer. When I was in college, I heard a quote attributed to the choreographer Pina Bausch: "Art can be anything. The cosmos is large. I am just a discoverer." I have thought about this quote a great deal over the years, but I've replaced the word "art" with "life." I lost a lot along the way as I attempted to become a mother. I went from trying hard to make a new life to having to save my own to feeling like my life was over. There is so much pressure on women with regard to our reproductive selves that we face an enormous amount of guilt when we have an abortion, a miscarriage, or an unsuccessful fertility treatment. I've had all three. One goal of this book is to strip away the guilt women might feel and to normalize the discourse around these issues. Approximately one out of three women will have an abortion before the age of forty-five; as much as 25 percent of all clinically recognized pregnancies end in miscarriage; and the majority of IVF cycles fail (as high as 77 percent of cycles performed worldwide).[1]

In my research, I spoke with fertility doctors, health professionals, adoption counselors, and sociologists and found that many came to their fields because of a personal experience. Mindy Berkson is the founder of an infertility consultancy in Illinois, the seventh highest-rated state in the

United States for IVF use.[2] She started as a venture capitalist but stopped working after she had a daughter. One year later, when she wanted another child, Berkson told me, "I found myself in the world of infertility as a patient. I spent three and a half years trying to conceive. I felt very lost, not knowing what questions to ask or how to find resolution. I always wondered why there was no advocate for me. Subsequently, what I found as a patient in this industry was a passion. I married that passion with my venture background and created an advocacy niche."[3] Dr. Arthur Greil, a sociology professor at Alfred University in New York, told me: "My wife and I spent several years in the mid-eighties (we were in our early thirties) trying to get pregnant. A colleague of mine was also in the same situation. We were talking one day about needing a new research topic. I suggested adoption, and he said he'd rather do infertility."[4]

This book is about the wisdom I have gleaned by talking to experts and people around the country, as much as it is about my own journey to become a mother. I look at how delaying motherhood intersects with feminism, reproductive science, evolution, popular culture, global economics, female friendships, and governmental policies. I hope this book compels others to reexamine their notions of how families are built and of how we define ourselves—whether we become parents or don't. I especially hope that in writing this book I can arm others with the knowledge they need to make smarter choices about their futures.

CHAPTER 1

A WOULD-BE MOTHER'S LAMENT

Most women my age have a story to tell about miscarriage or infertility—their own or a friend's.

I got married at thirty-seven and was pregnant two months later. I think most women probably remember the exact moment they knew they were pregnant. I know I do. My husband, Jay, and I were in Budapest, working on a show that he directed and I produced. We were taking a break at the Szechenyi Baths, the largest medicinal baths in all of Europe. As I stood in the outdoor thermal bath with steam rising into the cool November air, I felt dizzy. My eyes couldn't focus. I thought, *Maybe it's the steam*. But later that evening, I couldn't look at a glass of wine, and the smell of cigarette smoke made me ill.

Then my period didn't come. Sitting next to Jay on the flight home, I looked at him differently. He wasn't just my husband and collaborator; he was the father of our child. When we got back to New York, we went to see my ob/gyn, and there, on the ultrasound screen, was a fetus. My doctor said it was around eight weeks old. Jay and I listened to the heartbeat together and gazed at the screen at what looked like a real baby. We saw the tiny thing bounce a little, and we thought we saw it wave.

I immediately told everyone. I was beaming and convinced I was showing already. I was excited to tell my mother because for once I was doing what she wanted—I had finally gotten married and was going to have a child. She was in Sri Lanka, where I was born, when I broke the news. She asked if she could tell her family, and I said yes. At a holiday dinner, she stood up and announced, "There's going to be a new member of the family." My aunts and uncles—her seven siblings—were horrified because they thought she meant that she was marrying again (my father had passed away in 1994). They were relieved and overjoyed to find out that I was going to have a baby.

A few weeks later, Jay left the country for a month to teach an acting workshop in Salzburg. It was fine for him to be away, or so I thought, in those early stages of my pregnancy. I had friends to lean on and arranged for one to take me to my first trimester screening. I'm not usually prone to anxiety, but I was shaking with nerves the night before the visit. My teeth chattered, even though the heat was on. I felt paralyzed and couldn't call anyone. My brain was buzzing. I drank a cup of warm milk to calm myself down and eventually drifted into sleep.

My friend dropped me off at St. Vincent's Hospital in New York, which has since closed. The waiting room had a lumpy, dark-pink carpet and chairs with burgundy floral upholstery. In a surreal moment, Thom Filicia from the television show *Queer Eye for the Straight Guy* walked by. He was touring the hospital with the staff and talking about redecorating. I smiled and hoped the place would be redone by the time I had my baby.

In the ultrasound room, I had a sudden urge to go to the bathroom. I saw a tiny spot of blood on my underpants but didn't think anything of it. I sat in the reclining chair until the doctor arrived. As he put the scanner on my belly, I felt something was wrong because he was quiet and avoiding my eyes. Then he said, "I'm so sorry. There's no heartbeat." He called my ob/gyn, who told me to come to her office right away.

When I got on the 2/3 subway at 14th Street, I thought, *I can get through this*. Being in contact with other people, strangers on the subway, forced me to hold it together. *What point would there be to breaking down and crying in front of them?*

Almost twenty years before—when I went to have an abortion, walking into a clinic past protesters holding bloody baby dolls and crudely made posters of embryos, with two friends on either side of me locking their arms into mine for support—I couldn't have predicted the journey I would take when I tried to have a child. I didn't feel good about having an abortion, but at that time, my studies were more important. Also, I wasn't in the right place in my life to have a child. I wasn't in a steady relationship, and I was too young.

As I progressed through my twenties, finding a partner and having a child were not priorities. That was the path of my mother's generation, which my peers and I sought to avoid. Our mothers even encouraged us to be different from them. As Isolde Brielmaier, an art curator based between Savannah, Georgia, and New York City who had a child at the age of thirty-nine, said, "My mother had both me and my brother while she was in her late teens and early twenties, so she really encouraged me to live life to the fullest and focus on my own dreams and development before thinking about having children."[1] Laura Dawn, a Brooklyn-based creative director, said, "My mother frequently told me kids would 'ruin my life' and encouraged me to get an education and get out of Iowa."[2]

Almost every woman I spent time with was focusing on everything but settling down. I had one close friend from high school and one from college who were in their twenties when they had children. Today, they are still in the minority among my good friends. I always loved kids and hoped to have them one day, but first I wanted to have a career and earn my own money. I didn't want to have kids without the right partner, and it took me until my mid-thirties to find that person.

According to a Pew study that was conducted in 2008, approximately 18 percent of women in America do not have children by the end of their childbearing years. That year, there were 1.9 million childless women between the ages of forty and forty-four, compared with 580,000 in 1976.[3] A few years earlier CNN reported an "epidemic of childlessness" sparked in part by women adopting a "male model of single-mindedness" when it came to their careers.[4] I wouldn't say that I was single-mindedly focused on my career. In my case, it had as much to do with circumstance—I wasn't focused on identifying a partner; I didn't put myself in situations where I was likely to meet one; and he didn't magically appear.

I frequently performed with two theater companies that toured around the world, so I was never at home for long stretches of time. As a result, I spent my late twenties and early thirties having a series of short-term relationships, none of which lasted more than a few months. In my thirties, I began to long for stability. I was tired of being on the road, so I started producing films and events. But I never met the right guy.

Only after Jay and I got together, when I was thirty-five, did I seriously think about starting a family. We didn't, however, have the most romantic beginning. We met in November 2006 when a friend who worked at the theater where Jay was directing a show dragged me to a bar on East 7th Street and 1st Avenue in Manhattan. She wanted to introduce us, I thought, for work reasons because we were in the same field. As the night wore on and people got drunker, we all wanted to dance. Because you couldn't do that anymore in most New York bars—since former mayor Rudy Giuliani passed the cabaret laws, which prohibited dancing in bars without a license—we went to the theater and danced on Jay's set. He loved to dance as much as I did, and suddenly he went from being a director to a handsome man. I thought he looked like a mix of Beaker from *The Muppets* and a young Orson Welles. Throwing caution to the wind, we spent the night together. The next morning, there was no awkwardness. We shared a towel and toothbrush and were instantly comfortable with each other. But he had to leave for Cambridge, where he was a professor. We walked under the Williamsburg Bridge to where it would be easy to hail a cab. When he stooped a little from his tall height and looked into my eyes, I was hooked.

I didn't see him again for three months because he was out of the country directing a show. When he got back, our occasional e-mail exchanges became more frequent. In June 2007, I started seeing him more and more while he developed a show in New York. Every time I saw him felt better than the time before—which I took as a sign that this relationship might stick. By August 2007, I was referring to him as my boyfriend.

December 14, 2007, was a cold night, and we tried to hail a cab after leaving a holiday party near Union Square, but the M14D bus came quicker. The M14D takes a peculiar route: it goes all the way east on 14th Street, then it snakes its way through Alphabet City until it reaches FDR Drive and takes a right on Delancey Street. I often take it to get to my apartment on the Lower East Side, and looking out the window, I can see the transition from the prosperous neighborhoods west of Third Avenue to the projects along the East River. Most people who take that bus live in one of these projects. They're usually old, or they have kids. On this particular bus, even though it was close to midnight, a child around three years old was awake, making amusing noises and faces in our direction. Jay and I were entranced. He was the cutest kid we had ever seen. We started talking about how much we liked kids and how we'd like to have them, but we wanted to get married first. By the end of that bus ride, we were engaged.

I love telling people I got engaged on the M14D bus.

Around that time, Jay and I had also started working together. It was a big step because I had never collaborated with a director I was dating. Every time I worked with Jay, I said it would be my last time. We had different approaches. He worked best from chaos; I needed everything in order. We exasperated each other; we fought. But then the work turned out beautifully, and we would decide to work together again. We got a huge rush from what we did together. Producing fills my brain 24/7 with other people's stuff, but when the show or film is complete, I have a great product to share with the world.

A friend's father, after seeing one of our shows, said that I was Giulietta to Jay's Fellini. He had actually known the famous Italian director and his muse, so it meant something to hear this remark. He also said, "Giulietta was tough, too." I wondered if he was implying that I was tough. Later, I looked up Fellini and Giulietta. She was his wife and the star of four of his films. She had one miscarriage, and their son died two weeks after being born. After that, she was told she couldn't have children. The couple stayed together until Fellini died in 1993, and Giulietta died five months later.[5]

When I emerged from the subway near my doctor's office after finding out I had miscarried, I called my friend who had dropped me off at St. Vincent's. She lived close by and arrived within fifteen minutes. I had been numb in the interlude between hearing the news and seeing her; I had been inured by contact with strangers on a train, but as soon as I saw her face, I broke down. I felt loss in a way I had never experienced before, and now someone who knew me could help me understand. It turned out that she had had a miscarriage, too, before going on to have three kids—I hadn't known that about her. My friend sat with me in the room as the doctor explained what had happened and what I needed to do. The doctor told me that I should have a D&C (dilation and curettage) to remove the fetus and surrounding tissue. In that moment, when I was emotionally a disaster, my doctor offered a clinical analysis and a game plan.

I am by nature a can-do kind of person. It's what makes me good at my job as a producer. I focus on the tasks at hand, anticipating what others might need. I strip the emotion out of action so that I don't get too worked up and can keep everyone around me calm, feeling like they are well taken care of. It's a skill I perfected at an early age—the ability to assess a situation rationally and store emotions away.

I have a vivid memory from my childhood of holding a stuffed white bunny with pink ears and crying as I watched my father and mother fight. This recurred many times during my parents' marriage, although my bunny was eventually retired. As I got older, I got bolder and intervened, sometimes actually standing in between my parents. Life felt disjointed and surreal—there was conflict at home, but no one else saw it. It wasn't conflict all the time; mostly it was quiet, with each of us doing our own thing in our own worlds in the same house. Also, my father was a good dad. He and I would talk a lot after he got home from work at Long Beach Community Hospital, where he was a psychiatrist. We had similar interests: in books, science, and music. I admired him because he was totally self-made, a poster boy for the American dream who had put himself through medical school and provided for his family.

But there were times when I told him off for the way he treated my mother, and once I called him a bastard to his face. Those memories pain me now because I deeply loved him, but I felt I had to stick up for my mother. There was no way to rationalize his physical violence toward her. She gave everything to him and her family, and she deserved the world.

My parents were stuck in an unhappy marriage. They hadn't chosen each other; the marriage had been arranged by their mothers, who knew each other through the Catholic Church. As individuals, my parents were kind, attractive, and generous, but together they were sometimes toxic.

For most of my growing up, I shunned the idea of settling down. I didn't have a good example to aspire to.

Telling my mother about my miscarriage was almost more difficult than having the miscarriage. I knew that she would take it even harder than I did. She had wanted a grandchild so badly; it was a point of pride for her to tell her friends and relatives. Now she had to tell them the bad news. When I called her, I spoke steadily, but she couldn't see the tears running down my face. I told her, "I had a miscarriage, but it's okay." My mother caught her breath, then said, "What?" After a pause, during which I heard her choke up, she asked, "What did the doctor say?" I said, "What could she say?" Later, I found out that after we hung up she sat on her bed and sobbed.

My husband had been in rehearsal in Salzburg when I got the news, so my mother found out before he did. I didn't want to disrupt his rehearsal. Later, I texted him, "Call me," and within a minute, my phone rang. "It didn't go so well." "Why? What happened?" "There wasn't a heartbeat." "Oh, sweetie. I'm so sorry." It felt cruel to have to talk about this with him on the phone.

It took me a while to get over the shame of telling people I was no longer pregnant. I had thought I was good to go. I had seen the baby, and it had waved. I had already started imagining what it would look like, how I would always focus on making it feel loved and part of a happy home. I thought Jay and I would be great parents. What kind of a child would come from an Iowan farm boy and a Sri Lankan city girl? What amazing things would a child from two creative, passionate parents do? On the one hand, I was uncertain about bringing a child into this world—how it would alter our creative, peripatetic lifestyle. Other times, I thought about what a friend once told me: that having a child helps you forget about the world.

During the follow-up after the D&C, my ob/gyn tried to console me. "You have time," she said. And I believed her, even though in the back of my mind, I knew my window of time was shrinking. I didn't worry too much because it seemed like most women I knew were having kids later. I was thirty-seven and had many friends who were having babies naturally at forty, forty-one, forty-three. I thought I could be like them.

As Barbara Ehrenreich, the feminist author and activist, has so wisely written, we prefer positive spin to more difficult narratives.[6] We live for our aspirations, focusing on what is possible and going for it rather than what is probably not possible. In my case, I held up as examples the friends of mine who were successful in having children in their forties, rather than the many more who were not. I didn't know much about the inner lives of those who were childless, and they didn't talk about it.

After my miscarriage in January 2009, it took three months for my period to return. By October, almost the same time as the year before, I was pregnant again. I proceeded more cautiously this time, telling only my closest friends during the first trimester, not getting my hopes up. I was also mostly away from the social whirl of New York because I was spending more time in Cambridge, Massachusetts. I had transferred all my medical care there because I now had insurance through Jay's teaching position. My doctor wanted to monitor me closely because I had had a miscarriage, so I had ultrasounds scheduled two weeks apart. The first one was fine. It was too early to detect a heartbeat, but there was a sac and fetal pole. My husband was again out of the country for work, so I was alone. Teaching and directing workshops in Austria was his regular gig, and he made good money from it. Sometimes I went with him, but I chose not to go for the second year in a row because I was pregnant, again.

The night before the second ultrasound, I got scared—the kind of scared I felt as a child imagining ghosts and monsters lurking in the shadows or under my bed. Jay and I lived in an old house built around 1870, so the house made noises, plus Cambridge has a reputation for hauntings. I tried to go to the basement to do laundry, but I was too scared to make it down the stairs.

After the ultrasound, I could tell by the nurse's face that something was wrong. There was a heartbeat, but it was slow. The nurse avoided my eyes.

I spent the next two weeks taking it very easy. I didn't lift anything heavy. I slept a lot. I ate yams, avocados, blueberries, walnuts—foods that I had read were good for pregnancy. But then toward the end of that time, I stopped feeling pregnant. Maybe it was a hormone crash. I felt *un*pregnant, very abruptly, and the next ultrasound confirmed that there was no heartbeat.

The chance of losing a pregnancy after the heartbeat has been detected is less than 10 percent, so I told myself I must be very unlucky, even though I would later learn that I was far from alone. In the United States, while approximately four million parents welcome babies every year, around one million lose their babies before they are born.[7] That figure accounts for about 15 to 25 percent of recognized pregnancies, but if you factor in pregnancies that are not recognized, where the woman miscarries before knowing she is pregnant, the miscarriage rate could be much higher.

As women age, our ovaries are more likely to produce eggs that are not viable. The logical reason for my miscarriage was that I was getting older. By the end of my second pregnancy, I was close to thirty-nine. The conventional wisdom is that women are born with a finite number of eggs (approximately two million), and they decline in quality as we get older. The number of eggs at our first menstrual cycle is around 300,000 to 400,000. By age thirty, we're down to between 39,000 and 52,000 (13 percent of the eggs we had at puberty). By age forty, we're down to between 9,000 and 12,000 (3 percent of the eggs we had at puberty)—and not all of those eggs are viable.[8] The rate of egg loss increases around age twenty-eight and even more rapidly by age thirty-five. In addition, many of the eggs are aneuploid, meaning they have an abnormal number of chromosomes, which makes a successful pregnancy far less likely and increases the possibility of birth defects.

I didn't learn about this at home, in school, or at my doctor's office. I found the information on my own, after being devastated a second time.

My ob/gyn ran a pathology of the tissue after the D&C, and a chromosomal abnormality was confirmed. Subsequently, Jay and I had blood tests to check whether our DNA was incompatible, and I had a blood test to check for signs of ovarian aging. Everything came back normal. We just had to try again.

After two miscarriages, I had begun to think that maybe there was something wrong with me. *Maybe it's my fault.* I've done so many things in my life to tempt fate: living off of breakfast cereal and fast food as a child, starting to smoke in college. I began to see my whole future not working out, and I was scared.

I've made many mistakes, but I own them. I have many regrets, but I'm happy. But I shudder to think about the choices I made when I was willfully oblivious to their impact on my fertility.

When I was in boarding school at Phillips Academy Andover, I began making myself throw up—not after every meal but after most of them. I vividly remember when I learned how to do it. I heard two older girls making strange noises in the bathroom of my dormitory. The doors to their stalls were closed, but I could hear one saying, "Oh, my god," and shrieking like a harpy. As we left the bathroom, they looked at me and said, "Do you want to try?" One had a jug of water. They were swigging from it and puking. I was naive and thought they were cool—older, upper-class white girls. I didn't know that moment would change my life, at least for many years to come. I often wonder if I hadn't come across those two girls, would I have become bulimic anyway?

Undoubtedly, I had psychological scars relating to the unhappiness in my home because of the conflict between my parents. In addition, I had an uneasy relationship with food growing up. My mother fed me Sri Lankan rice and curry, which at the time I didn't like—although now I crave it. She would mold the food into balls and coax them into my mouth, where they would sit for an inordinately long time until I gave up and swallowed.

I had never thought of myself as fat, but I wasn't thin. In high school, I was surrounded by skinny, preppy white girls, and I was a misfit—not because I behaved badly, but because I just didn't fit in. The bulimia wasn't intentionally a way to lose weight as much as it was a way to consume and release. When I was in junior high school, I had studied the classics, both Latin and Greek. I had learned about the vomitorium, where ancient Romans threw up after binging at a feast. *People way back when used to eat and throw up. What was the problem?* (Vomitoria were actually hallways in amphitheaters and not where people went to throw up, but the misconception had been planted in my brain by my ancient history teacher.)

The bulimia got better when I started college at Harvard, but then I migrated to another habit. Halfway through my freshman year, I was having an iced chocolate at Café Pamplona in Harvard Square with a girl who was smoking. I told her I wondered what smoking felt like, and she gave me a cigarette. She looked hesitant as she slipped it out of her pack but didn't stop herself or me. She showed me how to hold it and gave me a light. I liked it. Then I got addicted.

When I read Caroline Knapp's memoir *Drinking: A Love Story*, I grasped something about myself I never had before. Knapp talks about how addictions can twin. With her, it was anorexia and alcohol. With me, it was bulimia and cigarettes. Both were ways of controlling my body. The bulimia was made easy by the free buffet at every school meal. I didn't binge-eat. I only sometimes had seconds. Nonetheless, I hated the feeling of being full. I preferred to be empty, lighter, less sluggish.

With cigarettes, there was the social aspect—many of my friends smoked, too. We ate together in the smoking section of the dining hall. Nowadays, the social aspect of smoking is practically nonexistent, since you can't smoke in restaurants and cafés anymore. Today, when I see people smoking on the street, I'm amazed that something that so clearly kills people—around four million a year—is legal. It took me a long time to quit the habit, and maybe I got out too late. Maybe it's not just age but my smoking that made my eggs unviable. I would later learn that eating disorders can throw off your fertility by impacting nutrition intake and hormonal balance, and that smoking can damage your eggs and reproductive organs and increase the risk of miscarriage.

After my second miscarriage, I avoided getting pregnant for about a year by monitoring my fertile periods and using the withdrawal method. I didn't want to go through another year in some stage of being pregnant, miscarrying, and recovering. Also, I didn't want to be pregnant again unless Jay was going to be in town for a long stretch of time. His absence during the two miscarriages had put a strain on our interactions, and over the next few months he was going to be directing a few shows in addition to being up for tenure. Moreover, I was riddled with doubt. *Why did I want to have a child? What were my motivations?*

As time passed, my doubts subsided, and I knew I wanted a baby. I thought I would be a good mother. Also, I thought it would soften me, give me a reason to cut back on my workaholism. Because I was now forty, I decided to be methodical about trying. By now I knew that my time was running out. I made an appointment with an ob/gyn in Cambridge at a nearby hospital, where I thought I would get more full-service care than at the university clinic. I talked with my new doctor about my desire to have a successful pregnancy, and he ordered a pap smear and blood tests. At a subsequent appointment, he told me all my tests came back great and suggested that I "go for it." He also put me on Clomid, a fertility drug that stimulates hormones to enhance ovulation and the release of eggs. He said the drug would give me a boost because of my age.

Soon after, I left for Sri Lanka. I was going to visit the city of Jaffna in the north for the first time in thirty years, now that there had been an end to the brutal civil war that had claimed tens of thousands of lives. I didn't know what I'd find, but I knew it would be an emotional journey. I bought a small, green cloth-bound journal at a gallery and store in the capital of Colombo, so I could document my experience.

I had gone to Sri Lanka primarily to attend my cousin's wedding. Such occasions are the only opportunities for my large extended family to come together from all over the world—Singapore, America, Australia, and England. In my mother's generation, the family would get together for baptisms, but like so many of our generation, my cousins and I were late bloomers. The first and last wedding among my cousins had been mine, three years before when I was the ripe old age of thirty-seven.

It deeply troubled my mother that she didn't yet have a grandchild. My cousin's wedding gave her the perfect chance to nag me about it. She was worried I would break the chain: I was the first-born of my generation, as was she, as was my grandmother, as was my great-grandmother. Now that my female cousin was getting married, my mother's line's primacy was at stake. I might have made it first to the altar, but what if my cousin beat me to the maternity ward?

A few days after the wedding, my mother, Jay, and I left for Jaffna. We had to get special clearance from the Ministry of Defense, and we flew in a fifteen-seat air force plane from Colombo. Sri Lanka had been embroiled in the longest civil war in modern Asia, and my last name is clearly Tamil, the ethnic minority. I was worried that the army guys would treat us badly, but I was struck by how kind everyone was. Sri Lanka had a lot of healing to do, but people did seem to want to get along.

When we landed in Jaffna, I immediately felt like I was in a familiar place despite the obvious devastation—the worst I had ever seen up close. Whole areas had been bombed out; some neighborhoods felt like ghost towns. But I was amazed at how much I remembered from my last visit when I was eight. Jaffna was frozen in time; the war had cut it off from the outside world. There was the same ice cream shop, the same temple. Even the smells were the same, entirely different from polluted and congested Colombo.

With my mother, Jay and I visited a home for nuns. I come from religious stock, even though I am not religious myself, and my family supports various Catholic institutions and charities. My mother asked the nuns to pray for a grandchild. To my dismay, she even told them I'd had a miscarriage. They looked at me with sad and sympathetic eyes—these women who had chosen never to have children themselves.

A few years before, I would have been horrified, but now, I wasn't embarrassed. I thought, *My mother doesn't even know about the second miscarriage.* I hadn't told her, mostly because she had taken the first miscarriage so hard. I didn't want her to get upset about something that had happened and couldn't be changed.

The day after seeing the nuns, we went to my grandfather's old school. The students had prepared a parade to welcome us. My grandfather had become a successful businessman in Colombo, but he remembered his roots and contributed to his alma mater. His children—my mother and her siblings—continued to fund the school.

After the parade, there was a luncheon where I met various teachers and administrators. I heard stories about how much the war had affected everyone's lives. One teacher had lost his mother in the war; another teacher had lost seven family members. I wished that the children at this school would never know the pain their parents had endured, the devaluation of life. Yet, I was struck by how much hope and generosity these people exhibited, despite their losses.

Later, one of the teachers invited us to meet his friend who taught at a local university. When I reached his office, I was overcome with nausea. I tried to hide how I felt for as long as I could, but I finally had to excuse myself and go to the bathroom. Feeling faint, I told them I had to leave and went back to the house where we were staying.

I must have been pregnant then.

When I got back from Sri Lanka, I didn't have any more episodes of nausea, but I hadn't gotten my period either, so I took a pregnancy test. It came out positive—it had been our first attempt to get pregnant in a year and a half. I scheduled a visit with my ob/gyn, and he wanted to monitor me closely. When my blood results came in, he called, saying, "You did it!" My hormone levels were where they should be. I was ecstatic.

When I arrived for tests two days later, I knew the technician hadn't looked at my chart because she asked me if this was my first pregnancy. When I told her that I'd had two miscarriages, she stiffened. I imagined the burden she must feel because of the possibility that she might have to deliver bad news. I felt sorry for her when I should have been feeling protective of myself. I could see the screen, and there was a sac but no embryo. She said it was too early to see anything anyway.

That afternoon, my blood tests came back, and they were encouraging. A nurse called to say, in a very upbeat voice, that my hormone levels had risen since the last test. I really liked this new nurse who had a warm and reassuring tone. She told me to come back in two weeks for another ultrasound.

At the follow-up, the dour technician greeted me. *Why wasn't she smiling?* She walked my husband and me into the room and said, "You must be nervous." I was outraged on the inside: *That is so not the thing to say to me right now.* But I didn't say that. I said, "Yeah." The screen looked the same as the last time. Nothing seemed to be growing inside me. She left the room to speak to the radiologist. A young female doctor came into the room saying, "I'm very sorry." She said my doctor would call me. The warm and reassuring nurse wasn't there that day. I needed her in that moment. I should have been sent straight from the ultrasound room to her or another nurse's office to talk about what had just happened, but instead I was sent home.

Jay and I walked to our car. I got into the passenger seat and doubled over in tears. I had failed once again. I was having extreme thoughts. *I can't bring a new life into this world, so why am I here at all?*

Twenty-four hours went by without a call from my doctor. My previous doctor in New York would have called me within an hour. Impatient, I left a message for the nurse, who rang back a few hours later. She apologized for my being sent home. She said that should never have happened and the mistake would be discussed among the staff. I complained that my doctor hadn't called yet. She told me that he had reduced his hours. I said, "Maybe I should switch doctors?" She said, "Tanya, I am sorry you have to go through this." I said, holding back tears, "I feel like an old pro."

But really, there is no way to be a pro at losing a baby. Having a miscarriage was familiar, but the circumstances were different each time. My head was in a different place. The first time, I was shocked. The second time, I was disappointed but not shocked because I had been worried from the start. The third time should have been a charm. I had cut down on existing commitments to minimize stress. I had embarked on a clean and healthy lifestyle with a diet of pregnancy-friendly foods, like salmon and dark leafy greens—instead of the chili-cheese fries that Jay and I used to indulge in at a bar near our house. I stopped drinking completely. I was mentally and bodily ready. Even so, I had failed.

After my third miscarriage, I was scheduled to have a D&C on August 31, 2011. At 7 a.m., Jay drove me to the hospital along an idyllic stretch of the Charles River in Cambridge. The sun was bright, the sky a perfect blue.

Jay held my hand as the technician put in the IV. When the doctor was running late and the IV was getting uncomfortable, he fetched a nurse. He waited during the D&C procedure until I was out of the operating room. He was there for me in ways that he hadn't been before when he was out of the country for the first two D&Cs. The love I felt from him made up for my feelings of loss.

The rest of the day is a blur. Either I left walking, or I was in a wheelchair. I think I was in a wheelchair. After I got home, I went straight to bed. The anesthesia had worn off, and I wasn't tired. But I was paralyzed by the feeling: *it is done*. While I slept, Jay went to pick up the antibiotics. The doctor had also given me a prescription for Vicodin, but I told Jay I didn't need it.

After I woke up, I wished I had the Vicodin. I wasn't in pain, but I wanted to forget. I went downstairs to where Jay was working on his computer and begged him to go back to the pharmacy and pick up the medication. He said I didn't need it if I wasn't in pain and he would worry if I took it. I was angry, but I don't remember what I said. I went upstairs. It's true that I didn't need Vicodin, but the last place I wanted to be was in my head. *I have nothing to show for everything I have been through. I am so unlucky. It looks like I might never be a mother. Will Jay still love me? Will he think I am withered and old?*

As time went by, I grew more comfortable telling people about what had happened. When I met new people, they often asked, "Do you have kids?"

I used to say, "No," but now I started saying, "No, but we've had three miscarriages." Occasionally people's reactions were puzzling. I could see their mood drop, like I was burdening them with this information. They had no words with which to reply.

Usually, however, the person had a story, too—their own, their friend's or mother's or sister's. A world of miscarriage opened up to me. My husband found out that even his mother had had a miscarriage between his second and third brothers. He hadn't known until she told him after hearing about mine.

Why did it take my having three miscarriages and talking about it to find out that a dozen of my friends had had miscarriages, too? In some cases, I discovered that a friend had also had multiple miscarriages. But then, I rarely talk about the fact that I had an abortion even though many women I know have had one.

"Even in this era of compulsive confession," as the author Peggy Orenstein, who has dealt with miscarriage and infertility, put it, "women don't speak publicly of their loss. It is only if your pregnancy is among the unlucky ones that fail that you begin to hear the stories, spoken in confidence, almost whispered. Your aunt. Your grandmother. Your friends. Your colleagues. Women you have known for years—sometimes your whole life—who have had this happen, sometimes over and over and over again. They tell only if you become one of them."[9]

And there are so many of us. Women between thirty-five and thirty-nine have about a 25 percent chance of miscarrying; women ages forty to forty-four have about a 40 percent chance of miscarrying. Even under thirty, the chances of miscarrying in any given pregnancy are around 12 percent.[10] My sex education teacher never talked about these facts, and mothers still don't talk to their daughters about it, so we don't grow up aware of it. Then when you're pregnant, doctors don't prepare you for miscarriage. When women do have one, they often don't talk about it because it's personal, embarrassing, painful—or because they are at a loss for words to describe the experience. The word itself has negative connotations (a miscarriage of justice, for example) and feeds into our feelings of failure.

A 2009 survey of infertility patients by pharmaceutical giant Schering-Plough revealed that 61 percent hide the struggle to get pregnant from friends and family. Barbara Collura, executive director of RESOLVE, the national infertility association, said that generally people, including some of her own volunteers, are unwilling to share their story. As a result, she argued, "because we have so little patient advocacy, we have so little prog-ress."[11] When I look back, I see all the ways I didn't prepare myself for having a child, either through poor habits or work/life choices. Although I can't say for sure that my attempts to become a mother would have taken a different route or been timed differently, I could have been more prepared for the realization that thirty-seven was simply too late to start trying.

In January 2012, superstar Jay-Z revealed in a song that his wife, Beyoncé, had had a miscarriage before giving birth to their daughter. This move shocked the mass media but got people talking about the subject of miscarriage in general. If a public figure like Jay-Z can be open about miscarriage, can't we all be? Or is it a tragedy that should be kept private? If more public figures shared their experiences with miscarriage and infer-tility, perhaps they would inspire people to be more open and share sugges-tions for how to cope.

On September 10, 2011, I saw the doctor in Cambridge who had performed the D&C. She conducted a pelvic exam and said that I had "healed beautifully" from the procedure. She encouraged me to see a specialist and have a recurrent miscarriage workup. I was now among a minority of women who have had two or more miscarriages. Less than 5 percent experience two consecutive miscarriages, and only 1 percent experience three or more.[12] The positive news was that since I could get pregnant, the chances were good that I could still have a baby. In fact, even after three miscarriages, a woman has a 72 percent chance of having a successful pregnancy.[13] But, she clarified, "the biggest factor for you is going to be your age." Words of death to me. So different from the words of my former ob/gyn, who said, after my first miscarriage at the age of thirty-seven, "You have time."

The next day, September 11, my phone beeped with an alert to "announce your pregnancy." As soon as my third pregnancy had been confirmed, I had downloaded a number of apps, like Sprout and BabyCenter. I plugged in the date of my last period, and the apps estimated my due date and scheduled reminders for various milestones. I had forgotten to delete them.

When the alert came on, I didn't feel sorry for myself. Whenever times are hard, I remind myself, *Hey, it could be worse*. But still I was sad, and I was grieving. The alert was a painful reminder of what could have been.

On that day, when I should have been celebrating getting past the first trimester, I took a walk to clear my head. I noticed more families huddling together than usual—maybe because it was the tenth anniversary of 9/11, when our collective future seemed to be in jeopardy. I saw parents sitting on benches with their children and reading to them. It was hard not to remember exactly what I was feeling on that day ten years ago when the world exploded. Because I lived in New York, it felt like war was everywhere and close. I couldn't see myself bringing a child into that world. Also, I was just thirty and without a steady boyfriend.

In 2011, the world was not that much better. War was still everywhere; injustice was an everyday occurrence; and the economy was a mess. But I felt more of, for lack of a better phrase, *the power of the people*. I felt it in the anticorruption protests of the activist Anna Hazare in India and in the massive marches for democracy during the Arab Spring. I felt it with the increased reach of the Internet and how freely we communicated with each other. I could engage with the 2011 world more than I could have with the 2001 world.

Plus, I loved being forty. I felt like I was who I wanted to be, and I had the right partner in my husband. But being forty meant I could no longer escape certain immutable facts. At the age of fifteen, a woman has a 40 to 50 percent chance of conceiving per cycle. At thirty-five, that number drops down to 15 to 20 percent. By the time she's forty-five, she has only a 3 to 5 percent chance.[14]

More women are waiting longer to have children, and more women aren't having them either by choice or by circumstance. The number of women ages forty to forty-four who remain childless has doubled in a generation, going from 10 percent in 1976 to 20 percent (approximately two million women) in 2006.[15] According to the 2010 National Survey of Family Growth by the Centers for Disease Control and Prevention (CDC), 6 percent of women ages forty to forty-four were deemed voluntarily childless, and another 6 percent are involuntarily childless. And it isn't just an elite white woman's problem. Rates of childlessness grew more sharply among nonwhites than whites from 1994 to 2008, with childlessness rates among black and Hispanic women jumping by more than 30 percent.[16] In the 1970s, it was the Baby Boom; now, it's what the Census Bureau has referred to as the Delayer Boom.[17]

D'Vera Cohn, a senior writer at the Pew Research Center, explained on National Public Radio that there were several reasons for the decline in birth rate for women over forty.

> One is there's an increasing acceptance and tolerance of childlessness. There are other options open to them that weren't available a decade or two ago in terms of careers. And of course, contraception is now much more reliable than it was for many of these women's mothers. There is also a substantial group of women, though, who cannot have children, and I don't want to leave them out. To some extent, their inability to have children may be due to another social factor, which is [that] women are postponing childbearing until older ages. And in some cases if you wait too long, that closes the door. And you may come to accept not having a child at the same time as you're medically unable to do so. So where does that get you on the voluntarily/involuntarily scale?[18]

It's a tragedy that more career women of my generation are unable to or are choosing not to have kids, because we would be great role models for our kids. We are more independent and more educated than our mothers' generation. Many of us started panicking about our biological clock in our mid-thirties, and maybe that was too late. We thought either it would work out or that reproductive science would come to our rescue, but the statistics don't support this mentality. As the CDC pointed out in its 2009 report on Assisted Reproductive Technologies (ARTs), the single most important factor affecting the chances of a live birth through ARTs is a woman's age. At age forty, the chance is 18.7 percent; at forty-two, it's 10 percent; at forty-four, it's only 2.9 percent.[19]

I didn't think about that reality when I was growing up or even later during my college years when I was pondering my future. My generation was going to be different from that of our mothers. We were reaping the benefits of feminism. No one was going to tell us what to do, and we could control our bodies. But crucial information was missing, and we didn't know to seek it out: We have a finite supply of eggs, and if we wait until we are in our late thirties to start having kids, many of us may be disappointed.

However, there are many women for whom delaying motherhood does work out. In a June 2013 article for the *Atlantic*, Dr. Jean Twenge, a psychology researcher, investigated the connection between advanced maternal age and fertility. Around the time of her divorce at the age of thirty in 2002, she felt overwhelmed by articles, books, and advertising that trumpeted the risks of delaying motherhood. When she dug deeper into the statistics, however, she found that some of the warnings were based on outdated data "from a time before electricity, antibiotics, or fertility treatment" and that newer studies showed that women in their thirties who had sex regularly during their fertile periods were almost as likely to get pregnant within a year as women in their twenties. Twenge herself eventually remarried and had three children after she turned thirty-five, giving birth to her third baby at the age of forty.[20]

It's important to balance these optimistic scenarios with the heart-breaking ones. In my situation, I had sex regularly and got pregnant easily in my late thirties, but the pregnancies didn't stick. By the time I sought expert help, my window within which to have a biological child had shrunk to a few years. For other women who also begin pursuing motherhood in their late thirties and early forties, they are really not giving themselves much time to make their goal of having a biological child attainable. Twenge acknowledges this fact: "The bottom line for women, in my view, is: plan to have your last child by the time you turn 40. Beyond that, you're rolling the dice, though they may still come up in your favor."[21]

We go to kindergarten at the age of five, high school at fourteen, and college at eighteen. These steps give us the tools to prepare for adulthood. Why don't we think of having children as a time-sensitive endeavor in an equally logical way? We're told that we should get a mammogram at forty and a colonoscopy at fifty, but there are no standard recommendations about fertility, such as "you should consider freezing your eggs by age twenty-eight." This advice would have been viewed as controversial because egg freezing was considered experimental until 2012. Now, with improved techniques, fertility experts would recommend freezing your eggs in your late twenties. In the world we actually live in, this option often comes to women's attention only after their egg stock has already begun to degrade in their late thirties and early forties.

We're not conditioned to feel the urgency of fertility. Hilary Grove is a thirty-seven-year-old partner at a Boston-based financial firm. She said that when she was growing up, no one ever talked to her about fertility. The most information she was given was that "eating disorders could cause infertility." Hilary was always told it was no big deal to wait to have kids, but now, as she struggles to have a child, she wishes someone had told her to take an egg reserve test every year once she turned thirty.[22]

What we are doing—having kids in our late thirties, forties, and even fifties—is a new frontier, and we don't know what the long-term effects are going to be. We've been referred to as the "sandwich generation," taking care of small children and aging parents at the same time.[23] What will be the effect on our children of losing their parents between the ages of ten and forty instead of between thirty and sixty? Many of our kids won't even know or remember their grandparents.

Julia Chaplin, a journalist and fashion designer who had a daughter when she was forty-one, said, "I wasn't ready to have a kid until I was forty. But lifecycle-wise, around thirty-two to thirty-five would have been better because I will be sixty when my daughter is twenty. Plus my mom is in her seventies now, and it's hard for her to really help out although she really wants to. My sister had a kid at age twenty, and my mom, who was in her fifties then, practically raised her son. I think that's how nature intended childcare."[24]

In my own family, my grandma has been the person I enjoy the most, and she's still alive. Although the average life span is longer than it was a hundred years ago, my mother would have to live to 104 to be around when my kid is forty, if I had one. What will be the effect of a grandparent-less generation?

Forty years ago, people predicted the world would crumble under its own weight. On October 31, 2011, the world population surpassed seven billion. Around that time, there were dozens of articles about demographics and the future. Improvements in food production and technologies have resulted in longer life spans, but fewer people are being born, especially in the developed world. Global birthrates have dropped by 45 percent since 1975, with the average number of children born per woman declining from 4.7 to 2.6 by 2010.[25] In many parts of the globe, lower fertility rates are a direct result of urbanization and family planning programs, as well as better education, health, and economic prosperity. The decline is desperately necessary for the ecological balance of our planet, but this balance can be in jeopardy when replacement rates, at which people die versus are born, fall below 2.1. In 1960, the US birthrate was 3.65; in 1970, it was 2.48, and by 2009 it had sunk to 2.05.[26] According to the United Nations Population Fund, there are seventy-five countries in which the fertility rate is below 2.[27]

Roderic Beaujot, a demographer at the University of Western Ontario, said, "With a lower fertility rate, the aging of the population is inevitable.

You have less people at the bottom of the [age] pyramid and with people living longer you have more people at the top of the pyramid."[28] By 2030, more than a third of the population in a number of Western states as well as some Asian countries, such as Japan and Korea, will be aged over sixty-five.[29] Who's going to take care of the aging population if there aren't enough young people around?

In the pages to follow, I tackle such questions and examine the root causes for how the trend of delaying motherhood took hold of my generation. I also discuss if in fact we were deceived, by whom, and what we can do about it. Along the way, I will tell you what happened to me during my journey to have a child. After my miscarriages, I considered many options from IVF to adoption. The book I have written is the book that I needed. Would I have read it in my teens or twenties—if my mother had given it to me, if a friend had talked to me about it, if a teacher had assigned it? I'd like to think so.

With all my pregnancies, I was struck by how suddenly they progressed from feeling real, like there was definitely something growing inside me, to feeling unreal. I felt like someone had died, but no one had. I felt like I was sick, but I wasn't. My quest to become a mother began to feel quixotic. By the third attempt, I was angry. My education, parents, doctors, and peers had encouraged me to delay motherhood, and I felt stupid. The language of the biological clock has been around for decades. We just don't take it seriously now because there are so many other messages that work against it and because it suits us to ignore what we would rather not hear.

CHAPTER 2
WHAT IS THE BIG LIE?

The Big Lie is that women can do what they want on their own time-tables. I heard it after my first miscarriage, at thirty-seven, when my ob/gyn said, "You have time." The Big Lie is that women can delay motherhood until they are ready emotionally and financially, until they have their careers figured out and have found the perfect partner, and that if they have trouble, then science will find a way to give them a child. But is it a lie or a willing deception?

Like most women, I grew up without ever really learning the most basic facts about the impact of delaying motherhood. I could have educated myself, but how was I supposed to know to look for information? I remember being told how babies were made when I was in fifth grade; I raised my hand and said, "Is there any other way?" I was taught how to avoid getting STDs in high school (back in 1984, HIV was entering the public consciousness and warnings to use condoms were everywhere). Then, as a freshman in college, I heard about the destructive effects of recreational drugs during "Freedom from Chemical Dependency Week." Along the way, no one ever bothered to mention what would happen to my fertility as I got older.

As a child growing up in America, I felt free. I wanted to be different from my mother, who had an arranged marriage and didn't have a job. Her life and that of her friends seemed to be confined to shopping, cooking, talking on the phone, and driving the kids to school. I thought of my mother as weak. It wasn't fair at all, but that was what I thought. I often witnessed my parents fighting—but they stayed together, even though I occasionally wished they would get divorced. I thought of my mother as the victim because she was the one who sometimes got physically hurt. I learned from this that women had to stand up for themselves because they couldn't rely on others to defend them.

When I was a teenager, my mother did have the courage to call a divorce lawyer, and I went with her to the appointment. But in the end, she didn't pursue it. Where would she have gone? How would she have supported herself? I decided then that I would be different. I would be independent. That was when I became a feminist. But I didn't think it would stop me from being a mother.

I have found myself wondering lately about the connection between feminism and my generation's decision to delay motherhood. Did feminism devalue motherhood? Did it lure us to impossible expectations? Did it lull us into complacency? Or did it create a world full of new possibilities that enticed us to wait until it was too late? As feminist author Amy Richards has written in her book *Opting In: Having a Child without Losing Yourself*, "The initial tension between feminism and motherhood developed because the former advocates the pursuit of independence, while the latter is based on dependence."[1]

During my childhood, Marlo Thomas, a TV star who played a single career woman in *That Girl*, was my feminist role model. "Unfortunately for my mother," she said in an interview, "she was raised at a time when women gave up their careers to be wives and mothers. I think in those early years when she was having babies, she didn't really notice it, that she'd given up anything . . . but then as time went on she started to look for herself again and she couldn't find herself. And I think I knew always that my mother was sorry she gave up her career. . . . I stored that away . . . and I've always felt guilty about that. I've always felt she gave up her life [to be a mother]."[2]

No one told us *not* to become mothers while pursuing our ambitions. Rather, they focused on telling us what *else* we could do. In 1972, Marlo Thomas launched *Free to Be You and Me*, an album, book, and TV special that benefited the Ms. Foundation for Women (where I would work after college). She felt that most children's books reinforced sexist stereotypes, and she wanted to create an alternative. She wanted kids to know that anyone—girl or boy—could achieve anything. That same year, the first issue of *Ms. Magazine* was published. The editors expected it to languish when it came out in January, so they called it the Spring issue, to give it a longer shelf life. To their surprise, 300,000 copies sold out in eight days.[3] Also that year, the Equal Rights Amendment, originally drafted in 1923, was finally passed by Congress (although it would fail in 1982 to be ratified by the required thirty-eight states), and Title IX banned sex discrimination in schools.

In January 1976, *Ms.* ran an article titled "Over 30? Over 35? Over 40? How Late Can You Wait to Have a Baby?" which, as science writer Gina Maranto has pointed out, "was among dozens of pieces appearing in *Vogue, Harper's Bazaar, Glamour, Cosmopolitan, Good Housekeeping, McCall's, Redbook, Essence, Ebony,* and *Ladies' Home Journal,* all of which dealt explicitly or implicitly with the phenomenon."[4] The phenomenon in question was a new move for women to put off childbearing until they had found their place in the world and cemented their careers.

In 1979, when Susan B. Anthony dollar coins were first minted, I got my first period. I was eight years old. I thought I was sick when I saw the blood, but I knew enough to be ashamed. I was two years away from sex education in school, and I hadn't heard any other girls talking about their periods, so I felt unprepared and alone. Two family friends in their twenties happened to be staying with us, and my mother asked them to talk to me. I remember one of them saying, "A period is what happens when you can make babies." I was shy, so I didn't ask any questions. But I was also perplexed and embarrassed. Eventually, in sex-ed class in fifth grade, I learned the mechanics of how babies are made, but no one ever suggested that it was a finite endeavor. Ten years may have been a little young to start thinking about our reproductive futures, but since we were learning about the process of making babies, we could have been told that we reach our peak fertility in our twenties and that our egg quality would begin to decline rapidly in our thirties. But that wasn't part of any course.

Before my generation, women were told what to do first by their parents and then by their husbands. They were told when to marry and whom to marry and when to have children. Their education was not a priority, and they were strongly dissuaded (if they could afford it) from having a career. World War II brought more women into the workforce, but there was a backlash in the 1950s, after the men from the military returned home to resume their prewar jobs, which forced women back into their homes as wives and mothers.

In 1960, half of all women were married by the time they were twenty.[5] But they were beginning to chafe at the bit. Then, in 1963, Betty Friedan wrote *The Feminine Mystique* and articulated what so many women had been feeling: "We can no longer ignore that voice within women that says: 'I want something more than my husband and my children and my home.'"[6] As feminism gained strength, it opened up opportunities for education and employment and urged women to stand on their own two feet.

When the Pill became legal in 1960 and abortion in 1973, women gained more control over their bodies. We finally had choices and the power of self-determination. In a sense, I was part of the first generation to benefit from all of this. We took a lot for granted. My friends and I could go to college. The colleges were co-ed. We could get jobs. We could be financially independent. In this world of possibilities where we could do anything, did we really want to have kids at twenty-two? When we were growing up in the 1970s, we didn't have TV shows like *Sex and the City* or *Girls*, but we did have *That Girl* and *The Mary Tyler Moore Show*, and neither of the main characters had or wanted kids. When I was in college, the most prominent feminists were Susan Faludi, bell hooks, and Gloria Steinem, none of whom had children at the time.

For me and for most of my friends, the big question after graduating from college wasn't whether or not to get married; it was whether to get a job or go to graduate school. Second-wave feminism had given women the freedom to do whatever they wanted in the world. In step with that message, in vitro fertilization (IVF), which was successful for the first time in 1978, gave us unprecedented control over our reproductive futures. Feminism dovetailed perfectly with science, and the two fed off one another. But this cozy partnership allowed for a serious omission: women have a finite amount of time in which to have a child, and no amount of independence can change that fact.

As the journalist and science writer Liza Mundy has written, "The tension IVF exposes is between pro-choice groups that have encouraged the idea that women can indefinitely control their childbearing, and newer infertility groups made up of women who, sadly, know better. Biology sometimes is a destiny, and women's groups are going to have to figure out how to accommodate that essentialist truth."[7] Pamela Madsen, the founder and first executive director of the American Fertility Association, put it more directly: "I cringe when feminists say giving women reproductive knowledge is pressuring them to have a child. That's simply not true. Reproductive freedom is not just the ability not to have a child through birth control. It's the ability to have one if and when you want one."[8] Forces of nature do not bend to feminist principles.

My generation became the guinea pigs for pushing the limits of repro-ductivity. By the nineties, when we were in our twenties, we were in a femi-nist euphoria. I entered my senior year of college in 1992, which has been dubbed the "Year of the Woman." That year, four women entered the US Senate, bringing the total number of women senators to six. We had, in Hillary Clinton, a First Lady with a distinguished legal career who'd aroused the ire of conservative women with her declaration that she wasn't going to stay in the kitchen and bake cookies. Janet Reno became the first female attorney general, Madeleine K. Albright the first woman secretary of state, and Ruth Bader Ginsburg brought the number of women on the Supreme Court to two.

A few years after I graduated from college, I worked as the assistant youth coordinator for the Nongovernmental Organization (NGO) Forum on Women, which was held in 1995 in Huairou, China. I met former "comfort women" (who had been forced into prostitution) from Korea and women from Catholics for a Free Choice. I remember vividly when Hillary Clinton arrived backstage in a perfect pink suit to give her speech. I heard her say from the podium: "If there is one message that echoes forth from this conference, let it be that human rights are women's rights and women's rights are human rights." It was exhilarating stuff.

I ended up in New York after the conference, doing follow-up meetings and assistant editing the papers that had been presented in China. The city became my urban playground. Work was rewarding and I had fun. I joined the Wooster Group, a multimedia theater company, and started acting in experimental shows. I didn't think much then about the fact that I was delaying motherhood, and I had many friends of like minds.

In a study of the growing population of single women published in the *Atlantic*, Kate Bolick pointed out, "From 1970 (seven years after the Equal Pay Act was passed) to 2007, women's earnings grew by 44 percent, compared with 6 percent for men. Women are also more likely than men to go to college: in 2010, 55 percent of all college graduates ages 25 to 29 were female. . . . Motherhood itself is no longer compulsory. Since 1976, the percentage of women in their early 40s who have not given birth has nearly doubled."[9]

This doesn't mean that marriage and motherhood are not still aspi-rations among younger women. The "Ultimate College Girl Survey," conducted online by Her Campus Media, surveyed nearly 2,600 college women in the classes of 2012, 2013, 2014, and 2015 from 677 different colleges and universities. An overwhelming majority of respondents to the survey expressed a desire to be married by age thirty and to have children "at some point" in the future. More than a third said that they'd like to have their first child between the ages of twenty-eight and thirty.[10]

My friends and I rarely talked about children. We were busy changing the world, becoming doctors, professors, actors, producers, writers, lawyers, artists, and who had time to think about wet diapers and baby food? So we pushed off decisions. Dating was fun, and the Pill was readily available. We were looking for boyfriends, not future husbands. Most of my friends first started thinking about getting married when they hit thirty—not with any urgency, but that was when the topic started to come up. We knew we should do it, eventually, if we wanted to have children. But we figured we had time. And we enjoyed our freedom too much to want to give it up.

"Today's young women feel redeemed by possibility," Peggy Orenstein writes in *Flux*, which chronicles the experiences of women in what she calls a "half-changed world." "Feminism has been passed down to them as an ethic of personal potential. They were weaned on the mantra 'you can be anything you want to be.'" The problem is, it's hard to focus on self-actualization if you have to take care of your kids. Cooking dinner, facing mounds of dirty laundry, and endlessly cleaning up other people's messes isn't what comes to mind to most women of my generation when we think of how to live up to our full potential. In the back of our minds, we might want to be mothers, just not too soon. Like so many feminists, Orenstein urges young women "to take advantage of this period of unencumbered time, until recently enjoyed solely by men, in which to live independently, explore career opportunities, enjoy friends and lovers, establish the self."[11]

I was definitely following her advice. Plus I was rejecting the traditions of my Sri Lankan heritage, rebelling against arranged marriages, and hoping to avoid the fate of my mother. When I looked at her and other mothers around me as I was growing up, I didn't see the women I wanted to be. They gave up so much for their families. The last thing I wanted was to be trapped at home with a crying baby or shuttling kids to afterschool activities. Besides, I barely knew anyone around my age who had a child. One friend from college got married and had a baby when she was twenty-six, and she almost disappeared from our social scene. A few Sri Lankan girls I grew up with had gotten married and had kids in their twenties, but they weren't close friends. Those twenty-something moms were freaks. *How could they settle down before pursuing their dreams?* That's what I thought then. Now I know many women who are freaked out because they *can't* have a child. So where did it all go wrong? When did all of that independence turn into a liability?

In 1970, barely one in a hundred births were to women aged thirty-five and over. By 2006, that number had jumped to one in twelve.[12] And buried in that statistic are the many women who tried desperately to have a child and couldn't because they had waited too long. Dr. Pasquale Patrizio, the clinical practice director of the Yale Fertility Center, told me that IVF shared some of the blame for this. "The growing popularity of Assisted Reproductive Technologies (ARTs) has given women the false impression and wrong sense of security that female fertility may be manipulated at any stage of life, an erroneous assumption that can result in irreversible future infertility and disillusionment."[13] He told me that a recent US study found that women thought they'd get pregnant when they "felt sufficiently 'stable' so that it would not disrupt their lives. . . . A general reluctance to become mothers and raise a child on their own has kept these women looking for the right relationship well into their thirties and forties while their chances of becoming pregnant quickly diminished."

Like many of my friends, I confronted mixed messages at home. Did my parents want me to be a doctor? Or did they want me to be a mother and stay home to take care of the kids? Growing up I watched the *Brady Bunch* and *Little House on the Prairie*, shows in which the men provided for their families. But I also watched *Wonder Woman* and the *Bionic Woman*, shows in which the women kicked ass while being preternaturally attractive—and they weren't mothers. My mother was an amazingly attentive parent, and she worked hard to give my brother and me a positive and productive childhood, despite the conflicts between her and my father. She took care of us tirelessly and selflessly. She heroically drove us an hour each way to school every morning. She made sure we studied every day. But I didn't want to follow my mother's path or the path of other mothers I met. I thought I would be a doctor, like my father, or a scientist, and kids would come later, if at all. It wasn't a conscious decision but a deduction.

I always liked children and thought I'd be a good mother, but I knew I didn't want to have a child on my own. I also didn't want to be tethered to the wrong man. It was hard to find the right partner, especially living in New

York City, where everyone is looking over her or his shoulder for the next best thing. Since there was no one in my life when I was in my twenties and early thirties who could possibly be Mr. Right, I kept myself busy with my education and career. I completed a Master's in Regional Studies–East Asia at Harvard University, then balanced performing in shows with working in various jobs, including as a research associate at the World Health Organization and an office management consultant at a doctor's office. It's not that I didn't try to find a partner. It's just that the men I dated always turned out to be wrong.

Until I met my husband, Jay, when I was thirty-five. He was kind and sensitive, with an encyclopedic knowledge. We could stay up all night talking about any number of subjects, from theater to politics to popular culture. We liked to walk aimlessly and discover new neighborhoods. I often wish I had met him sooner. In her book *Woman: An Intimate Geography*, science writer Natalie Angier mentioned a woman, Hope Phillips, who had been twice married and divorced, and then when she was forty-five, she met a man with whom she finally wanted to have kids. Phillips said, "It was ironic, as though God were kicking me in the teeth."[14]

I met Soon-Young Yoon when she was the UN Liaison for the NGO Forum on Women in China in 1995. She married Rick Smith when she was in her thirties, and they worked in different countries. Yoon had two miscarriages, and then, at the age of forty, she adopted a daughter. She is now the chair of the NGO Committee on the Status of Women in New York, and we meet for lunch every few months at a restaurant near her office by the United Nations. "If you look at the cost of educating a child in this country, it's not possible to have one until you have financial security," she told me when I asked her about her decision to put off having kids. "As a result, many women don't have children in their peak fertile years. In addition, if you like your lifestyle and don't want to make room for another being, you can wait until you are ready, which is often when you get older and worry about being alone. Women aren't prepared for that moment because there is little in this culture that tells us one day you are going to get older and feel alone."[15]

The language of the biological clock has always been around. I heard it many times, from nagging aunts and older friends. *It's time for you to settle down* or *It's time for you to have a child.* But it felt like an old-fashioned scold. Women's lives have changed dramatically in a generation, and I didn't feel like living up to old stereotypes. But maybe if I had been told instead *You have a finite number of eggs and if you wait to have children until you are thirty-five, you will have a much higher chance of miscarrying, of having complications during pregnancy or of having a child with birth defects—and that's if you are able to get pregnant at all*—I might have made smarter, more proactive choices.

Have women of my generation been falsely led by feminists to believe that delaying motherhood won't be a problem? Amy Richards, cofounder of the Third Wave Foundation, which is dedicated to youth activism, doesn't believe that feminism could be at fault. "I blame individual women for not doing their homework," she told me one day over tea at my apartment.

> It was more the medical establishment offering a false promise to women than feminists. I certainly think there was a false assumption out in the culture that if you weren't at the "right" place in your life at thirty, no worries, there were fertility treatments. I think the larger culprit here is the assumption of what it means to be "ready" to have kids. There is still too much emphasis on convention—marriage, money, homeownership. People wait because they don't have their life "in place"—but what that means is so subjective and misses the point that you can have everything in place and it might still not mean it's "good."[16]

And yet there is undoubtedly a subtext in the feminist message that it's more important to live a personally fulfilling life than to have kids. "I'm not sure I would have been strong enough to have children, to live that life, and come out the other end with an identity of my own," Gloria Steinem has said. "The way I came to think of it was that I could not give birth to both myself and someone else. It was a choice."[17]

"We went through an era where there was a lot of talk about women's bodies," Yoon told me over lunch one day, "but where was the conversation about motherhood?" She believes it's not that women didn't know the biological limitations of delaying motherhood. "But feminists were focused on a woman's right to get a PhD. Those who were advocating for work equalities were in fact ignoring the reality of what it takes to become a mother." Yoon's daughter is now twenty-five and in law school. "I'll tell my daughter if she doesn't go to law school, then she can get a PhD," she confided. "But I also want to tell her that she can and should think about how she might fit being a mother into that life. I don't want to be a grandmother too late!"[18]

In 2012, in a provocative article in *Newsweek* titled "Why Women Should Stop Trying to be Perfect," Debora L. Spar, the president of Barnard College, presented some revealing data on women in higher education and the workplace.[19] In 2009, wives outearned their husbands in 38 percent of American households. The following year they earned 47 percent of all law degrees and 48 percent of all medical degrees. By 2011, women accounted for 47 percent of the overall labor force in the United States and 59 percent of the college-educated, entry-level workforce.

And yet this progress has not made a deep impact at the top echelons in most fields. "As of 2012," Spar wrote, "women accounted for only 16 percent of partners at the country's largest law firms and 15 percent of senior executives at Fortune 100 firms. They constituted only 10 percent of the country's aerospace engineers, 7 percent of its Hollywood directors, and 16 percent of its congressional representatives." Spar pointed out that the number of working mothers rose from 45 percent of all mothers in 1965 to 78 percent in 2000, but women still did the bulk of the work at home, averaging around forty hours a week compared with twenty-one hours a week by men. One part of the feminist message seems to be sinking in—women are better educated now, and more of them are working, but that hasn't really changed the balance of power at home.

I decided to speak to Marianne Weems, cofounder of the V-Girls, a notorious feminist theater company that offered up feminist critiques of literary and art historical criticism. Now, Weems is artistic director of the New York-based theater company The Builders Association and a professor at Carnegie Mellon University. She is also a single mother, having decided at fifty to adopt a daughter.

> In the '70s, no American feminist could talk about their children without being seen as drowning in domesticity. That's the way the pendulum swung. It was black-and-white, one way or the other. I'm a diehard feminist. I don't think I could have done the things I've done if I'd had a child when I was younger. Even in my forties, I looked at younger women in their twenties who were having kids and thought, *You'll never be what you want to be.* However, I was also on the cusp of finding out that science had failed us, that for example I couldn't freeze my eggs the way men froze their sperm. What an unbelievable thing to hear you are too old to

have a child just when you are 100 percent ready to have one. Women like me are working to resolve this dilemma, figuring out how to live the feminist dream and incorporate children into our lives. If more choices for fertility had been evident when I was younger, I could have made more rational decisions without stepping outside of my career path or my feminist roots.[20]

If second-wave feminists had combined the language of "do anything" with a more scientific take on the biological clock, perhaps the ache among women of my generation for the child we can't have wouldn't be as profound. When peers in their twenties were having kids, we thought they were making bad choices by not prioritizing their own career ambitions, but when we look at them now, from the riper vantage point of our childless forties, we see that they have what we don't.

Would making women focus on their fertility be a setback for feminism? Would it be seen as an attempt to keep women in the kitchen? "I certainly don't think telling women to think in advance about their fertility would set women back—it's real," Amy Richards told me. "I think that education is a very pro-woman perspective."[21] Richards felt sex education should go deeper than including information about fertility and forms of family planning. She suggested, "I think it also has to be taught that not all women should have or want to have children."[22] It's not just about telling women we can freeze our eggs as a way to preserve our fertility; it's also about encouraging us to reimagine what our lives could or should look like. For example, we can choose to find the relationship before having kids or not, and we can choose to have kids or not.

Catherine Gund, who cofounded the Third Wave Foundation with Richards, believes that we need to change assumptions about how we build families in general and how we define family for ourselves. Gund has three kids with a female partner and one with a male partner. She's happy now as a single mom in her forties. She told me about seeing a baby wearing a onesie that said "MADE IN BED" on the front. She was amused in a way but also a little offended. Gund explained, "'MADE IN BED' presumes the fantasy of a romantic heterosexual relationship and follows from the adage that first comes love, then comes marriage, then comes baby in the baby carriage. That's not how a growing number of people's lives turn out, given queerness, adoption, fertility issues, single parenting, and so on. At this point, we need to be supporting a huge variety of families and the ways people make them."[23]

In 2001, the American Society for Reproductive Medicine (ASRM) launched a campaign to educate people about infertility. It created public service announcements on the impact of body weight, STDs, smoking, and age. Posters were placed on buses in New York, Chicago, and Seattle; and an informational website was launched. *Newsweek* ran a cover story about the campaign, which included signs that said "Advancing Age Decreases Your Ability to Have Children."[24] At the time, Dr. Michael Soules, the president of ASRM, said, "It's kind of like issuing a warning. It's our duty to let people know." Although the PSAs covered a range of influences on fertility, the ones highlighting delayed motherhood caught the most attention. Women's groups threw up their arms in outrage. Kim Gandy, then the president of the National Organization for Women, told *Newsweek* that the idea "you can choose what age you'll be to have your children is a ludicrous proposition for most women, as though you can simply snap your fingers and say, 'OK, I'm the right age,' and then have all the accoutrements magically appear—the stable relationship, financial stability, life stability."[25]

It's been more than a decade since that campaign, and the negative impact of delaying motherhood on fertility has become more painfully clear as my generation hits its fourth decade. The science is very real. "We haven't seen any real improvements in treating women over 40," Dr. Mark Sauer of Columbia University's Center for Women's Reproductive Care said, back in 2001. "You can't change biology."[26] Have feminist attitudes evolved over the past ten years to accept that truth?

Cheri Magid, a forty-three-year-old playwright and associate professor at New York University, has been married for many years. She didn't have a child, but not because she didn't want to. "I felt the pressure to 'make it.' I wanted to establish my life, and a child would have fundamentally disrupted my life. It's hard to figure out how to deliberately disrupt your life." She recalled receiving a letter from a fertility center a few days before she turned thirty-eight. The letter asked if she would consider freezing her eggs. Magid felt like Big Brother was watching her, knew where she lived, and knew how old she was. She said, "That's none of their business. When I was younger, I wouldn't have minded receiving a letter like that. But getting it at that age, it felt invasive and opportunistic."[27]

A lot of the messaging about fertility can seem tacky and market driven. *Fertility is a business, and here's our product: egg freezing. Maybe you should think about buying it.* I remember standing on a subway platform in Central Square in Cambridge, Massachusetts, and seeing a sign that said, "We're looking for a few good men" under a photo of a pretty woman with a come-hither look. It was an ad for sperm donors.

One of my friends, a Los Angeles-based filmmaker, had a son at the age of forty. She made an active choice to pause her career in order to become a mother. "I spent four years focusing on getting pregnant and then only worked for myself. The first directing job I took with someone else was when my son was six." She said she wasn't glad at all that she had delayed motherhood for so long. "I wish I had known the truth about a woman's fertility because I would have made it my priority to get pregnant earlier and have more children."

In July 2012, Anne-Marie Slaughter launched a firestorm with her essay "Why Women Still Can't Have It All" in the *Atlantic*. Using her personal experience working in the State Department while trying to raise two boys, Slaughter argued that the work/life balance for women in powerful positions is untenable because of the hours and expectations associated with a top professional career. At the heart of her essay was the argument that while women were traditionally expected to be far more present than men in their children's lives, this was something that was not thrust upon them so much as it was a reflection of an inherent inclination to respond more emotionally to their children's needs.

Her essay received more than a million hits and sparked dozens of response pieces. Commentators issued angry denunciations of various aspects of the piece, pointing to the irrelevance of the phrase "have it all," mocking Slaughter's unsympathetic voice as a successful, wealthy white woman, and condemning her message as antifeminist. "By positing that women are always going to be more conflicted than their male counterparts, without considering the unequal and unfair pressures on women," wrote Lindsay Beyerstein in a column for *In These Times*, "Slaughter is perpetuating the cycle of sexism: Women who do feel guilty will be less likely to reexamine their assumptions, and women who don't will be less likely to share their perspective (and thereby challenge our assumptions) for fear of being considered unnatural."[28] In a humorous spin on the debate, Stephen Colbert offered his advice for women who feel they shoulder too much of the burden at home: "Don't do that!" he said. "I don't!"[29]

A few months later, Hillary Clinton, for whom Slaughter had served as director of policy planning, was asked to weigh in on the debate in a profile that ran in the October 2012 issue of *Marie Claire*. "Clinton has very little patience for those whose privilege offers them a myriad of choices but who fail to take advantage of them," wrote Ayelet Waldman, who interviewed Clinton for the magazine. "'I can't stand whining,' she says. 'I can't stand the kind of paralysis that some people fall into because they're not happy with the choices they've made. You live in a time when there are endless choices. . . . Money certainly helps, and having that kind of financial privilege goes a long way, but you don't even have to have money for it. But you have to work on yourself. . . . Do something!'"[30]

These comments caused yet another controversy, though Clinton explained that she was not referring to Slaughter when she talked about whiners. And Clinton has made no secret of the fact that she shares many of Slaughter's views about the importance of asking society to do more to help working mothers. In 2010, she said, "We don't have enough support for maternal leave and the kinds of things that some of the European countries do. So we still make it hard on women to go into the work force and feel that they can be good at work but then doing the most important job, which is raising your children in a responsible and positive way."[31]

Slaughter wrote her essay in part as a response to Sheryl Sandberg, the COO of Facebook, who used her platform at a Barnard College commencement speech in 2011 to make the case for putting work ahead of family. Sandberg said she had "deep respect for my friends who make different choices than I do, who choose the really hard job of raising children full time, who choose to go part time. . ." but she encouraged women both to work and to be mothers without feeling guilty about making time for their families. In an earlier speech, she had lamented that when a woman starts thinking about having children, "she doesn't raise her hand anymore. . . . She starts leaning back." In March 2013, Sandberg published a book inspired by the speech called *Lean In* that went straight to the top of the *New York Times* bestseller list.[32]

As Sandberg writes in *Lean In*, "When arguments turn into 'she said/she said,' we all lose."[33] We are pitching ourselves against expectations—those we are conditioned to sense from society and those we impose on ourselves. These expectations can set us up for feeling like a failure. They can also set us up for resentment.

Strategizing for the work/life balance is indelibly connected to our goals for childbearing. However, if we don't completely know the reality of our fertility, we can't make adequately informed decisions. Although sometimes I feel stupid for how much I didn't know about my own fertility, I know that I am not alone. According to a 2011 survey of women in the twenty-five to thirty-five age range, 64 percent would seek fertility treatment if they were to have difficulty becoming pregnant, but many women aren't clear about what types of treatment are available. About half of women surveyed were familiar with IVF but overestimate its success rate, and many failed to recognize that the chance of success with IVF is affected by the age of the person whose egg is used (whether it is your own or that of a donor).[34]

"I think the primary reason that fertility preservation was not taught in sex education was two-fold," infertility consultant Mindy Berkson told me.

> First, options for fertility preservation were not readily available 10-plus years ago. For example, egg freezing is a relatively new process. Secondly, thirty years ago, women typically had completed their families by age thirty. The Baby Boomer generation was the first generation that proactively tapped the workforce, explored advanced educations and married much later in life. All of these factors contributed to delayed childbearing. Delayed childbearing ultimately drove up the rate of infertility and boosted a tremendous industry. With the increased industry demand came improved technologies, more options and advanced treatments. Now is the time for the educational message to catch up with the industry and history. Fertility preservation should definitely be a topic taught in sex education classes.[35]

Fertility preservation is not an option accessible to most women because it can cost thousands of dollars and is not typically covered by insurance. Nonetheless, presenting women with the facts and options is crucial. If someone—our mothers, a friend's mother, doctors, sex-ed teachers—had made an effort to educate us as teenagers about our fertility, we might have viewed our choices in our thirties very differently. Women should be taught about the life span of their eggs, about assisted reproductive technologies, and about the meaning of infertility. Sex education should be more than just preventing pregnancy and STDs.

In the early 1900s, Margaret Sanger was prevented from passing out pamphlets about contraceptive options because of the 1873 Comstock Act, which prohibited the distribution of any printed information deemed obscene. As the historian Jill Lepore wrote in the *New Yorker*, "[The Comstock Act] classified all sorts of printed material as obscenity and specified contraception as obscene so that it [was] illegal to send through the US mail information, even in a philosophical sense, about reducing a woman's fertility. . . . The courts ruled against her and said, 'A woman's right to life gives her the right to not have intercourse with a man.' Sanger's argument is that a woman has a right to have sex without fear of death [from childbirth]." Eventually, in the late 1930s, the American Medical Association ruled that doctors who were willing could and should give information about birth control to their patients.[36]

Like birth control, information about fertility and delaying motherhood should be promoted. Every young woman should be shown a chart of her overall fertility whether at school, a family planning center, or a doctor's office. She should know when her eggs are at their best and when their quality and number start declining. I didn't know the numbers, and if I had, I might have approached my thirties very differently. I might have gotten pregnant right after I met my husband when I was thirty-five instead of waiting two years, and I would have been more strategic about trying to get pregnant. I would have visited a fertility center after my first miscarriage, instead of waiting until I had had three.

Because of my experience, I tell my younger friends to start thinking about their futures, whether I think it might annoy them or not. Recently, I saw a friend before her wedding day. She is thirty-seven years old. A few months before, she had gotten pregnant but had an abortion because she wasn't ready to have a child even though she and her fiancé planned to have kids one day. On the inside, I was shaking my head and sad. But to her face, I told her about my experience; I told her some of the statistics; and I told her to try to have a kid as soon as possible because waiting until she's ready might be too late.

Women tend to visit their ob/gyns once a year, and each visit typically consists of just twelve minutes of conversation. Most women never discuss future pregnancy plans, age as an infertility risk factor, or infertility treatment options with their doctors. Among the women who do have those conversations, in most instances they initiated the discussion.[37] When I was a child, my mother often said, to my dismay, "Prevention is better than cure," but it's true. Doctors should be talking to us in advance about issues like miscarriage and infertility so that we're not shocked by our lack of awareness when those issues become a part of our lives.

Many feminists deliberately avoided the topic of motherhood because they were rebelling against its implied domesticity. But it's time that we reset the conversation and reconcile becoming a mother with also being a successful, independent woman. For starters, we need to get young women to answer these questions:

1. Do you want kids?
2. Under what circumstances?
3. If you answered "yes" to question 1 and "through natural delivery" for 2, then how will you build a life where having children is feasible and biologically possible?

*   *   *

You don't need to have all the answers, but you can be clearer on your motives and make decisions informed by science rather than in defiance of it.

CHAPTER 3

WHAT THE EXPERTS WISH YOU KNEW

D r. Carole Kowalczyk of the Michigan Center for Fertility & Women's Health has been working in fertility medicine for nearly two decades. She herself had a baby when she was just under forty. I asked her about her opinion of delaying motherhood: "Thirty-five is the new twenty-eight because women are more active and look better, because we take better care of ourselves. But our eggs are not following. It's amazing because a woman who is forty-something and looks younger—she doesn't understand why she can't get pregnant."[1]

Amy Richards, the feminist author, was told by her ob/gyn, "Thirty-eight is too late to wait to start thinking about whether or not you have children."[2] Meanwhile, when I was almost thirty-eight, my ob/gyn told me I had time. In *Budgeting for Infertility*, authors Evelina Weidman Sterling and Angie Best-Boss, both medical writers who dealt with their own infertilities, pointed out that this is not an unusual problem: "Don't get waylaid for too long at the gynecologist's office. Gynecologists have a bad reputation for saying you have plenty of time to get pregnant and not to worry."[3] Many, if not most, women I interviewed for this book knew their fertility declined as they got older, but they didn't know exactly when and how quickly. In the pages to follow, I look at the discrepancy between perception and reality with regard to fertility knowledge, at assisted reproductive technologies (ARTs) and the latest advancements, and at the need for more public information, research, and oversight.

Medical professionals themselves get confused about fertility facts. In Dr. Lillian Schapiro's novel, *Tick Tock*, about a doctor dealing with infertility, the main character thinks as she begins IVF: "I remembered how depressed I had been after a lecture in residency when they told us that fertility actually declined at 30, not 35. Why didn't anyone mention that on your first day of medical school? Why had I taken time off between college and medical school to enjoy life and live a little? It was too late now. The super-size needle would be my penance for two years spent away from the grindstone, going to clubs that didn't open until midnight, hanging out with neighbors, seeing all the latest movies on opening night, and never missing an aerobics class."[4]

The lack of awareness can place extra pressure on those specializing in fertility medicine. Dr. William Kutteh, director of Fertility Associates of Memphis in Tennessee, said that delayed motherhood has had a significant impact on his practice. He has noticed he spends "more time explaining natural decline in fertility, [has] more frustration for patients who have little knowledge of natural fertility, [and deals with] more folks having unrealistic expectations thinking that they will be the exception."[5]

Fertility issues affect approximately 10 percent of the world's population and cut across socioeconomic and cultural lines. According to the World Health Organization, infertility rates have been fairly stable since 1990, and "almost 50 million couples worldwide were unable to have a child after five years of trying."[6] US federal data from 2006 to 2008 suggest that among childless married women aged fifteen to thirty-four, 14 to 15 percent report fertility problems.[7] Around one-third of women aged thirty-five to thirty-nine have fertility problems, while 64 percent of women aged forty to forty-four years old do.[8]

Pregnancy rates have changed dramatically over the past few decades, with rates among younger age groups radically declining and rates among older ones radically rising. A National Center for Health Statistics report stated that for US women in their early twenties, pregnancy rates fell nearly 18 percent from 1990 to 2008.[9] The average age of women giving birth for the first time rose from 21.4 years in 1970 to twenty-five years in 2006.[10] The rate of first births for women in their thirties and forties has surged—quadrupling since 1970.[11]

The age group having the most babies is women aged thirty to thirty-four, and the number of women having their first child after age thirty-five continues to jump dramatically, from one in twelve in 2006 to one in five in 2012; in 1970, it was only one in a hundred.[12] Women aged forty to forty-four had the sharpest increase in pregnancy rates of nearly

65 percent from 1990 to 2008.[13] According to the Centers for Disease Control and Prevention (CDC), about 8,000 babies were born in 2008 to women aged forty-five or older, more than double the number in 1997. Of these babies, 541 were born to women aged fifty or older—a 375 percent increase.[14] (These babies were most likely born from donor eggs.) However, overall, Americans have had fewer babies each year since 2008, with births falling to a twelve-year low in 2011, leading to the smallest population gain since World War II.[15] These trends have resulted in a new landscape of when and how we do or don't make babies.

Navigating this terrain can be confusing, especially when we aren't adequately prepared with essential facts about fertility. According to Lindsay Beck, the founder of Fertile Hope based in Austin, Texas, for cancer patients whose treatments threaten their fertility, "infertility is [now] where breast cancer was in the 1970s—completely in the closet. In my experience, it's a much lighter atmosphere in the cancer waiting room than in the IVF waiting room. Cancer patients talk about antinausea drugs and what worked for them. They look at each other as a means of support. For some reason, fertility patients tend to ignore each other in the waiting room."[16]

According to a study at the University of California, San Francisco, nearly half of respondents who became pregnant through IVF after forty were "shocked" that they even needed treatment. Thirty-one percent said they expected to get pregnant without difficulty at age forty. However, fewer than a quarter said they would have tried to get pregnant earlier if they had more information about declining fertility. Twenty-eight percent said that their mistaken beliefs were based on incorrect information from friends, doctors, or the media. About a quarter of participants said their beliefs stemmed from messages they had received since adolescence about preventing pregnancy.[17] Judging from my experience after I tried to have a child and from the experiences of many of my friends, I believe the findings of the UCSF study are applicable to the larger population.

A Fertility Centers of Illinois public survey showed that only 18.2 percent of respondents accurately guessed how many couples are affected by fertility, and 28.1 percent didn't know that fertility declines rapidly in women after age thirty-five. In addition, 68.4 percent of survey respondents weren't aware that as part of a couple, both men and women are equally likely to be infertile.[18] In a study of US university students, 83 percent of women and 91 percent of men thought the age at which women experience a slight dip in fertility is older than it is (in reality, it happens between age twenty-five and twenty-nine). Two-thirds of women and 81 percent of men made the same mistake regarding the age at which fertility steeply decreases (after thirty-five); many thought it occurred after age forty, forty-five, or fifty.[19] These findings resonate with similar studies conducted around the world.[20]

Many doctors believe fertility counseling should be offered alongside contraception counseling, and the professionals have tried to sound the alarm at various times over the past few decades. There was a French study in the 1980s about the relationship of age and fecundity with respect to artificial insemination rates.[21] Numerous articles, including one by science writer Gina Maranto in the *Atlantic* in 1995, emphasized the correlation between delayed childbearing and infertility. In 2001, there was the American Society for Reproductive Medicine (ASRM) campaign on buses in the United States. In 2011, the Royal College of Obstetricians and Gynecologists (RCOG) in the United Kingdom advised women to complete their families between the ages of twenty and thirty-five during their "most fertile" years in order to avoid "regrets."[22]

Nonetheless, despite clear and accessible information about age and fertility, the confusion between reproductive science and reality persists. I contacted Dr. Pasquale Patrizio, the clinical practice director of the Yale Fertility Center, after reading about his research on ARTs and age in the journal *Fertility and Sterility*. He told me, "It is alarming to find women *surprised* to learn of their high risk status. A typical reaction: 'Doctor, what do you mean you cannot help me? I am healthy, I eat right, I exercise, and you are telling me that I cannot have my own baby?' This lack of awareness about the risks involved in delayed childbearing is unacceptable, and we as professionals have to intervene."[23] Women who delay motherhood are often stigmatized as "being selfish and unconcerned about starting a family," but Dr. Patrizio believes age-related infertility is a healthcare problem that should be addressed by doctors and society.[24] Journalist Sarah Elizabeth Richards, in an op-ed for the *New York Times*, explained, "In our fertility-obsessed society, women can't escape the message that it's harder to get pregnant after 35. And yet, it's not a conversation patients are having with the doctors they talk to about their most intimate issues—their OB-GYNs—unless they bring up the topic first. OB-GYNs routinely ask patients during their annual exams about their sexual histories and need for contraception, but often missing from the list is, 'Do you plan to have a family?'"[25]

Dr. Irene Souter, my doctor at Massachusetts General, is refreshingly straightforward. She is a few years older than me and has three kids of her own. Because she practices in Massachusetts, one of the few states that has mandated insurance coverage for fertility treatments, she has experience treating women from all walks of life. The one thing that surprises her patients, no matter what their background, is the sharp decline in fertility seen with advancing age. She thinks that women should be given honest information so that they do not overestimate their ability to conceive in their late thirties and midforties. I remember the feeling I had after Jay and I first met with Dr. Souter: *We are perfectly normal people. We're just old.*

Elizabeth Gregory wrote in her 2007 book *Ready: Why Women Are Embracing the New Later Motherhood*, "Today, both sides of the fertility spectrum get skewed in the media and the common lore. People seem to think simultaneously that *nobody* can get pregnant after 35 and that *everybody* can."[26] I started this chapter illustrating how women of the same age can be told either they do or don't have time to try for a child. Both messages cannot be correct, but if both are being spread, even among the medical community, it's no wonder that women get confused. Misinformation is a disservice and is sometimes hard to discern from real information. Amy Richards has written about a section in Susan Faludi's seminal work *Backlash* that "uncovered the backstory of a 1982 article that stated that women between the ages of thirty-one and thirty-five had a 40 percent chance of being infertile; the article failed to mention that this study was based on a sampling of women who were seeking fertility treatment because all were married to sterile men."[27] Disclosing that fact would have resulted in a very different reading of the statistic.

But we live in a society that can conveniently overlook the facts. We don't encourage kids to stop eating chicken nuggets and drinking sugary soft drinks, only to treat them later for diabetes. People keep smoking even though four million die a year from smoking-related diseases—and fifty million have over the past ten years.[28] Surely, educated people can make bad choices to engage in potentially risky behaviors. Nonetheless, it is imperative for society to make the correct data and information available to the general public so that positive changes can occur, even incrementally, and spread.

I live on the Lower East Side of Manhattan where Margaret Sanger (who would later found Planned Parenthood) was a nurse and saw firsthand the suffering of women who didn't have access to birth control information. We can apply this lesson to fertility knowledge. Mindy Berkson, the founder of Lotus Blossom Consulting in Chicago, has a decade of experience guiding couples through the IVF process and has struggled herself with secondary infertility (which means that a person was able to have a child but then has difficulty having another one). Berkson explained that awareness is key: "Women should know that fertility begins to decrease around age twenty-seven. By the time a woman reaches thirty years of age, 90 percent of the finite egg supply that she is born with is depleted. I think it is terms and statistics such as these that help women realize they cannot rewind the biological clock."[29] Dr. Kowalczyk said she urges women "to be respectful of their fertility and their goals in life. Time limits fertility because eggs age. . . . If family is important, factor it into your career path. Put that equation in there."[30]

Knowing the facts, though, doesn't mean we will stop delaying motherhood. Women will still have kids when they are emotionally, mentally, financially, and otherwise ready. Julia McQuillan, professor of sociology at the University of Nebraska, emphasized that planning for a family is not necessarily within our control:

> Regarding things that I wish were more widely known about infertility/ involuntary childlessness—I wish that people made the issue less about individual choices and more about societal structures. We could make structures and policies that make joint parenting or father involvement more serious, and then it would be more likely that the social world would be better structured to support all parents. Then women would not have to be as concerned about delaying for education or jobs. If we expected folks to combine education and/or employment with parenting—not just women but men, too—then we might structure the social world differently. For example, what if we had more daycares in workplaces? The way work/life structures, policies, and expectations are structured now have evolved over time—and involve social choices. Other cultures, other social times have made different choices. We could do a better job of working with biological clocks.[31]

Assisted reproductive technologies step in to help women deal with the aftereffects of a society that doesn't coordinate more logically with their biological clocks. However, women often don't realize that ARTs can't always help them reach their goals and that in fact, the odds of ARTs working for older women are much lower than they think.

The way I considered my options growing up was different from the generation before and after. When I was a child, sexual and reproductive freedoms had been revolutionized by the Pill and abortion rights. By the time I hit puberty, the primary focus in women's health was on deliberately delaying motherhood. For those growing up today, reproductive freedoms are being revolutionized again, in some opposite yet complementary ways to what I witnessed in the 1980s. Now the talk is about egg freezing, ovarian tissue freezing, sex selection, egg or embryo donation, etc. Young women can freeze their eggs as a kind of insurance against delaying motherhood—an option that was not yet perfected for me and my peers. Science writer Liza Mundy has argued, "Reproductive technology is mirroring social change, but it also enables and drives that change." She claimed, "In the twenty-first century the radical thing may not be to end a pregnancy, but to begin one."[32]

It's important for every woman, and man, to know the fertility basics, especially what happens to fertility over time. The facts can be articulated in a fairly simple paragraph like so: A woman is born with all the eggs she'll ever have: about 1 or 2 million, a number that continues to decline until menopause. During her reproductive years, she will ovulate perhaps 400 to 500 eggs, and the rest will die off. According to the American Fertility Association, the probability of conceiving decreases 3 to 5 percent per year after age thirty and at a faster rate after forty. Miscarriage rates soar as women age—from about 15 percent in women aged twenty-five to thirty, to about 40 percent in women over forty. According to the CDC, once a woman celebrates her forty-second birthday, the chances of her having a baby using her own eggs, even with advanced medical help, are less than 10 percent. At age forty, half of her eggs are chromosomally abnormal; by age forty-two, that figure is 90 percent. Her ovarian reserve decreases with age, and as the quality of eggs goes down, the chance of chromosomal damage goes up. Dr. Nicole Noyes of the New York University Fertility Center said our "prime" eggs occur between the ages of sixteen and twenty-eight.[33]

Communication about the fertility basics should be normalized. Mothers should talk to their daughters, friends should talk to each other, and doctors should be preemptive in providing the facts. I wish I had seen a chart of my fertility in my ob/gyn's office when I was in my twenties. The blog *Everyday Health* posted an article titled "10 Health Screenings All Women Should Have." It listed blood pressure screening (starting at age eighteen), cholesterol check (starting at age twenty), pap smear and pelvic exam (starting at age twenty-one or when sexually active), breast exam (starting at age twenty), bone density screening (starting at age sixty-five), blood glucose test (starting at age forty-five or when symptoms are present), colon cancer screening (starting at age fifty), skin examination (starting at age eighteen), and dental checkup (every year).[34] A fertility screening, starting at age twenty-one or when considering getting pregnant, should be added to that list. Women should understand that although they might not want to have kids now, they might change their minds as they get older. I certainly changed mine—when I was in my mid-thirties.

Trying to have children at a younger age does not mean it will be easy. A healthy woman's chance of getting pregnant naturally each month is about 23 percent up to age thirty-five, then it drops to 18 to 20 percent by age thirty-seven, and then to 5 percent in her forties. And as biomedical expert Dr. Henri Leridon explained in a paper for the journal *Human Reproduction*, "Under natural conditions, 75 percent of women starting to try to conceive at age 30 years will have a conception ending in a live birth within 1 year, 66 percent at age 35 years and 44 percent at age 40 years."[35] There are a host of potential problems at any age, with women of all reproductive ages being diagnosed with and seeking treatment for infertility. Twenty percent of all infertility diagnoses are "unexplained infertility."

Although infertility is traditionally seen as a female problem, more and more reports are emerging about the man's role. In fact, infertility cases are evenly accounted for by both male and female factors. Eighty percent of couples with unexplained infertility cannot conceive because of poor sperm quality, and sperm issues in general are the primary problem in 25 to 35 percent of infertile couples.[36] A sperm with damaged DNA is less likely to make a woman pregnant, and, if she does conceive, she is more likely to miscarry.[37] In Western Europe, male infertility procedures occur more frequently than female ones.[38] A study in Tanzania showed that 40 percent of Tanzanian men are infertile, while another study in India showed a 50 percent drop in the sperm count in men.[39]

Compounding the problem are indications that most men—as much as 80 percent in infertile couples—do not seek treatment. As Dr. David Walsh, the medical director of Sims Fertility Clinic in Dublin, Ireland, explained, "Women are collegiate in fertility issues; they'll discuss problems and treatments. Men are isolated. Women will talk about IVF but not many guys will go down to the pub and ask his friends 'have you tried ICSI?'"[40] (ICSI is intracytoplasmic sperm injection, an assisted reproductive technique in which a single sperm is injected into an egg.)

Both eggs and sperm are affected by various factors, such as age, poor diet, smoking, and alcohol. A Harvard Nurses' Health Study of 18,000 women over eight years found that "eating a slow carb (whole grain, vegetables, fruit and beans), whole food (in the state that mother nature created them), and mostly plant-based diet increased fertility by six-fold."[41] Being too thin or overexercising can interfere with ovulation, while being overweight can throw off your hormones and prevent conception. With regard to men, a study by Harvard Medical School found that a diet high in saturated fats produces significantly less and weaker sperm than a healthy, balanced diet. Being overweight can also increase the temperature of the testicles through the formation of fat cells in the groin area. Alcoholics have 30 percent fewer normal cells in their semen, and just one or two alcoholic drinks a day can increase your chances of having a low sperm count. Men who regularly eat junk food have a sperm count 43 percent lower than those with a healthy diet. Researchers at Hull University in the United Kingdom found that it takes up to five times as long for a man over forty-five to get a woman pregnant than if he was under twenty-five.[42]

Despite this possible increased difficulty in aiding conception, according to US government statistics, the birthrate of fathers aged forty and older has increased by more than 30 percent since 1980.[43] The growing group of older fathers could be affecting the gene pool. Recent studies have shown the potential links between advanced paternal age and birth defects or developmental issues.[44] An article in *Nature* magazine concluded that the number of genetic mutations that can be acquired from a father increases by two every year of his life, and doubles every sixteen, so that a thirty-six-year-old man is twice as likely as a twenty-year-old to bequeath de novo mutations (alterations in genes that are present for the first time in a family) to his children. A study of hundreds of families with autism found that spontaneous mutations can occur in a parent's sperm or egg cells that increase a child's risk for autism, and that "fathers are four times more likely than mothers to pass these mutations on to their children."[45] The risk of having an autistic child jumps from 6 in 10,000 before the father reaches thirty years old to 32 in 10,000 when he's forty—a more than five-fold increase. When he reaches fifty, the risk goes up to 52 in 10,000.

In 2001, a groundbreaking study concluded that men over fifty were three times more likely than men under twenty-five to father a schizo-phrenic child. A 2003 Danish study of 7,704 schizophrenics came up with results similar to the 2001 study.[46] Nonetheless, Evan E. Eichler, a pro-fessor of genome sciences at the University of Washington in Seattle, urged caution to the *New York Times*: "You are going to have guys who look at this and say, 'Oh no, you mean I have to have all my kids when I'm 20 and stupid?' Well, of course not. You have to understand that the vast majority of these mutations have no consequences, and that there are tons of guys in their 50s who have healthy children."[47]

Increased research about the relevance of paternal age and maternal age to fertility could result in better awareness and treatments. Studies on worms and mice have indicated that we might be able to delay the aging of eggs by manipulating genes that influence protein and cell quality or by adding supplements like Coenzyme Q10 that help rejuvenate eggs.[48] In addition, products have appeared on the market to help men and women take their fertility into their own hands at home, away from the doctor's office.

One company, ContraVac, based in Charlottesville, Virginia, devel-oped a product called SpermCheck Fertility so that men could test their own sperm. SpermCheck is the only FDA-approved home sperm test and became available in stores in 2012. For women, Cambridge Temperature Concepts in the United Kingdom came out with DuoFertility, a patch that measures their temperature 2,500 times per day. The information is trans-ferred into a computer program that comes with the patch, allowing couples to track the ovulation process so precisely that it can instruct them about the exact moment they should try to conceive. The company claims DuoFertility is just as effective as IVF, successful in 39 percent of couples who try it. A SpermCheck kit costs about $40. DuoFertility costs about $700, which is 100 percent refundable if it is not successful after a year of regular use.[49] These at-home monitors are fairly new, and for many infertile couples, pursuing assisted reproductive technologies is still their preferred route.

In June 2012, Lesley Brown, who had given birth to the first IVF baby, Louise, in 1978 in the United Kingdom, passed away. April 2013 saw the passing of Dr. Robert Edwards, who with Dr. Patrick Steptoe pioneered IVF and was Brown's doctor. The advent of IVF, which these individuals championed, was a game changer that was not wholeheartedly welcomed. In an article in the *Atlantic* after Brown's death, writer Megan Garber explained,

> For many, IVF smacked of a moral overstep—or at least of a potential one. In a 1974 article headlined "The Embryo Sweepstakes," the *New York Times* considered the ethical implications of what it called "the brave new baby": the child "conceived in a test tube and then planted in a womb." (The scare phrase in that being not "test tube" so much as "a womb" and its menacingly indefinite article.) And no less a luminary than James Watson—yes, *that* James Watson [who codiscovered with Francis Crick the structure of DNA]—publicly decried the procedure, telling a Congressional committee in 1974 that a successful embryo transplant would lead to "all sorts of bad scenarios." Specifically, he predicted: "All hell will break loose, politically and morally, all over the world."[50]

Whether Watson's prediction proved true is up for debate, depending on which end of the political and religious spectrum you stand. However, since Lesley Brown's courageous pursuit of what had been termed a "hopeless" endeavor, more than 5 million IVF babies have been born.[51] According to RESOLVE, the national infertility association, approximately 44 percent of women with infertility have sought medical assistance, and of those who seek medical intervention, approximately 65 percent give birth.[52] In 2010, more than thirty years after he revolutionized reproductive medicine, Dr. Robert Edwards was awarded the Nobel Prize, which recognized his immense contribution to science. At that time, he said, "Nothing is more special than a child."[53] Today, between 1 and 4 percent of all babies in developed nations are born through IVF.

In 1986, there were only 41 IVF clinics in the United States, according to an industry registry. Then around 1987, vaginal egg retrieval, as opposed to going through the abdomen, took off and sparked the rapid rise of IVF.[54] By 1996, there were more than 300 clinics, an increase of more than 700 percent.[55] According to a report by the CDC on ARTs surveillance, in 2009, there were 484 clinics around the United States.[56] Currently, an estimated

60,000 babies are born in the United States each year as a result of IVF treatment. According to the Society for Assisted Reproductive Technology, in 2010, women younger than thirty-five went through nearly 40,000 cycles of IVF using fresh embryos from non-donors, while women between the ages of thirty-five to thirty-seven and between thirty-eight to forty underwent about 20,000 cycles for each age group, and those aged forty-one to forty-two underwent nearly 10,000 cycles.[57] It is important to note, however, that the majority of infertility treatments fail; as Miriam Zoll, author of *Cracked Open: Liberty, Fertility and the Pursuit of High-Tech Babies*, pointed out in her piece about delayed motherhood for the *New York Times*, CDC data show IVF failure rates as high as 68 to 79 percent in women ages thirty-five to forty, and 88 to 95 percent among women ages forty to forty-four.[58]

Although infertility strikes women of all ages, older women are more likely to pursue ARTs and be able to afford them. In the early 1980s, many clinics would not accept women older than thirty-five.[59] Then, between 2003 and 2009, the number of IVF cycles performed for women aged over forty increased by 41 percent—four times as fast as for women under thirty-five.[60] One clinic, the Center for Human Reproduction in New York, has a reputation as the "fertility center of last resort" and noted that the most dramatic improvement in pregnancy rates were observed in women at ages forty-four to forty-nine, where pregnancy rates increased to 10.3 percent.[61] However, research from doctors at the fertility clinic Boston IVF showed a much greater IVF success rate for women under thirty-five (65 to 86 percent) than for women over forty (23 to 42 percent).[62] The *New England Journal of Medicine* revealed that live birth rates from assisted reproductive technologies reliably decline with the mother's age, with optimal estimates declining from 74.6 percent for women under thirty-one, to 27.8 percent for women aged forty-one to forty-two, and down to 1.3 percent for those over forty-three.[63]

A 2009 study from the Sackler School of Medicine in Tel Aviv concluded that age forty-three seems to be a cutoff point for IVF with a woman's own eggs, which is viable with only 5 percent of women at that age.[64] However, other studies have shown that after age forty-four is more of a cutoff. Dr. Patrizio was part of a team that conducted a study of women aged forty-three years and older undergoing ART treatment using their own eggs. Their findings, as presented in the March 2013 issue of the *Journal of Assisted Reproduction and Genetics*, showed that overall clinical pregnancy and live birth rates were 8.3 percent for the forty-three-year-olds and 5.3 percent for the forty-four-year-olds. No pregnancies occurred among women aged forty-five and older.[65] An earlier 2005 Cornell University study surveyed women over forty-five who attempted IVF with their own eggs and also showed that none of them became pregnant.[66]

IVF for women of any age comes with risks. In a special report on National Public Radio, surprising data on the rise of multiple births was presented. Since 1980, the rate of twin births has jumped 70 percent. Twins are conceived naturally just 2 percent of the time, while for those women who get pregnant with fertility treatments the rate can be more than 40 percent. Two-thirds of this increase is specifically because of fertility treatments. With Clomid and other oral drugs, the chance of twinning is about 5 percent. With fertility drug injections, that chance jumps to between 10 and 15 percent.[67] The other third of the increase in twins is because more women over thirty are having babies. The female body normally releases one egg per month, but as women age, hormonal changes make them more prone to release two eggs.[68] Around 30 percent of women who undergo IVF have twins or triplets.[69] According to the National Vital Statistics Report, in 2003, one out of 18 births to women aged thirty-five years or older was a multiple delivery. The report explained that the increase is directly related to fertility treatments.[70]

American Society for Reproductive Medicine guidelines on embryo transfer have stated that no more than two embryos—and ideally just one—should be transferred into a women under thirty-five, but there was no government regulation of IVF until the 1990s.[71] Moreover, because IVF is expensive and arduous, most women do not choose single-embryo transfers—only around 7 percent of women under thirty-five in 2009 did so. They think they can increase their odds of having a successful pregnancy despite the clear disadvantages of having multiples.[72] Such births are high risk, especially because the babies are more likely to be born prematurely. Twins are six times and triplets twenty times more likely to suffer from cerebral palsy than single births. As a result, cerebral palsy is becoming more common in the United States, "even though," science writer Liza Mundy explained, "a traditional major cause of cerebral palsy, jaundice in newborns, has been all but eliminated."[73]

Ovarian hyperstimulation syndrome (OHSS)—the negative effects of drugs used to overstimulate the ovaries to produce more eggs for harvesting—is also a danger of fertility treatments. The ovaries can swell to several times their normal size, and fluid may leak into and accumulate in the abdomen. In rare cases, this can cause internal bleeding, pulmonary edema, or even death. A confidential inquiry into women dying during childbirth in the United Kingdom found that OHSS is now one of the biggest causes of maternal mortality in England and Wales.[74] In the United States, the National Institutes of Health asserted that high-dose stimulations lead to OHSS in 10 percent of IVF patients, with severe forms of OHSS occurring in 1 percent of IVF patients.[75]

A potential solution is pursuing "mini-IVF," where only two or three eggs are produced instead of as many as fourteen or fifteen. "Under names such as low-intensity IVF, eco-IVF and even patient-friendly IVF—a technique of in vitro fertilization is increasing in use with promises to be safer, cheaper, and easier on patients trying to have a baby," wrote Michelle Muniz in the *St. Louis Post-Dispatch*.[76] Mini-IVF also can save as much as $5,000 in medications.

Another risk of assisted reproductive technologies is birth defects, with studies showing that around 8.3 percent of children born through ARTs had defects, whereas only 5.8 percent of those not born through ARTs did.[77] According to the CDC, major birth defects occur in about three out of every hundred babies born in the United States. This information indicates that the corresponding figure for IVF babies is four in every hundred.[78] A team at Nanjing Medical University in China collected forty-six studies involving more than 124,000 children born through IVF or using ICSI. They found that the risk of having a birth defect was 37 percent higher than that for the children conceived normally.[79]

Those pursuing treatment might be older and thus more prone to chromosomal issues as the result of ovarian aging. In addition, ARTs help eggs and sperm to reproduce when they wouldn't have ordinarily survived. New techniques are beginning to mitigate the risks. For example, preimplantation genetic diagnosis involves thoroughly testing embryos for major chromosomal or genetic abnormalities. Genetically normal embryos are then frozen for a month or two before being thawed and inserted in the womb.[80] In addition, a team of researchers in Nottingham, England, released their findings in May 2013 about the promising development of using time-lapse imagery of developing embryos to determine which ones were least likely to have chromosomal abnormalities.[81]

A mother in the United Kingdom, Nicky, was a carrier of a rare cancer gene called Li-Fraumeni. Her doctors offered a treatment whereby her embryos would be removed, screened for the faulty gene, and put back into the womb. Her son, Tom, now faces only a 4 percent risk of getting a tumor instead of 50 percent.[82] And further techniques are in development for the future. In 2012, researchers at the Yale School of Medicine and at Oxford University identified the chromosomal makeup of a human egg by testing the cells that surround the egg, called cumulus cells.[83]

Around one in 6,500 children worldwide are born every year with mitochondrial diseases, of which there are about 150 types that can result in blindness, muscle weakness, and heart failure among other problems.[84] One mother, Sharon, lost all seven of her children to Leigh's Disease, a rare mitochondrial disease that affects the central nervous system and begins between three months and two years of age. Genetic therapies could save people like Sharon from their intense suffering.[85] For example, three-person IVF uses the core genetic information from the mother and father but transfers it into a donor egg that contains healthy mitochondria. Although it is still not clear if this technique could lead to a healthy baby, research shows that it can work in the lab.[86] OvaScience is one company developing the method of injecting mitochondria from "egg precursor cells." A trial of eighty women is under way, and the results are expected in 2014.[87]

Because of the risks and costs of fertility treatments, prospective parents should think through their options before they embark on their journey to have a child. They should anticipate how far they are willing to go and realize that treatment is not a guarantee. When I asked Dr. Sunday Pirkle of the Texas Fertility Center for her advice about fertility treatments, she said, "1) have an endpoint in mind, and 2) allow yourself to grieve the losses—that, in turn, allows you to move forward in a different direction that you might not have otherwise considered."[88]

One such direction is adoption, but too often adoption is seen as a last resort. Many people who struggle with infertility keep trying and trying until their chances to bear a biological child run out. Author Peggy Orenstein interviewed a forty-year-old prospective single mother who, despite a few failed attempts at becoming pregnant, was going to pursue using donor egg and sperm because she viewed resorting to adoption "like a failure."[89] In the *Huffington Post*, Kathy Bright, herself an adoptee, wrote about her friend's order of options for becoming a mother: "First, natural born. (Well, of course. Who wouldn't?) Then, fertility treatments. Then foster. Then adopt."[90]

People who wait too long to adopt might find that they are passed up in favor of younger adoptive parents. Beth Hall, the founder of Pact, An Adoption Alliance in Oakland, California, told me, "For infant placement, we generally do not work with families where there isn't at least one parent who is under fifty years old. Generally, expectant parents placing newborns have a range of younger families to choose from, and don't select couples where both parents are fifty or older. There are many difficult questions raised for the child when a newborn is placed with an older couple, or older single adult, especially if they are first-time parents." She said some of those considerations include the energy level of the parents as well as the likelihood that the parent would be alive to see the child through to adulthood. But even then, "if their parents live to an older age, these young people may be put in the position of dealing with issues of elder care at a time when they are just setting out in life as adults."[91]

Nancy Rosenhaus, the associate director of an organization called Adoptions with Love in Newton, Massachusetts, herself "went through several years of infertility and treatments in my early thirties and finally became pregnant. I decided that when I returned to work that I wanted to do something in the field of infertility. This is where I belong."[92] Drawing from her own experience, she now helps match prospective adoptive parents with children.

Victoria Birk Hill, the managing director of in Harmony, a Michigan-based wellness center, who also works with Dr. Carole Kowalczyk of the Michigan Center for Fertility & Women's Health, similarly went through years of infertility and treatments until a friend suggested adoption after her third failed IVF cycle. She was able to adopt through a friend who knew of a woman who was pregnant but unable to take care of the child. Birk Hill said, "I don't wish anything to change the adoption of my daughter, but I do wish that I had not been subjected to years of fertility pain and despair. It was a tough ordeal. Next to the death of my mother it was the hardest thing I had ever gone through."[93]

Swedish researchers compared outcomes for a variety of types of couples: those whose IVF treatment failed; those whose IVF treatment resulted in children; and couples who decided to adopt after unsuccessful IVF treatment. Quality of life was highest among couples who adopted children after unsuccessful IVF treatment and lowest among couples who remained childless after their IVF treatments had failed. The study showed that parenting is rewarding regardless of how one becomes a parent.[94]

Another advantage to adoption is the vast and thorough support system for prospective parents, as I have found among my friends who have adopted. Liza Mundy explained there is

> a huge, huge difference between the world of assisted reproduction, which is relentlessly profit-making, and the world of adoption, which is generally driven by organizations with goals other than money. Adoptive parents are supported for their entire lives. IVF patients are cast adrift. As the psychotherapist Jean Benward pointed out in a talk at the 2005 American Society for Reproductive Medicine (ASRM) conference, in adoption the client is "a child who needs a home, a family." Everything that's being done is being done in the service of that child and its needs. "All adoption plans have to be reviewed and formally accepted by a judge; all parents have to undergo home study, fingerprinting, background checks." Adoption is legislated by states, regulated, and socially accepted; moreover, there are resources available to the parents throughout raising the child. In contrast, sperm and egg donation is conducted largely out of sight, with little scrutiny and no provision by anybody for long-term support. At fertility clinics, parents using egg or sperm donation are given, at most, an hour of counseling.[95]

This situation is improving, thanks to organizations such as RESOLVE, the national infertility association, stepping in to provide more information and community for those pursuing ARTs. These resources, including psychological support, should be presented to the infertility patient during the very first visit.

Adoption certainly comes with its own obstacles. For example, government regulations can make international adoption prohibitive, and being matched with a child in the United States can be a difficult and even troubling process. I have a friend who with her husband has been trying to adopt for years. One agency she contacted asked if she was willing to be matched with a child of color because her goal would be much easier to achieve and also explained that a child of color is cheaper. Although my friend is open to a child of any color, she was offended by the agency representative and never called again. But her search continues. She has even started a Facebook page asking for people to contact her if they know of a child being given up for adoption.

A possible solution for potential adoptive parents could be found in greater collaboration between the ART industry and embryo adoption networks. There are upward of 500,000 frozen embryos leftover from IVF procedures in the United States. A small number of couples—perhaps a few hundred a year—donate their frozen embryos to other couples trying to have children. The rest are sitting in storage facilities across the country, and the number is growing by 4 percent a year.[96] Because of personhood bills, which prohibit the destruction of these embryos, and conservative groups like National Association for the Advancement of Preborn Children (NAAPC—a blatant riff on the civil rights organization the National Association for the Advancement of Colored People), frozen embryos are stuck in limbo.[97] Some organizations have offered embryo adoption services, like Nightlight's Snowflakes program, whose first adopted baby, Hannah, came from a frozen embryo in 1998; and in 2013, NASA research scientist Kelly Burke, age forty-five, went public about her recent adoption of a nineteen-year-old embryo after five years of failed fertility treatments.[98]

When I started at the Fertility Center, I was already considering adoption as a possibility, but like so many women, I wanted first to exhaust my options for having a biological child. Prior to settling on IVF treatment, I asked Dr. Souter about freezing my eggs just so I could have them in case my journey through ARTs became too long. I could have eggs on ice for a year or more down the road, when my internal eggs might be too old. But Dr. Souter told me it was already too late. "The success of the procedure has improved dramatically over the last decade, and egg freezing is an evolving technology that helps preserve reproductive potential, but it is by no means a guarantee for fertility."

This is true no matter the age of the mother. An article on the website My Fertility Choices says, "According to the American Society for Reproductive Medicine (ASRM), implantation rates of cryopreserved (frozen) eggs range from 17 to 41 percent, and clinical pregnancy rates (per transfer) range from 36 percent to 61 percent."[99] In an analysis by researchers from New York Medical College and the

University of California, Davis, of 2,265 frozen egg cycles undergone by 1,805 patients between 1996 and 2011, "Women whose eggs were frozen with the slow freeze method before age thirty had a greater than 8.9 percent likelihood of implantation per embryo; this declined to 4.3 percent for embryos from eggs frozen after age forty. For vitrification cycles, implantation declined from 13.2 percent for embryos from eggs frozen at thirty to 8.6 percent for embryos from eggs frozen at forty."[100]

Dr. Jamie Grifo, program director of the NYU Fertility Center in New York City, has done more than 1,100 frozen egg cycles since 2005 and recommends that the earlier the eggs are harvested, the better. "Ideally, the best results are under thirty-five, optimally in their early thirties," he said. In his studies of live birth rates from 2003 to 2009, the pregnancy rate among thirty-year-olds is 61 percent, but at age forty-four it drops to 5 percent.[101]

Egg freezing is being trumpeted as the answer to preserving a woman's fertility until she is ready to become a mother. In May 2013, journalist Sarah Elizabeth Richards released her book *Motherhood, Rescheduled: The New Frontier of Egg Freezing and the Women Who Tried It*, about women who have frozen their eggs. Richards herself spent about $50,000 to freeze her own eggs between the ages of thirty-six and thirty-eight (as of this writing, she had not yet attempted to use her frozen eggs).[102] Brigitte Adams, who froze her eggs in 2011 at the age of thirty-nine and runs a website called Eggsurance, said egg freezing is "the new birth control pill, an option that empowers women and increases their choices."[103] Industry experts have predicted that in time newer techniques using frozen eggs for in vitro fertilization will overtake traditional methods of treatment using fresh (nonfrozen) eggs. Pregnancy rates of frozen eggs versus fresh eggs are comparable and will continue to improve.

Dr. Pasquale Patrizio of the Yale Fertility Center has been researching the efficiency of IVF and cryopreserved eggs for a decade. He said that if you look at the number of babies born per number of eggs frozen and rewarmed, the rate is around 10 percent. Depending on the freezing method (slow freezing or vitrification, which uses chemicals to dehydrate the egg before it is frozen) the egg survival after thawing is between 70 to 85 percent. He explained, "If you freeze ten eggs, an average of seven to eight will survive the thawing. Of these, 65 percent (five to six) will become embryos and from these an average of one embryo will produce a live birth. So the final yield is about 10 percent implantation rate (one egg out of ten will result in a live birth). This rate *is similar* to the one obtained with fresh eggs (in the same patient population, younger than thirty-five)."[104]

Human sperm, 1,000 times smaller than the human egg, have been successfully frozen since 1955. The origins of egg freezing in fertility treatments go back to the late 1960s, with experiments on mice. The world's first baby from a frozen embryo was born in 1983, and the first baby from a frozen egg was born in 1986. In October 2011, Frozen Egg Bank Inc., run by medical director Dr. David Diaz, hosted the world's first baby reunion of seventy children born from frozen eggs.[105] However, for many years, the potential of egg freezing had been largely neglected because of the flawed preservation techniques. Ice crystals that damaged the egg were a risk during the previous slow freezing process, until vitrification was perfected. The cryobiologist Dr. Amir Arav of Israel applied successful vitrification techniques to the eggs of many animal species, and Dr. Masashige Kuwayama of Japan adapted Dr. Arav's ideas and applied them to human eggs. Dr. Kuwayama presented his findings in 2006 at the 22nd annual meeting of the European Society of Human Reproduction and Embryology, and the field of egg freezing research entered a new era of progress.[106]

Nonetheless, as with IVF in general, egg freezing does come with risks. I have mentioned, for example, ovarian hyperstimulation syndrome, which occurs when fertility medicines cause the ovaries to become swollen and can result in fluid leaking into the belly and chest area. In addition, freezing eggs is expensive, is elective (meaning it's not covered by insurance), and is not guaranteed. I have two friends who are now in their early forties who froze their eggs a few years ago, only to find that when they were ready to use them, none of the eggs had actually survived. And they had no recourse for getting their money back.

Although egg-freezing techniques have significantly improved over the past few years, my friends' experiences are a warning. As Dr. Ellen Greenblatt, medical director of the Centre for Fertility and Reproductive Health at Mount Sinai Hospital in Toronto, Canada, said, "If [women] stop worrying about the aging factor on fertility until they're beyond reproductive age, thinking that, 'Oh well, I've frozen my eggs,' and those small number of eggs don't lead to a pregnancy, that can be very devastating."[107]

From July 2005 to January 2011, there were 241 women who considered elective egg freezing at Reproductive Medicine Associates of New

York and received a counseling session. In 2005, their ages averaged thirty-nine years. Six years later, in 2011, the average age of women seeking this treatment was 37.4.[108] However, thirty-eight years is pushing the limits of the viability of the eggs.[109]

In 2004, the ASRM ordered that "egg freezing should only be provided as part of research studies with strict oversight, at no charge and only to patients with no hope of having genetic children."[110] Then, in 2012, the same organization said the procedure was no longer "experimental." Dr. Samantha Pfeifer, coauthor of that ASRM report on the sanctioning of egg preservation, said, "A lot of the women interested in this are in their late 30s and early 40s, and their chance of having a live birth is not as good as younger women. These older patients must be counseled on this. This is not a technology that says, 'Freeze your eggs so you will have more options down the road.' The best way to conceive is with your own eggs, through natural intercourse. There are no data that support this as a social mechanism to delay childbearing."[111]

In a PBS special following the ASRM report, Marcy Darnovsky of the Center for Genetics and Society said that removing the "experimental" label "would enable insurance companies to cover the costs for women who might become infertile because of cancer treatments, for example, but it's still an experiment." She expressed her concern that "a lot of fertility clinics, hundreds really, are already aggressively marketing this procedure for elective purposes, for what is sometimes called social egg freezing." Dr. Eric Widra of Shady Grove Fertility Center, the largest fertility practice in America with offices in four states including Washington, DC, agreed with Darnovsky's worries about the marketing aspects but believed from his experience that the technology is safe and effective. He emphasized that what's important is to monitor egg freezing "very closely as that is still a very young technology."[112] The long-term data doesn't yet exist.

According to an article in *Nature* in 2011, estimates said that fewer than ten babies worldwide have been born from eggs frozen for women aged thirty-eight or over. Moreover, it is estimated that fewer than 2,000 babies in general have been born from frozen eggs, about 400 of them in the United States, and many of them from donor eggs.[113] The first case of a pregnancy from egg donation occurred to a woman without ovaries in Australia in 1983. Now, even women in their sixties are having kids using donor eggs. In the future, scientists may be able to create eggs from our stem cells or donated amniotic membranes, but for now, the best chance for older women is to use eggs from a younger woman if they haven't frozen their own eggs in their twenties or early thirties.

Because of the lack of oversight and little to no requirement to report, statistics from egg-freezing clinics are scarce. As the *Nature* piece described, Briana Rudick, a fertility specialist at Columbia University, "contacted every clinic in the United States [in 2009], 64 percent of which responded. Of the 140 that provided data on their egg-freezing service and outcomes, forty-five had never thawed a client's frozen eggs. At least thirty clinics had no live births from the eggs that they had thawed, and eleven more had achieved only one live birth. Only eight respondents had managed ten or more live births."[114] Entrepreneurial individuals have taken the distribution of information into their own hands. For example, Brigitte Adams said she founded the site Eggsurance to create "a safe and welcoming community for women exploring or going through the egg freezing process to connect and share their personal experiences, find or review fertility clinics and gain knowledge to make informed decisions."[115]

Ovarian freezing has also become a hot topic but should not be considered a mechanism for fertility postponement. Only twenty-one live births have been reported worldwide and mostly in patients who had cancer.[116] At Children's Hospital of Philadelphia, researchers have frozen ovarian and testicular tissues taken from cancer patients as young as three. By the time these children are of reproductive age, the technology might be perfected enough to make it possible for them to have their own children.[117] Dr. Sherman Silber of St. Louis started offering the option to women who will pay the price, around $8,000. He said to NPR in December 2012, "If you say that we don't have evidence for ovary freezing working and that it's experimental, that's kind of baloney. It is not experimental anymore. It really is a very robust procedure."[118] However, many experts, including Glenn Schattman, president of the Society for Assisted Reproductive Technology, came out against doctors like Silber, arguing that they give women hopes that cannot be guaranteed. Schattman said, "It really should be reserved for patients that are at imminent risk of losing their fertility in the very near short term."[119] The procedure carries risks, as does any surgical procedure, and there isn't yet enough data to back up its promotion.

Womb transplants could be another new frontier worth exploring. The procedure has been carried out successfully in animals that then had babies.[120] Researchers in the United Kingdom have said womb transplants could be routine and inexpensive by 2020.[121] Dr. Mats Brannstrom of Gothenburg, Sweden, has performed four uterine transplants from mother to daughter.[122] Also, in early 2013, a woman in Turkey became pregnant using her own eggs with a transplanted womb.[123]

Assisted reproductive technologies were developed and have proliferated without the benefit of sufficient oversight of the ethical, sociological, and medical repercussions. They are like the Wild West of reproductive science. Dr. Geoffrey Sher, one of the country's most successful fertility doctors and the founder of the Sher Fertility Institute, has said, "Most of us have heard the saying often credited to Mark Twain, 'There are three kinds of lies: Lies, Damn Lies, and Statistics.' Well, unfortunately, IVF success rate reporting is a perfect illustration of this point."[124] As the 2011 article in *Nature* pointed out, fertility treatments have been among the quickest to leap from lab to clinic. "There's a history of moving forward quickly in reproductive medicine," said Laura Shanner, a bioethicist at the University of Alberta in Edmonton, Canada. "There are endemic problems of poorly done, poorly structured research."[125] Marketing techniques prior to adequate human testing poses obvious risks. Without ample research and the funding to support it, promising breakthroughs might never be properly realized. For example, stem-cell research could one day help infertile women "grow" new eggs.

But ART research often becomes complicated by politics. During the 2012 presidential campaign, it was revealed that three of Mitt Romney's sons might have used IVF to expand their families, but Romney's running mate Representative Paul Ryan, a staunch Roman Catholic, had cosponsored a Sanctity of Human Life act that claimed human life begins at fertilization and would have severely restricted IVF.[126] Personhood bills, like one passed in North Dakota in early 2013, could impede IVF. The Personhood USA movement has the potential to drive US-based research away from certain states or even abroad. Bernard Siegel, founder and director of the Genetic Policy Institute, said, "Any state passing a personhood measure would surely send the wrong message to the world. Do we prefer the Dark Ages or the promise of 21st century biomedical research?"[127]

While interfering with research that will improve ARTs, government at times ignores issues where it should intervene, such as the growing trend of gender selection in IVF. In China and India, where male babies are more desirable, gender selection can be used to prevent having girls. Interestingly, in the United States, it's the opposite. A clinic in Fairfax, Virginia, reported that 75 percent of its gender selection requests are for girls.[128] Shouldn't we be addressing the ethical issues of what it means to be able to determine the sex of your child? In addition, there are myriad social and economic problems that arise when the male-to-female ratio is thrown out of balance. For example, increased violence against women in parts of India is attributed to there being too many "missing" girls who have probably been aborted.

Another big issue is the regulation of sperm donation. In the 1980s, a eugenics enthusiast, Robert K. Graham, who had made a fortune inventing shatterproof eyeglasses, founded the Repository for Germinal Choice, to which he intended to lure Nobel Prize winners to donate their sperm. Graham was accused of being a Nazi and of trying to create a "master race." In the end, 229 offspring were born from the program's sperm donors—who were young scientists but not Nobel winners—before Graham died in 1997 and the Repository was shut down in 1999.[129]

More recently, a Bay Area man offered his sperm for free and was reported to have fathered an estimated fourteen children. FDA officials argued that he posed a threat to public health and fined him $100,000.[130] In 2011, the *New York Times* ran a story about a man who discovered that he had unwittingly become the father of seventy children because of poor regulations at a sperm bank.[131] In the United Kingdom, a British doctor supposedly fathered 600 children by surreptitiously using his sperm with patients at his own fertility clinic.[132] These situations seriously impact the gene pool, including the possibility that genetic defects could be spread more widely. With dozens of children sharing the same father potentially in proximity to each other, it is not impossible that these children might unwittingly mate—what some experts refer to as "accidental incest."[133]

Egg donation is also lacking enough oversight. Dr. Robert Klitzman, a professor of clinical psychiatry at Columbia University in New York, coauthored a study in *Fertility and Sterility* that looked at organizations recruiting egg donors. Dr. Klitzman and his colleagues viewed 102 websites for such organizations and found that 56 percent of them did not mention the short-term risks of egg donation.[134] In addition, the ASRM has set forth ethical standards, such as that donors should be at least twenty-one years old and should not be paid more than $10,000. Also, higher payments should not be given based on donor traits, such as blonde hair or a graduate degree. However, the guidelines do not carry legal authority and adherence to them is voluntary.

Many aspects of the infertility industry are needlessly confusing and complex. Part of the problem is that infertility, like much of medicine, is a liberal art as much as it is a science. A bigger part of the problem is that governments and medical institutions must issue more guidelines and enforce them so that we, the patients and consumers, don't feel like we have been deceived. Women and men are not adequately prepared for the physical, economic, and psychological costs of delaying childbearing. When they enter the world of infertility, as I did, the experience can be shocking and disillusioning. The controversies over ARTs highlight the need for better research, more widespread data collection, and more accessible information.

CHAPTER 4
DECISIONS, DECISIONS

When I walked into the Fertility Center at Massachusetts General Hospital on September 7, 2011—just a week after my third D&C—I was stuck in a continuum of loss. The first pregnancy had brought me joy then heartbreak. The second and third ones were accompanied by fear, which I suppressed until my anxiety was ultimately proven justified. One miscarriage felt like a disappointment; three felt like a curse. I began to mull over the mistakes I had made in my life and wonder if past or even occasional transgressions had resulted in my not being able to carry a baby to term.

All my life, I've put one foot in front of the other and prepared for various possible futures. I've seen the options and kept going with whichever one became most real. What I've done is not as important as what I will do. *But maybe what I've done is preventing me from having a child.* Becoming a mother was a role I shirked throughout my childhood, teens, and twenties. Then I met Jay, and motherhood seemed desirable and fun because I had a partner I wanted to have a child with.

Now he and I were sitting in the office of Dr. Irene Souter as a couple with fertility problems. My ob/gyn had warned me that the biggest obstacle to having a successful pregnancy would be my age. Why had I waited so long to see a specialist? Why hadn't my previous doctors referred me to one earlier? In a survey conducted by Merck (the pharmaceutical giant) and RESOLVE (the national infertility association) of fifty-seven participants, 91 percent of those seeing a fertility specialist wished that they had gone earlier.[1]

I remember the feeling of heaviness between Jay and me that day. We were in the world of infertility now. Our courtship and marriage had been so exciting and full of love, but the failed pregnancies came soon into our union and kept coming. A 2010 *SELF* magazine article on breaking the silence around infertility quoted a man named Jack who was pursuing fertility treatments with his wife: "It's almost impossible to convey what it's like to people who haven't gone through it. There's a feeling of despair and loss that you just can't quantify. So much weight is on the line, so many questions about genetics and identity and what it means to pass that down—or not."[2]

Is it worth trying so hard to have a child? What are Jay and I missing out on now by focusing so much on our fertility? Will he still love me if I don't have a child? How do I find the words to talk to him about this?

Several studies have found that the psychological impact of a diagnosis of infertility can be as devastating as a diagnosis of cancer.[3] The idea of not passing your genes on to a future generation or the evaporation of a long-held assumption of what your future would look like can feel like a death sentence. Science writer Natalie Angier has compared the two diagnoses: "Most women who attempt IVF are nearing the end of their patience and fecundity. . . . The chance of an older woman [41 to 42 years] giving birth to a baby conceived from her eggs through IVF is maybe 12 to 18 percent. If you heard that these were your odds of surviving cancer, you'd feel very, very depressed."[4]

After my third miscarriage, my mother actually offered to carry our child. I was touched but horrified. My mother was sixty-four years old! She said a friend of hers had suggested it. I thought it was pretty enlightened for Sri Lankan ladies to discuss an idea like this. In the United States, there have been at least four cases of women carrying their grandchildren. Angie Stockton of Georgia gave birth to her grandson when her daughter couldn't conceive.[5] Nonetheless, I rejected my mother's offer since I didn't think it would have solved the problem, which was that my eggs were old. I thought I still had a chance of carrying a child myself, so fertility treatments were my next tactic.

Because of my "advanced maternal age," I had started to think about egg donation. I also thought a lot about adopting, which was something I had fantasized about doing when I was younger. With so many unwanted children in the world in need of homes, why bring more children into it? If I went the adoption route, I would adopt from Sri Lanka. But I was also nervous about adopting. I'd heard stories about people who had arduous and disturbing experiences with the process. Also, before pursuing adoption, I wanted to try to have a kid with my and Jay's DNA. I wanted a child who looked like us. I wanted to see what happened when you mixed us up—an exotic Sri Lankan and a Midwestern farm boy.

When Jay and I walked into the waiting room on September 7, everyone looked depressed. There was no art on the walls. I wished they would make these places look more happy. In her office, Dr. Souter told me that because it was so soon after my miscarriage, I would have to wait until my period returned to begin the recurrent miscarriage tests. Jay would have to be tested as well, and we set up his blood work and semen analysis appointments for later that week.

When I spoke that afternoon to a friend in New York, she asked when I would next be in town. I told her that I no longer had control over my schedule because I couldn't predict when I'd have to be in Cambridge for medical tests. I had to call the doctor's office on the first day of my cycle and then go for blood work on the third and tenth days. Between the sixth and twelfth days, I had to have an X-ray test of the uterus and fallopian tubes—a hysterosalpingogram. I enjoyed rolling the word off my tongue even though the procedure was scary. I was reminded of saying the word "dolichocephalic" (having an elongated head) as a child. I had first seen the term in *The Hound of the Baskervilles*, the Sherlock Holmes book.

By October 13, I still hadn't gotten my period. It had been less than two months since my D&C, and periods can take anywhere from a few weeks to a few months to return. But I wanted to be back on a cycle so that I could take all the recurrent miscarriage tests before my rehearsals for a new show with Jay began in a few weeks. I called Dr. Souter's office and was asked to come in for a blood test in a few days if my period still hadn't come.

On October 17, I went in to have blood drawn. Many women, most with their partners, were in the waiting room. They all seemed older than me. That afternoon I received a message that, based on the blood work, my menses would arrive within the week, so there was no need to induce a period. If it didn't come in seven to ten days, then I was to call the doctor's office.

By October 20, still no period. The news came in that Gaddafi was dead in Libya. I watched the video of fighters chanting "Allah Akbar" and reveling in seeing his battered body. I didn't feel joyful; I felt disturbed that in victory these fighters were as bloodthirsty as their opponent. They enjoyed killing.

Now that I was trying harder to bring a new life into the world, I was even more aware of what was happening in the world. For years, beginning in 2001, I was an infrequent consumer of current events. I didn't subscribe to a newspaper and didn't have a television. Sometimes, I would look at news online. But by 2011, I avidly read the news, first thing in the morning on various apps on my phone, then later in the day on my computer.

On November 1, I had to go to New York to begin rehearsals. Two days later, around 2 p.m. during rehearsal, I really had to go to the bathroom. I saw blood. Because it was a Thursday and I had to visit the hospital on day 3 of my cycle, I would have to fly round-trip between New York and Boston both that Saturday and the following Saturday (day 10), if I were to make rehearsals—something I have always been proud never to miss. If I had gotten my period a week prior, it wouldn't have been a problem. If I had gotten my period on a Saturday, it would also not have been a problem because then I would have to come in on a Monday, when I didn't have to be at rehearsal. That night, I went online and bought myself very expensive last-minute flights, leaving around 6 a.m. from JFK and returning around 9:30 a.m. from Boston's Logan Airport. On November 5 at 4:30 a.m., I quietly kissed sleeping Jay—whom we agreed would stay behind since these appointments were just for routine blood work—on the cheek and took a cab to JFK.

On day 5 of my cycle, I began the Clomid Challenge Test. Although I'd taken Clomid before, I didn't really understand its effects, except that it is a fertility drug that stimulates the follicles. Evidently, the increased hormones can really mess with your emotions, but I wasn't warned about that by anyone at the Fertility Center. Dr. Lillian Schapiro, an ob/gyn who struggled with her own infertility, wrote a novel titled *Tick Tock* about, well, a doctor who deals with her infertility. When the main character is given Clomid, her doctor advises: "'Clomid can make you irritable, Amy,' he said with a laugh. 'You'd better warn your husband.'"[6] I didn't get that intel, and I wish I had because I know I wasn't myself in the rehearsal room or at home.

By November 10, I didn't feel the effect of the hormones as strongly as before. Maybe it was just exhaustion and extreme stress. I was noticing my body too much those days: the way it was not as fit around the middle and the dryness of the skin on my forehead. Every nerve and pore felt connected to each other. My upper right wisdom tooth was coming in, and I kept touching it with my tongue.

I went that night to a screening of *Connected*, a film by Tiffany Shlain. Her father, Leonard, a physician and scholar, wrote *Sex, Time and Power*, about human sexuality and evolution, in addition to many other ground-breaking books. Shlain's film is subtitled *An Autobiography of Love, Death, and Technology* and deals with her father's death, the lessons he passed along to her, and how we all should declare our "interdependence." As I watched the film, I was struck by its boundless optimism about the world's possibilities. I was humbled by what a bad mood I'd been in. I was embarrassed by my occasionally nihilistic thoughts, like *What was I trying to make a baby for?* and *What would it be like to disappear?*

What kind of world do we live in? I asked myself. Every time I thought of it, it made no sense. As Christine Overall, philosophy professor and author of *Why Have Children? The Ethical Debate*, has explained, the decision to have kids involves

> an ethical question, for it is about whether to bring a person (in some cases more than one person) into existence—and that person cannot, by the very nature of the situation, give consent to being brought into existence. Such a question also profoundly affects the wellbeing of existing people (the potential parents, siblings if any, and grandparents). And it has effects beyond the family on the broader society, which is inevitably changed by the cumulative impact—on things like education, health care, employment, agriculture, community growth and design, and the availability and distribution of resources—of individual decisions about whether to procreate.[7]

Did I really want to be a mother? And why does it feel like we have to jump through so many hoops to become one? Wouldn't it be great and logical if there were more support systems (like universal insurance coverage for fertility treatments) in place for those of us going through the process of having children and more support systems (like subsidized childcare) for those who are already parents?

At one point I had a free subscription to *Good Housekeeping*, and I actually read every issue. Ellen DeGeneres was on the October 2011 cover. I really like Ellen, so I immediately opened the magazine. In it was an article called "Crisis Control" by Mark Matousek, which began with boilerplate suggestions like acknowledging your pain, dialectical thinking, deep breathing, and yoga; but it ended with the concept of "Focus on Faith"— that the ability to turn one's confusion over to a higher power and to find solace in psalms is a boon when the chips are down.

But I've always had a hard time believing in God—not so much God as a concept but the institutions that have been built on Earth around God. I was born Roman Catholic. I was baptized and did my First Communion in a church my family has attended for decades. I got married in this same church, wearing a veil and saying the prayers. I liked the priests (there were three at my wedding) who conducted the ceremony; they are very good men. But I had the church wedding only to please my mother and her family. I didn't do it because I believed. I did it because I wanted to keep the peace. The truth is that for me, as a woman, I am offended by much of what the men who run the Catholic faith advise. Why can't women be priests? Why can't people have sex before marriage?

My pondering got me thinking about the problems women face in confronting their realities. Too often, they are expected to tough it out or turn to faith. Believing will help you have that child. Believing will ease your burden. I will live the life that I have been given.

But this is fatalism, I thought. *If you believe that, then you might as well believe that babies are dropped down chimneys.*

Those years of failing to become a mother had given me time to think hard about what I wanted. They had also sparked an intense desire for . . . I don't know, success at having a child. *Now, I want so much to have a child that I will be destroyed if it doesn't work out.*

When I went to Boston for my day 10 Clomid Challenge Test, my plane was delayed, so I arrived ten minutes late. It didn't matter though because I always ended up waiting for my name to be called. The waiting room was dotted with many different types of people. An African couple who spoke French. A lesbian couple. A blonde who looked very young, and a woman with gray hair who looked old. No one made eye contact with each other, which I'd come to realize was not unusual.

On November 14, I picked up a copy of *Metro* on my way to Massachusetts General for my last follow-up test, the hysterosalpingogram, or HSG. The front page announced, "WELCOME TO 2050." According to the article, we will have a stress-free future. Our cars will communicate with each other, so there won't be any more accidents. Robots will clean our houses. Our food will come from our rooftop gardens. And there will be two billion more people. The article didn't talk about the things that can't be changed, like women's biologies. Will we be able to have kids easily in our forties in the future?

The HSG was conducted by a doctor who looked like he was twenty. The nurse was jolly, and they both asked me questions about myself to distract me while they executed the uncomfortable procedure of sticking a catheter with a balloon up my vagina, inflating it, and passing fluid around my uterus to see if the machinery functioned well. The doctor asked what I did for work. I said I produced movies, and the nurse got excited. When the doctor went into the next room to speak to the technician, the nurse said she had an idea she wanted to talk to me about after I was done. The doctor returned and said that everything looked beautiful. I got dressed and was free to go, but the nurse wanted to escort me down the hall. She had a screenplay idea she wanted to discuss. In that moment, I didn't want to think about work or anything having to do with work. I felt incredibly weird having this conversation with her. She gave me her number and said to call her if I was interested.

On December 6, Jay and I went for our assessment with Dr. Souter. We had passed with flying colors. The various tests for things like a prothrombin mutation (which increases the chances of blood clotting) and cystic fibrosis had come back negative. My estradiol hormone level was elevated on day 3 at 73, and my follicle-stimulating hormone (FSH) level was elevated on day 10 at 13.9, but they were acceptable for my age and would not prevent me from getting insurance coverage, which would have been the case if my FSH level had been too high. The doctor's office would submit for the insurance, and once it was approved, we could set up a treatment plan.

On December 20, insurance approved, I met with Dr. Souter again to figure out the schedule. She said that treatment would help me conceive faster. She also wanted me to know that there is a higher risk for birth defects with IVF, but part of the reason for that is because the population is older. Based on my menstrual cycle, she said that I would start the Pill on January 24. I'd cycle, then the egg retrieval would happen on February 20 and the transfer on February 27. We had one issue, which was that Jay was due to leave for Hong Kong to direct a ballet at the end of January, but Dr. Souter said he could deposit his sperm at the cryobank.

We had to spend all of the next few weeks in New York, because our show was opening. The script raised the question that we might all be living in a computer simulation and was based on the novel *Simulacron-3* by Daniel Galouye, which partly inspired the film *The Matrix*. The theme of the show felt especially poignant at that time, when my worldview was in a state of constant reevaluation because of my fertility issues. In addition to producing, I was playing a role as the CEO of the company, RIEN Inc., which designed the computer simulation. The character called for me to be extra-mean. For inspiration, I watched a lot of Glenn Close in the television show *Damages*, in which she plays a murderous, conniving head of a cutthroat law firm. I had fun, but it was also scary to play someone so harsh, especially with what I was dealing with in my personal health life.

Jay and I struggled with each other on the making of the show, more so than ever before. I felt like he was second-guessing me on matters of production, and he felt I was too critical both of him and others on our team. We had fights, not a lot but enough that felt hurtful. By the time we got into tech though, the tensions calmed down, and the show was a big hit, our most successful collaboration ever. Nonetheless, I felt a strain on our interactions that I had never felt before, even with the ups and downs of the miscarriages and our working together.

Aside from the individual grief that a woman deals with when she struggles to have a child, infertility can be a huge psychological stressor on the man as well. As Dr. Paul Turek, a urologist at the University of California, San Francisco, explained: "Men are encouraged to work hard, shut up, be culturally invisible, to get the work done, and not complain, and deal with it. And so in a man's world, you see several reactions to infertility. You see deep depression, self-blame, and guilt. Lots of guilt. Or you see men brush it under the rug and have no idea of how to deal with it, and it comes back in a destructive way such as a divorce or something bad."[8]

Although ultimately Jay was cleared health-wise by the Fertility Center, there had been some concern about the round cell count in his sperm. He had to see a urologist, undergo further testing, and was put on antibiotics. He was definitely not happy about the scrutiny, and the extra appointments added stress to his already hectic life.

I wasn't thinking about the impact of the Fertility Center experience on my relationship, but when it was compounded with the intensity of building a show at the same time, the effect was obvious. I had been nervous. I had seen my future not working out before me. Physically, I was depleted. Mentally, I was confused. Who was this person I had become? Looking back, I wish I hadn't been so stressed during those months with all the back-and-forth to Boston, the scrutiny of the fertility tests, the Clomid, etc. I should have been enjoying my time with Jay, but time was not on my side, and I had to heed its call. We were still having sex regularly, but the experience of it felt different, partially because we were avoiding getting pregnant naturally. I still loved and craved physical contact with Jay, but intercourse felt more loaded.

In an Indiana University survey of men and women using IVF and seventy health providers, the responses showed that women undergoing IVF had significantly less sexual desire, less interest in sexual activity, and less satisfaction with their sexual relationship compared to women who did not require IVF. Nicole Smith, a doctoral student with the Center for Sexual Health Promotion at the Indiana University School of Public Health, said, "With assisted reproductive technologies, couples often report that they feel like a science experiment, as hormones are administered and sex has to be planned and timed. It can become stressful and is often very unromantic and regimented; relationships are known to suffer during the process."[9]

After the run of our show was over, on January 23, Jay drove the truck with the set, while I drove our car back to Boston. As I made my way from our apartment on the Lower East Side through Chinatown, I heard gunshots—they were announcing the Year of the Dragon. When I got home that afternoon, I discovered that my period had started—an auspicious day to begin. I called Dr. Souter's office to let them know, then picked up the Pill from the pharmacy.

I was really going through with it. There was no stopping the train now. I was one of many women for whom the technology had advanced too late. We were behind on the egg-freezing-is-no-longer-experimental bandwagon, and our consciousness-raising days preceded the time when how to get pregnant was as important as how to prevent getting pregnant. We didn't think through what would happen if we delayed motherhood to our late thirties, and we held onto the single-digit percentage points that tell us we might be able to have our own biological child through IVF.

Before Jay and I had begun at the Fertility Center, I had asked him if he still wanted a kid. He said yes, but he wouldn't feel like a failure if we didn't. I felt like we would be great parents together and that our child would do great things. Also, what about the great things *we* would do because of our child? I had read about a video game designer whose work was inspired by watching his son playing in the park. Jay and I are both artists, and we both work in theater. It was beautiful that we had found each other. Theater suited my belief about life—that it is ephemeral, temporary, and fleeting. As a child, the theater was perfect for me because as long as I was inhabiting someone else's world, I didn't have to live in mine—where my parents didn't get along and I was often sad at home. When I was in kindergarten, I was in *Snow White*. The lead part went to a blue-eyed, brown-haired girl named Jenny (there were four Jennys in my class . . . we had been born around the time of *Love Story*—the iconic film with a main character named Jenny). I played a tree and threw my whole body into inhabiting that tree. In seventh grade, I played a bag lady in a show written by the drama teacher. The drama teacher, who also directed the show, pulled me aside one day and told me I had talent. "You have the most marvelous and completely natural facial expressions." (From the time I was very young, I spent hours watching *I Love Lucy* and learned everything I know about facial expressions from Lucille Ball.) I wondered, *Dear drama teacher, if I'm so marvelous, why am I playing the bag lady and not the lead?*

Although Jay and I came from totally different worlds, we were both from homes where the parents tried to do the best they could but there was sadness between them. When Jay's parents split, he and his three siblings went to live with their mother. A year later, his younger and only sister died of Ewing's sarcoma at the age of twelve. Jay had been her bone marrow donor and during that time had to put his sports career on hold. He had been a junior Olympian high jumper. My parents stayed together but often fought. I remember one night my father ripping up all their wedding pictures after a heated argument. What does one do with memories like that? I loved both my parents and got along with them both, but I grew up thinking that my brother and I held them back because they seemed to be staying together for us.

It was a big leap for both me and Jay to get married, and now we were about to make another leap to start a family.

On February 11, 2012, I was getting ready for the IVF cycle to begin and was preparing to begin the fertility drug injections the next day. The autumn had been exhausting, going back and forth for various recurrent miscarriage workup tests. I'd given more blood over the previous few months than I had over the course of my entire life. I'd had medical instruments stuck inside me so many times that I had dissociated my vagina from being a sexual organ. Once the tests had been completed, at the beginning of December, I had been given the go-ahead. I was in great health and a good candidate for IVF. The assumption was that IVF would boost my chances because the doctors could preselect the strongest eggs and then embryos. Although the success rates at my age were less than 50 percent, I would know relatively quickly whether or not the pregnancy was viable. After months of evaluations, I was finally beginning my adventure in assisted reproductive technology. I had cleared my slate as much as possible for the following two months, so that I could focus completely on the process.

I spent the day preparing for the daunting schedule, which would be timed precisely according to my cycle. I read the instruction booklets that arrived with the delivery of drugs from Village Fertility Pharmacy; I watched the injection demo videos on the pharmacy website. I looked at an online fertility forum where women posted their IVF stories. The results were mixed, and the posts were punctuated with emoticons to illustrate their elation or despair. Many women had multiple failed attempts. One woman ended up with triplets.

I also looked online for "foods to eat during IVF" and was told to eat foods rich in folic acid like carrots, spinach, and pineapple (the latter of which contains enzymes that break down proteins and may or may not improve the success of embryo implantation). I was told to splurge on organic versus conventional foods; pesticides could or could not harm the fetus. I went to the store and bought groceries for a week.

To get to the hospital, I decided to drive even though it was an easy subway ride. It was a very cold morning (unusual that winter, which had made Cambridge feel like it could be the next Miami). The night before, a friend who was living with us asked if I wanted company. I had said no because it would be just a routine visit. There would be appointments down the road when I would need company.

A little before 7 a.m., I woke up and Skyped with my husband, who was in Hong Kong directing a show. With the thirteen-hour time difference, my day began as his ended. It had been three weeks that we had been apart, and we had a rule that one of us would visit the other if we were apart for that long. The plan was for me to go to Hong Kong as soon as I could once I had dealt with the initial IVF appointments. Until I could join him, checking in with each other first thing in the morning and last thing at night had become a reassuring routine.

I drove to the hospital with my IVF schedule and some fertility drugs that I wanted to ask about in my bag. As I signed in at the Fertility Center reception, I was struck by how many 2s there were that day: 2/12/12. *Maybe I'll have twins.*

In the waiting room, I picked up a *Vogue* with Meryl Streep on the cover and flipped straight to the feature about her. She talked about her passion cause, a National Museum of Women's History. I was surprised to learn there isn't one already. *When it is built, I hope it will include a section about reproductive technologies. That, to me, is one of the most important advancements between my generation and prior ones.*

My name was called by Annie, a familiar nurse with an Irish accent and a jolly vibe. She escorted me down the hall, asking, "What's your name and date of birth?" As she led me into the ultrasound room, she asked if I'd had a scan before. "Yes, of course, many times." She left me alone to take off my pants and settle onto the reclining gray vinyl bed. A doctor I hadn't seen before entered the room. He was white, American, probably in his fifties. His energy changed as he reviewed the screen. "Has anyone ever mentioned a cyst to you before?" "No." He measured my ovaries, counting two follicles on the left and three on the right. He asked Annie to call in the other doctor on duty. Annie left the room and returned with another doctor I'd never seen before, with an African accent and a youthful face.

I heard the words "ovarian cyst." The wand moving slightly inside me was such a familiar feeling.

The African doctor left the room, and the American doctor asked me to sit in the nurse's office. That day, Ellen was on duty. I'd spoken to her on the phone but had never met her. She asked if everything went okay. I said, "I don't know, but I have questions about the drugs. Should I ask?" She said, "Yes, let's get that started." I pulled the schedule from my backpack, and she reviewed the dates and tasks. She demonstrated how to prepare the Menopur (hormone) injection by sticking the needle into each of six vials, pushing the fluid into the vial, and sucking the liquefied powder into the needle. Then, she showed me, demonstrating with her leg, how to pinch my thigh and stab it with the needle and with a steady hand push the liquid into it.

Why is the doctor taking so long? Ellen registered the look on my face and seemed to know what I was thinking. She went to the doctor's office across the hall, and he came with her back to her office. I could tell by his face that he had bad news. "Ellen, can you set up lab work for Tanya so she can take care of it before she leaves?" He said I couldn't start the cycle until they figured out what was going on with the cyst. It was about three and a half inches in diameter. "You took the Clomid Challenge Test?" Yes. I did it in November. *Do I sense him making a connection between the Clomid and the cyst?* I wanted to know everything, but I asked, "Can the tests reveal anything good?" He said, "I like the way you put it, 'anything good.' Well, they could show that there is no hormonal activity, and then you can proceed. But we have to stop the process now until you and Dr. Souter can understand what is going on." "Okay," I said. He said, "You are handling this very elegantly." *What does he expect me to do, break down in tears?* "Thank you," I said. "Life sucks. What to do." He and Ellen smiled and laughed a little.

He shook my hand and left the room. Ellen typed the request for lab work into the computer. Instead of thinking about myself, I was thinking about the drugs that were sitting in my bag. *What do I do with them?* They had been delivered just the day before yesterday. *Maybe some of them will last, but the Lupron has an expiration date of April 25, 2012.* I said to Ellen, "You know, for the future, it might be good if you did an ultrasound before patients spend hundreds of dollars on fertility drugs." It was a combative thing for me to say, but I felt justified. She responded, "We can't know until we do the baseline ultrasound, which has to be on day 3."

But, I am thinking to myself, *I haven't had an ultrasound in two months.* The cyst wasn't there then. If I had had an ultrasound after being approved by insurance for treatment, only three weeks ago, would I have been spared the extreme letdown of that moment? I'm a producer. I thrive on the organization of things. Sometimes this mechanism kicks in at the expense of emotion, like right then when my frustration about the clinical aspects of the process were foremost on my mind. But the outcome was settled: *I cannot start today.*

I returned to the waiting room until a nurse with a Caribbean accent called me in for a blood test. She asked for my name and date of birth. "March 20." She said, "You won't have snow this birthday," referring to the strangely mild winter we'd been having. I thought, *And I won't be pregnant.* I told her, "Yes, the world is ending, but it feels good." We both laughed at my jab about the positive side of global warming.

Over the previous few months, anything could have gone wrong with the recurrent miscarriage workup. I could have had diabetes or blood clotting issues. I could have had weird allergies. My uterus could have been the problem. But I was in excellent health, and my machinery worked great. I had been ready to launch.

I had never imagined that a routine ultrasound at the beginning of the IVF process would destroy everything I had endured and had been mentally and physically prepared for. I was only supposed to be confirming that my ovulation had been suppressed. The following months had been set. The injections were supposed to begin that day, which was day 2 on my schedule. I was to take twenty units of Lupron (which suppresses ovulation) for three days, adding 450 units of Gonal-F (which stimulates the follicles) the next day, decreasing Lupron to 5 units on day 5, adding Menopur (a combination of FSH and LH, or luteinizing hormone) on the sixth day. On day 11, the male partner was to give his sperm. (Jay was away, but he had deposited his sperm at a sperm bank.) On day 13, I might have had to do an hCG injection (which triggers the final maturation of the eggs) at a specific time, after which I would stop the Lupron and Gonal-F. Day 14 would have been the evening prior to egg retrieval; I wouldn't have been able to eat or drink after midnight. And so on.

I asked the phlebotomist who took my blood sample when the results would be in. I would get a call that afternoon. I drove home and tried not to think about the future. I was glued to my computer, catatonic, waiting for the phone to ring. Everyone was talking about Whitney Houston who had died the night before. She had been my adolescence. I was more of a new wave and Prince girl in the '80s, but I loved Whitney Houston. I watched a video of her singing "I Will Always Love You." I hadn't cried at the hospital. I'd never cried in front of a doctor. But I started crying watching this video.

Around 2 p.m., my phone rang with the familiar "blocked" caller ID, and I knew it was the hospital. Ellen said my tests were normal, but unfortunately the doctor didn't want me to start the cycle. She set up an appointment with Dr. Souter for Tuesday, two days from then.

I wrote down questions in my little green journal from Sri Lanka, so I wouldn't forget them on Tuesday: *Why didn't they detect the cyst two weeks ago when I came in for the mock IVF procedure? Could the cyst have appeared in the last two weeks or could they have missed it two months ago during my last ultrasound? How many women develop cysts after taking Clomid? What about my insurance? I'm only covered until March 18, and I turn forty-one on March 20. Don't the coverage rules change after forty-one?*

The way I was feeling, I could have stayed home, shut down, and gone to bed. But instead I went to a friend's house to watch the Grammys. I wanted to see Adele sing for the first time since she had vocal cord surgery, and I wanted to see Jennifer Hudson perform a Whitney Houston tribute. I didn't tell my friend what had happened to me that day. I just wanted to enjoy myself. Also, I didn't really know what was going on. As a woman, when I hear "ovarian cyst" I think of scary possibilities, even though cysts are usually nothing. I didn't want my friend to worry.

The next morning, I distracted myself with tasks. My husband tried to reach me a few times on Skype, but I was too preoccupied to answer him. I was on the phone with Village Pharmacy, which was telling me that once the drugs leave the premises, they can't be returned. I left a message for Pam, my chief nurse at Massachusetts General. I spoke to my insurance company to see what would happen now that I wasn't starting IVF. *Will I be approved again?* Luckily, it seemed I would be. Since I had the insurance rep on the phone and wanted to focus on clinical things, I asked her about the bill I had received with the drug delivery. My total due was $166.57, but the prices didn't make sense; some drugs were $3.25, some were $40. She explained the cost breakdown. I paid a maximum of $8 for a Tier 1 drug, or generic; a maximum of $25 for a Tier 2, or brand name; and up to $40 for a Tier 3, or non-preferred medication. That parlayed into Diazepam costing me $1.32—a generic for which I paid exactly what it cost; Vivelle was $76.35 but cost me $40; progesterone cost me $8 but was actually $56.06; methylprednisolone also cost $8 but was actually $10.74 (not a big discount there); and then came the whoppers: Gonal-F cost me $25 but actually $3,299.87; the Lupron was $8 but was $173.19 (*okay, not so bad*); and the Menopur was $25 but was actually $1,899.66.

It seemed odd to pay more for a drug that cost under $100, like Vivelle, than one that cost over $3,000, like Gonal-F. But that's our insurance system. At least I lived in one of the fifteen states that mandates partial or complete insurance coverage of IVF.[10] That list was comprised of Arkansas, California, Connecticut, Hawaii, Illinois, Louisiana, Maryland, Massachusetts, Montana, New Jersey, New York, Ohio, Rhode Island, Texas, and West Virginia. I was surprised not to see Oregon, and I was surprised to see Texas.

America makes little sense with regard to fertility treatments, how much they cost and who can access them. If I had delayed motherhood in one of the thirty-five states that doesn't mandate IVF coverage, I would probably not have been trying to have a baby. In most states, I guess it is a pursuit of the wealthy, those who can afford the drug and procedure prices—the average cost for one cycle can range between $10,000 and $20,000.

After the call with the insurance company, I didn't understand even more the cost of healthcare in America. Maybe I could have done what some experts actually encourage: become an IVF tourist and visited an exotic destination where treatment was cheap. I could have finally visited India, where I had never been even though I often visited my native Sri Lanka, less than an hour away by plane. Infertile couples flew to India from everywhere to partake of the plentiful ART centers.

I was not prepared for the deep malaise that was settling in.

A 2004 study by Harvard Medical School showed that 40 percent of infertile women suffered from depression and 87 percent from anxiety.[11] According to a study of 202 women undergoing IVF at the University of California, San Francisco, there is a connection between IVF and depression or anxiety. "Of 103 women with a failed attempt, 60 percent had symptoms of a clinical anxiety disorder—up slightly from 57 percent before their IVF cycles. And 44 percent had clinical depression, which was up from 26 percent before treatment."[12]

I took a break from the phone and computer to play the piano, the Andante from Schubert's Sonata in A Major. Schubert was good music for my pensive mood. My brain was spinning with numbers, logistics, and IVF vacations, but I was going nowhere that day.

CHAPTER 5
THE LIMITS OF EVOLUTION

S ociety has evolved to encourage women to delay motherhood, but our bodies have not evolved to allow for that delay. Our periods arrive when we are girls, long before we should be having children, and menopause ends our fertility, long before our lives are over. In the pages to follow, I explore the impact of evolution on women's bodies and how it relates to the trend of delaying motherhood. In addition, I examine the specific life stages—menstruation, sexual activity, childbearing, and menopause—which can transform a girl into a woman into a mother into a grandmother.

In a discussion about delaying motherhood, it is essential to consider who shapes society, what laws and policies impact women's sexual and reproductive freedoms, and what factors affect gender relations. Therefore, I also look at how men and society have sought to control women's bodies and sexualities. If women are delaying motherhood because of institutional biases in place that compel us to prioritize other aspirations first, we need to understand the root causes of these biases and identify ways to alleviate them.

With assisted reproductive technologies (ARTs), older women may believe they have greater agency over their bodies, but the science doesn't greatly improve their chances of a live birth if they are using their own older eggs. As Harvard Medical School researcher Alan S. Penzias has said, "Even as effective as IVF is, it can't reverse the effects of aging. We cannot reverse the biological clock."[1] New advancements in ovary, egg, and embryo freezing suggest that in the future we may be able to bend nature more in our favor, but until those techniques are proven, perfected, *and* more accessible and affordable, we are tethered to the reality of evolution and biology.

Grounding this reality with an understanding of feminism is crucial.

The research has had to be reevaluated to temper academic principles originally established by men—which science writer Natalie Angier has amusingly characterized as "higgamus, hoggamus, Pygmalionus, *Playboy* magazine, eternitas. Amen."[2] In other words, the original theories on evolution and biology have propagated negative stereotypes and harmful, gendered behavior. Accepting biology in no way means accepting those theories, too. As the historian Gerda Lerner told the *Chicago Tribune* in 1993, "In my courses, the teachers told me about a world in which ostensibly one-half the human race is doing everything significant and the other half doesn't exist. I asked myself how this checked against my own life experience. 'This is garbage; this is not the world in which I have lived,' I said."[3]

In *Woman: An Intimate Geography*, Angier showed how the female body is "part of the answer, is a map to meaning and freedom." She wrote, "Woman, the bowl, the urn, the cave, the musky jungle. We are the dark mysterium!"[4] And she cited Mary Carlson of Harvard Medical School who "coined 'liberation biology' to describe the use of biological insights to heal our psychic wounds, understand our fears, and make the most of what we have."[5]

Puberty is a tumultuous experience—a sign that we are not children anymore, and today, both boys and girls are reaching it at younger and younger ages. Early puberty in girls was first documented in 1997 and has been established by several subsequent studies.[6] A November 2012 issue of *Pediatrics* presented evidence that boys also are developing sexually at an earlier age—about nine years old among African American boys and around ten years old among non-Hispanic white and Hispanic boys. The lead author of both the 1997 and 2012 studies was Marcia Herman-Giddens of the University of North Carolina's School of Public Health. She said, "The changes are too fast. Genetics take maybe hundreds, thousands of years. You have to look at something in the environment. That would include everything from (a lack of) exercise to junk food to TV to chemicals."[7] A link between early puberty and developmental issues has not been documented for boys, but early puberty in girls has been linked to lower self-esteem, more depression, and more eating disorders.[8] (In my situation, perhaps there was a link between my anxiety over getting my first period at eight years old and my susceptibility later to bulimia.) Sonya Lunder, a senior analyst with the Environmental Working Group, said, "The overall concern is that by hastening puberty you're actually shortening childhood. The real impact of this is not only on future fertility" but also that puberty is a "physiological change in your brain."[9]

Caitlin Moran, a hilarious feminist author, has written about her experience: "There's crazy shit breaking out all over the place. Bleeding and masturbatory experimentation are the very least of it. The transformation of my body from something that does little more than poo and do jigsaws into a magical department store that will, one day, vend babies takes up nearly all my time and worry."[10]

When I myself got pubic hair, I was disgusted. I went to my parents' bathroom, grabbed my father's razor, and shaved off the hair. (I was happy to read in Moran's *How to Be a Woman* that she did the exact same thing.)

With her period, a woman receives a message that her fate is sealed as a child-bearer. As Angier has described, "There is no clearer rite of passage, no surer demarcation between childhood and adulthood, than menarche, the first period. When people talk of the indelibility of a strong memory, they speak of recalling exactly where they were when Kennedy was shot or the *Challenger* space shuttle exploded. But what a woman really remembers is her first period."[11] Moran wrote about hers: "'My first period started: yuk.' I write in my diary. 'I don't think Judy Garland ever had a period,' I tell the dog, unhappily, later that night."[12]

I remember vividly when I got my period. I saw the blood on my underpants and didn't know what was happening. I just thought it was something bad. Maybe I was sick; maybe I was dying. For two days, I wrapped my underwear in lots of tissue and hid them at the bottom of the garbage can. My mother found them when she was cleaning the house. Where I come from, Sri Lanka, when a girl gets her period, it's a cause for celebration. My parents bought me five gold coins to cash in or turn into jewelry at a later date. But I firmly rejected the idea of throwing a "period party." Nonetheless, my mother told all her friends, and I felt humiliated. The worst part about that time was when she said to me, "Now the boys will come after you," as if when a girl gets her period, she emits a magical scent that attracts the opposite sex.[13]

The menarche ritual has occurred throughout history and continues in many cultures today. In the 1991 book *Blood Relations*, the anthropologist Chris Knight pointed out that "menstrual rituals were among the first and most important rites performed by early humans."[14] In some cultures, the rituals have been brutal. Among the Loango of East Africa, girls were confined to dark huts and prohibited from letting their feet touch the ground or allowing their eyes to see the sun for two years. In New Ireland in the South Pacific, girls were also confined—in dark cages and for four years.[15]

In the book *Sex, Time and Power: How Women's Sexuality Shaped Human Evolution*, the physician and scholar Leonard Shlain described how menstruation taboos "served to strip political power and autonomy from women." Among the Bribri Indians of Costa Rica, a menstruating woman was "forbidden to come near a male's hunting weapons or touch any food or utensils." In the Jewish Orthodox tradition, the period of *niddah*, during which a woman is considered impure, is marked by five days of menstruation followed by a week. Husbands and wives sleep in separate beds, and the man cannot touch her or even take care of her when she is sick unless there is no one else to help.[16]

Historical medical writings abound with morbid and even scary depictions of women's bodies. Angier explained that Victorian "scientists were astounded by the ovarian cycle. . . . Some were simply fascinated by it; others were disgusted by it. All wrote gothically of it, and found in the monthly follicular rupturing and oozing yet another reason to pity the fair, better, bruised, and battered sex." For example, she mentioned that Havelock Ellis, the British physician and social reformer who studied human sexuality, "saw the monthly release of an egg as a 'worm' that 'gnaws periodically at the roots of life.'"[17]

In modern times, negative portrayals of menstruation have persisted. But could there be reasons to appreciate our periods?

For some, periods are certainly a curse, accompanied by debilitating cramps and headaches. But for others, periods are not a big deal. Once I became an adult, I began to find mine reassuring. When it arrives, I feel like my body is working.

Angier, citing Margie Profet, an evolutionary biologist at the University of Washington, described menstruation as an adaptation: "It is a product of design, the designer in this case being that greatest and most unpretentious of deities, evolution by natural selection."[18] A striking element of that design is the length of the cycle, approximately 29.5 days, which correlates to the interval between two new moons. As a result, a menstruating woman can have a hyperawareness of the passage of time, marked by the cycle between her periods. In fact, there is much evidence, as presented by the feminist author Barbara Walker, to show that men prized women's wisdom, which they associated with menstrual blood: "The Norse god Thor owed his enlightenment to bathing in a river of menstrual blood. Odin was similarly gifted with shrewdness because he stole and drank the wise blood from the Mother Goddess, a myth quite similar to the Hindu god Indra's theft of knowledge from the Primal Matriarchs via their menstrual blood."[19]

Another positive design element is cryptic ovulation, meaning that women don't outwardly exhibit when they're ovulating. As Leonard Shlain explained, "In the majority of primate species, a female in estrus displays spectacular physical manifestations as ovulation approaches. Her vulvar sexual skin (best seen from behind by the male) blushes a flaming red and swells with edema fluid, sometimes impressively."[20] However, we humans not only don't signal when we're ovulating, but we also (for the most part) wear clothes that conceal our genitalia. In addition, we can have sex every day of the year, unlike some species that can physiologically *only* have sex when they're ovulating.

Angier asserted, "We are carnal beings whose sexual activity far exceeds any reproductive needs. . . . We are not helping our offspring or our mates or the whole damned race; we are helping ourselves. Let us help others too. When your daughter or niece or younger sister runs to you and crows, 'It's here!' take her out for a bowl of ice cream or a piece of chocolate cake, and raise a glass of milk to the new life that begins with blood."[21]

I guess I should have let my parents throw me that period party.

As we approach puberty and increasingly thereafter, we start to think about sex, perhaps fantasizing about movie stars and musicians. With me, it was Duran Duran. I painfully swooned over John Taylor and sometimes Simon Le Bon. I would have taken any of the Durans, really. I also thought I was meant to be with one of them because they shot the music videos for "Hungry Like the Wolf" and "Save a Prayer" in Sri Lanka. I remember feeling tender when my puberty began, like I was caught unaware and had to hide. I remember boys as being aggressive by comparison. For instance, during a sleepover at our house, a boy tried to screw my Baby Alive doll—which had orifices through which it could be fed and through which it could go to the bathroom. I was traumatized.

Angier explained that "the brain of a prepubertal girl is primed to absorb the definitions of womanness, of what counts and what doesn't, of what power is and how she can get it or how she will never get it."[22] I needed to learn from our close relatives, the bonobo apes, whose females defend each other from sexual targeting even though the males are stronger. But I am glad I'm not a sow. Did you know that the term "male chauvinist pig" came about because male pigs spit a steroid compound on the female to cause her to spread her legs and freeze?[23]

Natalie Angier challenged patriarchal notions of the sexual passivity of women. As she wrote, "Women are said to have lower sex drives than men, yet they are universally punished if they display evidence to the contrary. . . . How can we know what is 'natural' for us when we are treated as unnatural for wanting our lust, our freedom, the music of our bodies?"[24] The anthropologist Barbara Smuts has written, "It seems premature to attribute the relative lack of female interest in sexual variety to women's biological nature alone in the face of overwhelming evidence that women are consistently beaten for promiscuity and adultery. If female sexuality is muted compared to that of men, then why must men the world over go to extreme lengths to control and contain it?"[25]

In general, human females have the capacity to orgasm more intensely than any other species. Despite this advantage, girls are not conditioned to take pleasure from sex. As Peggy Orenstein has written, "Most young women are profoundly alienated from their bodies at sexual initiation; they're rarely privy to adequate information, and less than half have masturbated."[26] Citing the work of sociologist Marcia Douglass and anthropologist Lisa Douglass (authors of *Are We Having Fun Yet?*), Orenstein noted that "less than a third of women experience orgasm regularly in sexual encounters, while seventy-five percent of men do."[27] Women need to take control of the paradigm, because as Orenstein explained, "there's a critical connection between sexual agency and a lifelong sense of self."[28]

The pleasure of sex is tempered by the treacherous experience of childbirth. The anthropologist Nancy Burley has theorized that sexual signaling disappeared in human females because childbirth was so painful; it was better for women not to know when they were ovulating.[29] In February 2012, I attended a conversation between the artist Laurie Anderson and the neuroscientist Dean Buonomano about the fallibility of memory and the brain. A question came up about how women supposedly have a reflex that enables them to forget the pain of childbirth so that they continue having children. Buonomano said it's a miracle we're all still here considering how grueling it is to have us.

Maternal mortality increased as our brains continued to expand over time—tripling in size over the last 2.5 million years. The pelvic girdle remained relatively unchanged, so women had to deal with the severity and high probability of tears and lacerations during delivery. Many women died during the process. Fortunately, science stepped in—through cesareans, prenatal testing, epidurals, and birth control—to make childbirth less perilous for women.

Aside from the way we deliver babies, the way we conceive babies is also complicated, with the need for a sperm to meet an egg. Why we reproduce the way we do is a mystery. As Angier wrote, "The study of the origins of sex is a vigorous discipline, with a plethora of proposed justifications and a dearth of proof for any of them."[30] However, a key reason for reproducing sexually is survival. In human beings, the first evolutionary milestone is surviving to a reproductive age; the next one is successfully mating with the opposite sex. Reaching the second milestone is the more challenging endeavor. By combining the genes of two individuals, we improve the overall gene pool.

Although both men and women confront the difficulties of conceiving a child, a woman typically releases one or maybe two eggs per month, while a man produces 3.6 billion sperm, each of which is capable of fertilizing an egg. Moreover, as women age, we increasingly face the glaring disparity between men's and women's fertility spans. As Leonard Shlain put it, "The puzzling installation of a biological alarm clock set to ring at an ungodly early hour in our species alone is all the more baffling when compared with the absence of a similar device in men."[31] He added: "Instead of knowing she is fertile right up to the time she dies, she becomes acutely aware that her biological clock will stop ticking at not the stroke of midnight but more like six-thirty or seven o'clock in the evening. Just when the party is really getting interesting, and she has finally figured out how all the participants interact, the pumpkin coach arrives. This, then, is the cruel double bind for women."[32]

Natalie Angier wrote, "There's a principle in evolutionary thinking called the naturalistic fallacy—making the mistake of assuming that what is, is for the best."[33] That our eggs run out is not the best for women who have delayed motherhood. Assisted reproductive technologies have stepped in to remedy our evolutionary deficiency, but they are not guaranteed to work, and they carry their own risks for adding to evolutionary issues.

The phenomenon of delayed motherhood could ultimately impact evolution. Liza Mundy wrote in her 2007 book *Everything Conceivable* about how ARTs are changing the world, "Evolution is being thwarted." By facilitating the passing down of genes most likely to succeed, evolution is guided by the "survival of the fittest," but in Mundy's opinion, ARTs are allowing for problems to be "admitted in the gene line that Nature would have headed off at the pass."[34] She asserted, "Assisted reproduction may someday make the human race better. Then again, it may make the human race worse."[35]

While the risks for having a child born with developmental disorders or birth defects do increase with advanced parental age, implying such children may make the human race worse is myopic and ignores the wisdom and joy these children contribute to the world. For example, writer and life coach Martha Beck, writer Priscilla Gilman, and artist Kelle Hampton have given us beautiful memoirs about having children with special needs.[36] In particular, Beck acutely captured the dilemma over her decision to proceed with her pregnancy after discovering her son would have Down syndrome: "I am very much afraid of being caught in the firestorm of controversy over abortion, genetic engineering, medical ethics. It worries me to think that I will be lumped with right-to-lifers, not to mention every New Age crystal kisser who ever claimed to see an angel in the clouds over Sedona."[37]

Controversies aside, Mundy's point about the long-term outcome of changes in the gene pool as a result of ARTs is worth considering. The discussion could also include a look at the repercussions of letting women transfer three, four, five, or more embryos and carrying all of them to term, saying it's "God's will."

On the positive end of the debate, there are certainly ways in which older parents can benefit society. For instance, ART kids tend to have motivated parents—people who were determined to become parents despite considerable emotional, financial, and physical tolls. I see this among many of my friends, including single mothers and same-sex couples, who had to be more intentional in their pursuit of parenthood.

Also, parents who struggled more to have kids could be more attentive to the needs of their kids. A 2012 study in the United Kingdom—where the first IVF baby was born in 1978 and where the number of mothers over forty who gave birth almost doubled between 2000 and 2010—showed that the children of older women are less likely to have accidents or need hospital care. They also develop a broader vocabulary from a young age and achieve higher scores on IQ tests in a range of measures up to the age of five.[38]

A US study showed that the offspring of older fathers could be genetically programmed to live longer because older fathers pass along longer telomeres, which curb the deterioration of chromosomes.[39] As Mundy has pointed out, "Both because of what it can do and what it can't, assisted reproduction is affecting human evolution in contradictory ways, driving us forward and backward at the same time."[40]

Dominique Bousquet, a lithe and youthful-looking forty-four-year-old, asked me, "Do you think we will evolve so that we can have children later? Because so many women are pushing to have children later, then our bodies will adapt?"[41] Bousquet is a New York-based masseuse who married and divorced once in her thirties. At the age of forty-three, she found the perfect mate. For the first time, she thought she would like to have children. She'd read or heard about women in their late forties having biological children, so maybe that could happen for her?

But menopause is a biological process that evolution is unlikely to change—at least anytime soon. There are theories that menopause evolved 1.5 million years ago. However, such theories cannot be proved because ovaries don't leave fossils behind.[42] A chimp goes through menopause around forty and dies around forty-five, while a woman, according to Leonard Shlain, "undergoes menopause at a point in her life when she still has many remaining years of health, vitality, and strength."[43] Most mammals ovulate until they die. Contemporary human females live longer than most mammals (bowhead whales are an exception, with a life span of around 150 years). Despite currently being the longest-living terrestrial mammal, a woman stops ovulating earlier than other female mammals.

While some aspects of aging occur at varying times and to varying degrees, and some can be delayed for decades, menopause is unchangeable. According to Angier, "Whatever a woman does, however rigorously she attends to her health, at the half-century mark, give or take a few years, she will go into what the renowned evolutionary biologist George C. J.

Williams called 'premature reproductive senescence.'"[44] A woman's reproductive system, unlike other systems within her body, is programmed "to shut down operations considerably before closing time," said Shlain.[45] Some have theorized that this is because we simply live longer than our ancestors. Alison Galloway, an anthropologist at University of California in Santa Cruz, argued: "I don't think there's anything beneficial about menopause. I don't think it's been selected for. It's the result of our recent expansions in our lifespan. We outlive our follicles."[46] If we died in our forties and fifties, the original ratio of fertile years to life span would be logical.

However, menopause could have been meant to occur well before the natural end of a woman's life—thus, it is an evolutionary benefit. For instance, the Hadza of northern Tanzania live in some ways how human beings did in the Pliocene and Pleistocene periods during which *Homo sapiens* evolved. In cultures like that of the Hadza, grandmothers are very important; older women are necessary repositories of knowledge for how to survive. Rather than dying when their eggs run out, many Hadza women keep going past menopause.[47] Aside from this anthropological evidence, it could be that menopause arrives to shut down the reproductive mechanism while we still have enough energy—having and rearing kids is an exhausting and, again, potentially deadly endeavor. Menopause could be a way of ensuring that there are grandmothers to help out. Among the Hadza, for example, grandmothers help take care of the young while the mothers go foraging and the fathers hunt. Julia McQuillan, professor of sociology at the University of Nebraska, explained, "Regarding evolution, aging, and the long time periods in which adult women cannot be pregnant (I call these 'post-reproductive' years), there are some anthropological studies about the importance of grandmothers for the survival of grandchildren."[48]

In my family, I am the eldest grandchild, and I have a close and fun relationship with my grandmother, even though I don't see her that much because she lives in Sri Lanka. She became a grandmother at the age of forty-six—a few years older than I am now. Today, with more women delaying childbearing, especially college-educated women, more women won't be grandmothers until they're in their seventies—or even older.[49] It's hard to qualify this fact as good or bad for society, but it does result in kids having less time to benefit from their interactions with their grandmothers.

Taking this into account, menopause makes sense, allowing us to transition from the metabolically expensive activity of childbearing to the golden years of grandmothering. Thus, the problem is not with biological evolution but with cultural evolution, where women's relationships to their sexuality and reproductive freedoms become complicated.

While women have greater agency over their lives and careers, they have had to fit into a society structured by and for men, around men's needs, and based on men's schedules. In the past, women were so engaged with bearing and raising children that they didn't have the freedom men did to shape society. The anthropologist Sherry Ortner, in her 1974 article "Is the Female to Male as Nature Is to Culture?" explained how women are associated with nature because of their reproductive systems and childbearing. Men have an antagonistic relationship to nature because of their need to conquer it. This inclination has been attributed in part to testosterone and its impact on aggressive tendencies.[50] Men's desire to control culture and society fuels their desire to control women. Natalie Angier explained it this way: "As recently as the nineteenth century, physicians argued that the uterus competes directly with the brain for an adequate blood supply. Thus any effort a woman made to nourish her mind through education or career could come only at the expense of her fertility."[51] As Dr. Horace Bigelow wrote in 1883, "Excessive education 'is accountable for much of the sterility and physical degeneracy of American womanhood.'"[52]

On a visit a few years ago to Sri Lanka's Peradeniya Botanical Gardens in the lush city of Kandy, I was amused to discover that pineapple trees have genders and visibly manifest their sexual differences. The male had protruding, long phallus-like growths, and the female had what appeared to be breasts. In general among humans, however, the line between maleness and femaleness is thin, and before we are born, the sexes are not far apart. We all start in the womb as females until hormones differentiate us into male or female. As we reach middle age, we come closer together again, hormonally speaking, when men's estrogen levels rise and women's decline. The word "hormone" comes from the Greek for "messenger"— our hormones direct us toward one gender or another.

Carl Linnaeus, the Swedish taxonomist, introduced the term "Mammalia" to name our class, linking us to our identification with our breasts, the mammary glands. He named our species *Homo sapiens*: man of wisdom. Thus, physically we are tied to our lactating mothers, but mentally we are tied to our reasonable fathers. This separateness was used to keep women in the dark. As Angier described, "Thinkers of the Enlightenment advocated the equality and natural rights of all men, and some women of the time, including Mary Wollstonecraft and Abigail Adams, John's wife, argued that women too should be given their due rights—enfranchisement, for example, or the rights to own property or divorce a brutal spouse. The husbands of the Enlightenment smiled with tolerance and sympathy. . . . Through zoology and the taxonomic reinforcement of woman's earthiness, rational men found convenient justification for postponing matters of women's rights until woman's reason, her *sapientia*, was fully established."[53]

In the foraging and hunting cultures of old, women could exercise more control over a man's access to her, but then culture was reconfigured in a way that was deleterious to women's status. The anthropologist Sarah Blaffer Hrdy has noted, "I am convinced that male control over productive resources needed by women to reproduce lies at the heart of the transformation from male-dominated philopatric primate societies to full-fledged patriarchy."[54] Men were necessary to help provide for the young. A bond between a man and a woman, like a marriage, was necessary for survival. Women went from being foragers to being possessions and protected. The first slaves were women, "and the impetus behind slavery was the possession of nubile wombs."[55]

Another example of the weakening of women is that when a woman married, she was forced to leave her tribe and live with her husband's family, which meant she had to adapt to unfamiliar surroundings. Also, women often came with a bounty to attract the man. Many cultures today continue the practice of dowry. I had one—a house near my grandmother's in Sri Lanka, which would be gifted to whomever I married, but after the war began in the early '80s, my parents gradually gave up the dream that we would live there. Eventually, we sold the house to a relative, and my dowry was never replaced.

Misogyny and patriarchy are manifestations of men's desire for control. Before the advent of paternity tests, men uniquely faced the risk of paternal uncertainty, which was exacerbated by cryptic ovulation and internal female fertilization. According to the author Rebecca Hannagan, Charles Darwin, for all his chauvinism about men being "active and ardent" and women being "passive and reclusive," "attributed a more important evolutionary role to females than did most evolutionists for nearly a century after him: female choice in sexual selection. Since females bear the greater parental investment through pregnancy and lactation, they have more to gain from being highly selective about with whom to mate than do males."[56] Women exercised control over mating choice and thus could arouse in men the desire to control women's reproductive independence.

As Leonard Shlain asserted, "Misogyny is a disdain for women and denigration of the values commonly associated with the feminine. Patriarchy is a set of institutionalized social rules put in place by men to control the sexual and reproductive rights of women."[57] Throughout time, men have sought ways to control women's sexual and reproductive freedoms. As Shlain explained, "A man's control of the former ensured that he could relieve his intolerable itch on terms favorable to his sex; control of the second assured his place in posterity."[58]

Every day we read about how misogyny and patriarchy persist in various forms. Throughout the world, women live with a constant fear of violence. According to a National Intimate Partner and Sexual Violence Survey conducted by the US government in 2010, one in four women reported having been beaten by an intimate partner, and one in six women have been stalked. Nearly one in five women said they had been raped or had experienced an attempted rape at some point, while one in seventy-one men had.[59]

During the Arab Spring in 2011, an army doctor in Egypt was accused of performing forced "virginity tests" on women detained by soldiers. In 2012, he was acquitted. While I was working on this chapter, on December 16, 2012, a twenty-three-year-old female physiotherapy student was raped and tortured by a group of six men on a bus in New Delhi, India; she eventually died from her injuries. Despite having had a female head of state (Indira Gandhi, who served a record four terms from 1966 to 1977 and then again from 1980 until her assassination in 1984) and passing a new anti-rape law in 2013, India is reputed to be one of the worst countries in the world for women's rights.

The hideous rape became a rallying cry for protesters—both men and women—throughout India to call for better protection of women. In the city of Amritsar, a group carried a sign saying, "DON'T TELL UR [sic] DAUGHTERS NOT TO GO OUT. TELL YOUR SONS TO BEHAVE PROPERLY."[60] Although the practice is not to name rape victims publicly, the victim's father came forward and asked that she be named. "My daughter didn't do anything wrong, she died while protecting herself," he said. "I am proud of her. Revealing her name will give courage to other women who have survived these attacks. They will find strength from my daughter."[61]

This tragedy in India was during a time of relative peace. During war and in areas of conflict around the world, rape and violence against women is highly prevalent and rarely prosecuted. There have been reports of babies as young as six months being raped in the Democratic Republic of the Congo. What will it take to stop the madness? The UN envoy on sexual violence in conflict, Zainab Hawa Bangura, argued that it has to be a "massive liability to commit, command or condone sexual violence in conflict."[62] Any conflict resolution, whether in Syria or Mali, has to include sexual violence prevention. Following from this idea, laws on rape and violence against women around the world have to call for stricter punishment and accountability.

In February 2013, the US Senate expanded the reach of the landmark Violence against Women Act of 1994. Encouraging the House to take action as well, President Barack Obama said, "Delay isn't an option when three women are still killed by their husbands or boyfriends every day. Delay isn't an option when countless women still live in fear of abuse, and when one in five have been victims of rape. This issue should be beyond debate—the House should follow the Senate's lead and pass the Violence against Women Act right away. This is not a Democratic or Republican issue—it's an issue of justice and compassion."[63]

Control over women's bodies is a seemingly eternal flashpoint and political quagmire. States across America from Montana to New Jersey to Texas have cut or eliminated government-funded family planning programs. According to RESOLVE, the national infertility association, in 2012 alone there were efforts to get personhood ballot initiatives—which seek to define that life begins as early as at conception—in at least eight states.[64] In February 2013, North Dakota, rated the worst state in the United States for women, passed a personhood bill that could shut down the state's one abortion clinic and threaten family planning programs. Such personhood bills could restrict access not only to birth control and abortions but also to fertility treatments. Sara Stoesz, the CEO of Planned Parenthood of Minnesota, North Dakota, and South Dakota, denounced what she perceived as "politicians inserting themselves into the private medical decision-making of women and families in our state."[65]

In 2012, we saw a toxic combination of ignorance and bias in male politicians' and political commentators' remarks on women's issues. Radio personality Rush Limbaugh called Georgetown University law student Sandra Fluke a slut for asking for insurance coverage for birth control: "What does it say about the college co-ed Susan Fluke [sic] who goes before a congressional committee and essentially says that she must be paid to have sex—what does that make her? It makes her a slut, right? It makes her a prostitute. She wants to be paid to have sex. She's having so much sex she can't afford the contraception. She wants you and me and the taxpayers to pay her to have sex."[66]

Also in 2012, Todd Akin, a Republican congressman from Missouri, said that rape does not result in pregnancy when he attempted to skirt answering a question about whether abortion is justified in cases of rape: "It seems to be, first of all, from what I understand from doctors, it's really rare. If it's a legitimate rape, the female body has ways to try to shut the whole thing down."[67] While his use of the word "legitimate" is despicable, if Akin had been talking about ducks, he might have had a point. Apparently some breeds of ducks, where there are very aggressive male ducks that rape often, have developed incredibly complex vaginas with multiple false channels, so that they can in fact contract their vaginal muscles to send unwanted sperm away from their eggs.[68] But human females have not yet acquired that self-protective trait.

Limbaugh and Akin were subsequently taught a good lesson in the 2012 election cycle—one during which Obama and Mitt Romney mentioned women nearly thirty times in their last presidential debate. A record number of women were elected to Congress, with eighty female members of the House joining twenty members of the Senate. Some of these female Congress members believe that if more women serve, more problems will be solved. Democratic senator Claire McCaskill, who defeated Akin in Missouri, asserted, "By nature we are less confrontational and more collaborative. Not only do we want to work in a bipartisan way, we do it."[69]

How do gender relations and cultural evolution play out in other areas, and how might they impact women's aspirations for motherhood? At the college and graduate levels in the United States, women outnumber men and earned 60 percent of all bachelor's and master's degrees awarded in 2010. Men are now more likely than women to hold only a high school diploma.[70] However, women comprise only 33 percent of faculty at doctoral-level institutions. A 2010 article in the *Washington Post* highlighted the difficulty of motherhood in tenure-track positions based on a study conducted by a group of researchers from Barnard College: "The tenure system of academia is uniquely incompatible with the biological clocks of working women."[71] In a piece for the *New York Times*, Mary Ann Mason wrote that when she was dean of graduate studies at UC Berkeley, "Should I wait until I get tenure to have a baby?" was the question female graduate students asked her most.[72] With doctorates generally awarded in a student's early thirties and tenure coming approximately seven years later, women face having to sacrifice either career or motherhood. As Mason noted, "Among tenured faculty 70 percent of men are married with children compared with 44 percent of the women."[73]

Earlier, I cited Martha Beck's memoir about having a son with special needs. Part of Beck's challenge was balancing motherhood with a life in academia. She wrote, "Back then, even the potential for motherhood was most definitely a blot on the credibility of female students and staff. I had several friends who obtained abortions when accidental pregnancies threatened to scuttle their academic progress. One woman I knew decided, with her husband, to abort a planned pregnancy when a crucial three-day exam was scheduled near her due date. I don't know whether she even asked if the exam could be rescheduled. That sort of thing simply wasn't done—especially not for 'personal reasons.'"[74]

Priscilla Gilman, who was earning her doctorate when she had children, wrote in her memoir, "In choosing to get pregnant while still in graduate school, without a completed dissertation or a job, I was taking a huge professional risk. . . . At the time I first became pregnant, only one other female graduate student in my department had had a baby (three children later, she left the profession), and almost all of the female professors had waited until securing tenure before trying to conceive. I was aware of the ominous studies and statistics showing that having children dramatically reduced a woman's chances of receiving tenure."[75]

When it comes to higher-level faculty in math-intensive fields, such as chemistry, physics, mathematics, engineering, and computer science, women are especially scarce.[76] Larry Summers, while president of Harvard

University—and coincidentally a mentor to Facebook COO Sheryl Sandberg—sparked a controversy over women in science when he claimed during a 2005 speech that "the general clash between people's legitimate family desires and employers' current desire for high power and high intensity, that in the special case of science and engineering, there are issues of intrinsic aptitude, and particularly of the variability of aptitude, and that those considerations are reinforced by what are in fact lesser factors involving socialization and continuing discrimination. I would like nothing better than to be proved wrong, because I would like nothing better than for these problems to be addressable simply by everybody understanding what they are, and working very hard to address them."[77] He was arguing that the dearth of women in high-end scientific positions couldn't simply be because of discrimination. As he said earlier in his speech: "If there was really a pervasive pattern of discrimination that was leaving an extraordinary number of high-quality potential candidates behind, one suspects that in the highly competitive academic marketplace, there would be more examples of institutions that succeeded substantially by working to fill the gap."

Many lambasted him as implying that women were not as good as men at science and engineering. Nancy Hopkins, a professor of biology at Massachusetts Institute of Technology, was at the speech and walked out in protest. Later, on Amy Goodman's radio show *Democracy Now!* Hopkins said, "He gave three reasons that he felt explained the small number of women that we see at the top of science and engineering, and the first one was, they have babies, and the second one was these aptitude differences. And I really found it so inappropriate, in coming from the President of Harvard University, that I felt I should leave, so I did."[78]

However, acknowledging the problems that exist before women get to the stage of qualifying to teach at the highest levels could be a means for more effectively devising solutions. Dr. Sally Ride, the late pioneering female astronaut, spoke to the *New York Times* about her opinions on the dearth of women in math and science, which she believed was due to early conditioning. Her answer was "to set up science programs all over the country meant to appeal to girls—science festivals, science camps, science clubs—to help them find mentors, role models and one another."[79] More recently, Reshma Saujani, the daughter of two engineers, founded Girls Who Code with financial support from tech giants like Google and Intel to address what she saw as the dire paucity of women in computer science classes. Saujani, whose parents were refugees from Uganda, explained, "I saw the ability of technology to either enhance poverty or reduce it, and I saw girls not getting the same opportunities boys were. Back in the '60s, you didn't have gender parity in law or medicine, but something happened and women started opting into these professions. We have to do that in computer science."[80]

As in academia, the landscape in the general workforce is mixed with regard to gender parity. In 2010, women held 51.4 percent of all managerial and professional positions, up from 26 percent in 1980.[81] However, in the corporate sector, women are only around 15 percent of the top executive levels and account for only about 4 percent of the CEOs at Fortune 500 companies.[82] A 2011 study by Deloitte found that women made up just 12.2 percent of the boards of directors at more than 1,700 US-listed companies.[83]

Now, women outnumber men in the American workforce, and nearly three-quarters of the 7.5 million jobs lost in the depths of the Great Recession between 2007 and 2009 belonged to men.[84] In 2010, nearly a quarter of women earned more than their husbands, up from 4 percent in 1970. While women contributed 6 percent of US household income in the 1960s, now they contribute more than 40 percent.[85] However, in many areas, women continue to earn less than men. In 1990, women in the United States earned around 72 percent on average of what men earned when working year-round full time; in 2012, that figure rose to about 77 percent.[86] In 2011, the median weekly wage for full-time female workers was $684, compared to $832 per week for men.[87] Among doctors as well, studies have shown that women are paid less, about $168,000 on average versus $200,000 for men. Moreover, according to a *New York Times* article, female doctors tend "to be in lower paying specialties, have fewer publications, work fewer hours and hold fewer administrative leadership positions."[88]

In a piece for *Slate*, Hanna Rosin pointed out that the official Bureau of Labor statistic of women earning 77 percent of what men do for full-time work is different from the often-cited and erroneous statistic that "women make 77 cents to every man's dollar." Men more typically exceed working the official thirty-five full-time hours than women do. However, if we look at both women and men working forty hours per week, then women actually earn around 87 percent of what men earn. (Among African Americans, the gap narrows even further to women earning about 91 percent of what men earn.) Rosin cautioned against focusing wage equality into "tidy, misleading" statistics and encouraged broadening our perspective to understand why, for example, male and female MBAs earn around the same amount right out of school, but ten to fifteen years later, the gap in salary widens to as much as 40 percent, "almost all of which is due to career interruptions and fewer hours."[89]

The stories above illustrate that when it comes to sexual, reproductive, and economic freedoms, we need feminism more than ever. With misogyny and patriarchy continuing to rear their ugly heads, feminism is as important today as it was during its peak in the '70s and '80s. Caitlin Moran explained: "What is feminism? Simply the belief that women should be as free as men, however nuts, dim, deluded, badly dressed, fat, receding, lazy, and smug they might be."[90]

Feminism inspires us to ask ourselves, "Is that all there is?" It inspires us to join together to advocate for change. As Debora L. Spar, president of Barnard College, wrote, "Making a world that is better for women also demands that women work together. In its earliest incarnation, feminism was about communal action and goals; about giving women the power to shape not only their reproductive lives, but also their destinies and that of the world around them. Over the decades, though, this collective goal has been lost, replaced by the individual struggles that now compel most women."[91]

Natalie Angier asked, "Who says that feminism and evolutionary biology must inevitably spit on each other's slippers?"[92] The anthropologist Ernst Mayr told her that human beings are no longer evolving genetically. If this is the case, Mayr said, then evolution "from this point on will have to be cultural evolution rather than genetic evolution."[93] Angier agreed with Mayr and wrote an article for *Natural History* magazine about his opinions. Readers were outraged, but understanding the interplay of science, society, and our bodies can help us make better choices for moving forward.

In the future, we might in fact be able to manipulate our fertility span. Professor Nick Bostrom, director of the Future of Humanity Institute at Oxford University, delivered a 2005 talk at a conference hosted by TED (Technology, Entertainment, and Design—a nonprofit dedicated to "Ideas Worth Spreading"). Bostrom discussed how we use modification technologies, like contraceptives, contact lenses, vaccines, etc., to rewrite human nature. Future technologies, he argued, will be used further to transform the human condition and to enhance human capacity.[94] As Dr. Anders Sandberg, also from the Future of Humanity Institute, told the BBC, "I think mid-century, I would be rather surprised if there wasn't a lot of implants and enhancements around. . . . Eventually you reach the point where you can start doing things that normal people can't do."[95]

An example of where we are heading in this regard is that with some of the reproductive technologies in progress, we can envision how we might graft our younger selves onto our older selves. New studies have shown that ovary transplants can remain effective for at least seven years and "raise the possibility of being able to stop menopause and allow women to delay motherhood."[96] In addition, the biologist and science writer Dr. Aarathi Prasad has said, "The mood of scientists . . . looking to the future is we will either technologically or scientifically evolve out of the menopause."[97]

But for now and likely for many years to come, we have to work with the bodies we have. We can push them only so far, and science can help us get only so far beyond our natural capabilities. As Dr. Al Yuzpe, of Vancouver-based Genesis Fertility Centre, has pointed out, "I've been in the field of infertility for 42 years, and we've seen an evolution. The one thing we've never been able to overcome is the effect of female age."[98]

Our biologies might be fixed, but our societies are not. We can adapt and make changes that alleviate the constraints of the physical world. As Angier proposed, "We need a little culture here, a little education and deliberation. Cultural evolution works pretty well. Culture has a way of becoming a habit, and habits have a way of getting physical, of feeding back on the loop and transforming the substrate."[99] Take, for instance, seat belt requirements or public smoking bans. Seat belt laws have saved thousands of lives, have prevented thousands of injuries, and have saved the United States billions of dollars annually as a result.[100] Because of restaurant and workplace smoking bans, cardiac deaths, when measured in a specific neighborhood, have shown the potential to drop by 17 percent and heart attacks by 33 percent.[101]

With regard to women's rights and specifically to parenting, Amy Richards has pointed out, "The changes wrought by feminism were often subtle and so integrated into our daily lives that younger people have no reason to know that the women's movement paved the way. We have baby seats in grocery carts, diaper-changing stations in men's and women's restrooms, schools that don't segregate for boys and girls for sports, tax deductions for child care expenses . . . feminism's investment in parenting is undeniable."[102]

These are some of the abundant examples of how public education campaigns combined with policy reform can result in new patterns that benefit society. By taking a hard look at how evolution—both biological and cultural—and delayed motherhood affect each other, we can identify ways to make the situation more sustainable. We can ensure more prepared generations of prospective mothers.

CHAPTER 6

BABY MADNESS AND THE MEDIA

On April 1, 2013, I came across a story about forty-three-year-old Jennifer Lopez and her twenty-five-year-old boyfriend Casper Smart having a baby via IVF and a surrogate, who was being paid $5 million. *Wow!* I thought.

Turned out it was an April Fool's joke.[1]

A few days later, the media reported that Halle Berry was pregnant at the age of forty-six with her second child and that it was "the biggest surprise" of her life.[2] This story was real. The first question that came to my mind was, *Is she using a donor egg?* But none of the various articles mentioned that she might be pregnant through assisted reproductive technologies (ARTs).

When we're talking about anyone—celebrity or otherwise—it's not our business how she got pregnant. This is an intimate, private decision, and we can't expect people to share that level of detail. Nonetheless, realistic media portrayals of the way pregnancies happen (or don't) when the mother is older can have a positive influence by encouraging honest conversations about delayed motherhood. Celebrity culture has a big impact on popular opinion. As Amy Richards, the feminist author who is on the board of advisors for MAKERS, an online archive of influential women's stories, said, "What people are willing to believe when it comes to celebrities is crazy!"[3]

Baby coverage in the mainstream media has reached a fever pitch. Alessandra Stanley, the chief television critic for the *New York Times*, explained, "In today's 24-hour tabloid culture, signs of celebrity baby bumps, morning sickness and secret surrogacies are as closely monitored via Telephoto lens and Minicams as engagement rings and cosmetic surgery scars. Nothing is private anymore, and everything about celebrity parenthood is up for grabs and public exposure."[4]

We've gone from the '70s feminism of "Hey, you don't have to be a mom" to babies being a status symbol. In tabloid magazines such as *Us Weekly* and on TV shows like *Access Hollywood*, we see stars choosing to have children whether (like Reese Witherspoon) or not (like January Jones) they have a partner. We also see more coverage about women becoming mothers when they're older. We see Kelly Preston having a baby at forty-eight, but we don't hear if she used her own egg or a donor egg. Celebrities and the media could be more responsible with the information they spread and could be powerful allies in destigmatizing issues like infertility.

From reality TV to *People* magazine (which has a special section called "Moms & Babies" on its website), baby making is popular entertainment. When is this type of entertainment harmless, and when is it damaging? In the pages to follow, I explore media culture on the topics of mother-hood, feminism, and infertility, and end with a call for more honesty and responsibility.

During my first appointment with Dr. Souter, she cautioned me about my chances of having a successful pregnancy. She said women might not have realistic expectations regarding their chances of live births because they watch Hollywood stars and older women in the public eye getting pregnant in their forties. Dr. Souter asked, "How do we know how they got pregnant? Did they require aggressive treatments? Did they have to resort to donor eggs?"

On December 10, 2011, a few months after this appointment, I woke up to numerous stories about Michelle Duggar's miscarriage—on CNN, Reuters, in *People*, etc. Duggar had a reality show on cable channel TLC called *19 and Counting* about her having baby after baby (the name of the show changed depending on the number of kids, e.g., *17 and Counting*, *18 and Counting*). That same evening, I turned on the television while making myself dinner. The Duggars were on *Extra*, the celebrity news show. A few seconds later, Jennifer Aniston was on, addressing pregnancy rumors—she wasn't.

Next, I watched *Access Hollywood*, cohosted by Maria Menounos, whom I remembered had frozen her eggs earlier that year. About that decision, Menounos had said on national television, "We're so wrapped up in our work and time goes by so quickly. I'm having fun, I'm living my dream. I had a couple of different colleagues approach me in the last two or three years and say, 'Don't do what we did and wait until you are forty and forget to have kids.' I realized I could be a candidate."[5] The *Daily Beast* has reported that Diane Sawyer, the anchor of ABC's *World News Tonight* who first married at the age of forty-two, tells women who work for her to freeze their eggs as soon as possible, before they hit forty when it might be too late.[6]

The media fuels a public fascination with women's fecundity and fertility. The more births—as with Duggar and "Octomom" (Nadya Suleman, who had octuplets through IVF after already having had six children)—the better the spectacle; the more extreme the age, the more the public will notice. For example, MTV had a hit with its reality show, *16 and Pregnant*, while the October 3, 2011, issue of *New York* magazine ran a story titled "Parents of a Certain Age" about women in their late forties, fifties, and even sixties having their first children (the provocative cover depicting a gray-haired pregnant woman would later win Cover of the Year from the American Society of Magazine Editors).

Through the years, there have been many news items about older dads: Rod Stewart became one at sixty, Paul McCartney at sixty-one, Julio Iglesias at sixty-three, etc.[7] But even with recent studies showing the link between advanced paternal age and an increased risk of various disorders, older dads aren't new or shocking. Older moms, however, are a relatively recent phenomenon because ARTs have made their pregnancies possible. Dr. Pasquale Patrizio of the Yale Fertility Center said that because of the rise of ARTs, women feel that their fertility may be manipulated at any time, and "the problem is exacerbated due to images of celebrities who seem to effortlessly give birth at advanced ages."[8]

Science writer Liza Mundy has written about how misleading it can be for the public to see older female celebrities getting pregnant without knowing if they had the help of fertility treatments, egg donation, and the like. In her book *Everything Conceivable*, Mundy pointed out that we've seen Jane Seymour pregnant at forty-four, Susan Sarandon at forty-six, Holly Hunter at forty-seven, and both Geena Davis and Wendy Wasserstein at forty-eight.[9] Mundy highlighted the story of Joan Lunden, who had twins in 2003 at age fifty-two but didn't reveal that they might have been conceived through donor eggs. Perhaps she implied this was the case when she said to *Ladies' Home Journal* that she wanted to send a message to readers: "I don't want them to feel that they can't achieve what we have if they can't produce their own eggs. I want everybody to understand that however they make their families doesn't make any difference."[10]

It's not just public figures who conceal their use of donor eggs; women in general do. Mundy cited a 2004 study that "found that 40 percent of egg-donor mothers did not plan to tell their children or were unsure what to do."[11]

In addition to older celebrity moms in the news, younger stars seem more thrilled than ever to talk about their opinions on and desires for motherhood. In 2012, pop music sensation Adele announced at the height of her fame that she was going to take a time-out to focus on her relationship and start a family. Meanwhile, during an interview with Oprah, Lady Gaga proclaimed, "I want kids. I want a soccer team. I want a husband. I don't want to have one kid. I want to have a few." Caressing her imaginary pregnant belly, she said, "I want to experience that."[12] One night, when I was watching *Extra*, the hot news of the evening was whether reality star Snooki (of *Jersey Shore* fame) was pregnant. When asked about Snooki's pregnancy, the singer Rihanna remarked, "We are women. We have kids. We're reproductive machines. That's what we're here for."[13]

Feminist author Caitlin Moran was once a music journalist with *Melody Maker* in the United Kingdom. She wrote, "When I interviewed, say, Björk or Kylie Minogue, the last thing on my mind was asking them if they wanted children. After all, I never asked Oasis or Clive Anderson if they did." But she said her editors would press her to ask.[14] Nowadays, however, many female stars don't seem to need much prodding to comment on this subject.

When asked about feminism, though, they can be less forthcoming and even defensive. Katie McDonough, assistant editor of *Salon*, put together a list of female public figures who "won't cop to the F-bomb." Pop star Katy Perry has said, "I'm not a feminist, but I do believe in the strength of women." Yahoo! CEO Marissa Mayer has said, "I don't think that I would consider myself a feminist. I think that I certainly believe in equal rights. I believe that women are just as capable, if not more so in a lot of different dimensions, but I don't, I think, have sort of the militant drive and the sort of, the chip on the shoulder that sometimes comes with that." Even Madonna, whom I would think would be an über-feminist, has said, "I'm not a feminist, I'm a humanist."[15]

In the April 2013 issue of British *Vogue*, Beyoncé gave her reaction to the F-bomb: "That word can be very extreme. . . . But I guess I am a modern-day feminist. I do believe in equality. Why do you have to choose what type of woman you are? Why do you have to label yourself anything? I'm just a woman and I love being a woman. . . . I do believe in equality and that we have a way to go and it's something that's pushed aside and something that we have been conditioned to accept. . . . But I'm happily married. I love my husband."

In *New York* magazine, journalist Maureen O'Connor defended Beyoncé, saying she is clearly a feminist in her actions and words and that her discomfort with the word is influenced by the way the media baits the issue. In O'Connor's opinion, "Women who have a vested interest in being popular—i.e., celebrities—are still afraid of the word 'feminism.'" Some seem to think being a feminist means you are against men. Taylor Swift has said, "I don't really think about things as guys versus girls." Lady Gaga has said, "I'm not a feminist. I hail men, I love men."[16]

Gwyneth Paltrow has also downplayed feminism as somehow interfering with being a good wife. In a March 2012 interview in *Harper's BAZAAR*, she said she gave the following advice to a girlfriend: "This may not be feminist, but you have to compromise. It's been all about you and you're a big deal. And if you want what you're saying you want—a family—you have to be a wife, and that is part of the equation. Gloria Steinem may string me up by my toes, but all I can do is my best, and I can do only what works for me and my family."[17]

These negative depictions of feminism dishearten me, because, as I've argued elsewhere in this book and as numerous feminist authors have explained, feminism is about arming women with choices, access, and information so that they can make better decisions and pursue their ambitions. Moran explained: "I do understand why women started to reject the word 'feminism.' It ended up being invoked in so many bafflingly inappropriate contexts that—if you weren't actually aware of the core aims of feminism and were trying to work it out simply from the surrounding conversation—you'd presume it was some spectacularly unappealing combination of misandry, misery, and hypocrisy, which stood for ugly clothes, constant anger, and, let's face it, no fucking."[18] Nonetheless, feminists, as with any type of person who identifies with a particular cause—LGBTQ activists, human rights activists, etc.—come in all shapes and sizes. You *can* be the good wife and the good feminist, too.

In her book *Lean In*, Facebook COO Sheryl Sandberg explained her own conversion to feminism after shirking the word for much of her youth. "Social gains are never handed out. They must be seized. Leaders of the women's movement—from Susan B. Anthony to Jane Addams to Alice Paul to Bella Abzug to Flo Kennedy to so many others—spoke out loudly and bravely to demand the rights that we now have. . . . Looking back, it made no sense for my college friends and me to distance ourselves from the hard-won achievements of earlier feminists. We should have cheered their efforts. Instead, we lowered our voices, thinking the battle was over, and with this reticence, we hurt ourselves. Now I proudly call myself a feminist."[19]

In contrast to the negative portrayals of feminism, other celebrities inspire people when they open up about topics like motherhood, single motherhood, and adoption. For instance, Padma Lakshmi, host of TV's *Top Chef*, chose to be a single mother when she had her daughter, Krishna. Lakshmi said, "I don't feel alone at all in parenting my daughter. Krishna has a whole other side of her family who loves her, too. And so Krishna is parented by me, but also by her grandmother and aunts and cousins and uncles and friends."[20]

TV actress Mariska Hargitay has been very open about her adoption of two toddlers when she was in her forties. She knew the odds of having a successful pregnancy were slim and went straight to adoption to add to her family, which already included one biological child.[21] Madonna, Charlize Theron, and Sandra Bullock have also publicized the joys of adoption—moreover, they adopted as single mothers. Filmmaker and actress Nia Vardalos has taken the cause even further by writing a book, *Instant Mom*, about her journey to adoption. She went through ten years and thirteen IVF attempts. Vardalos told the TV show *Access Hollywood*, "During my process of trying to be a mom I rarely talked about it, I kept it inside. I had a feeling of shame that is inexplicable to me now."[22]

Actor Hugh Jackman has spoken often about the journey taken by him and his wife, Deborra-Lee Furness, through multiple miscarriages and IVF attempts. In a sit-down television interview with Katie Couric, he said, "It's almost secretive, so I hope Deb doesn't mind me bringing it up now. . . . It's a good thing to talk about it. It's more common, and it is tough. There's a grieving that you have to go through."[23] The couple ultimately adopted two children. UK-based pop singer Lisa Stansfield has talked about her experience pursuing three unsuccessful rounds of IVF when she was in her forties. She eventually decided to abandon the idea of becoming a mother.[24] In 2012, Taiwanese star, singer, and actress Hebe Tian shocked fans with her announcement that she was freezing her eggs. She said, "I plan to do it when I turn thirty next March, but I still think it's better if love would blossom naturally instead."[25] In India, Bollywood star Aamir Khan revealed that he and his wife, Kiran, had a baby born through IVF to a surrogate mother.[26]

"Stars . . . they're just like us." This is a popular feature in *Us* magazine that hilariously sends up the daily routines of celebrities. There's Reese Witherspoon carrying her groceries, or Sir Paul McCartney pushing his own luggage cart. Extrapolating from this concept, I believe when celebrities open up about their struggles to become parents, they're not just *like* us, they are doing a public service, helping others in their position to feel less alone. As Leigh Blickley, an associate editor at *Huffington Post* Celebrity, has pointed out, "Countless numbers of celebrities have struggled to have children on their own, whether it's due to medical reasons, age or personal choice. Stars like Nicole Kidman, Giuliana Rancic, and Sarah Jessica Parker have been open and honest about their battles with infertility and have discussed how gestational mothers changed their lives."[27]

In the same vein, the more stars talk about miscarriage, the more normal that word will become. Gwyneth Paltrow has revealed she had a miscarriage. Jay-Z revealed in a rap song that he and Beyoncé had a miscarriage. Ann Romney, wife of 2012 presidential candidate Mitt Romney, has also revealed that she had a miscarriage, between her fourth and fifth sons.

Fertility-related stories are increasingly prevalent on reality TV. Bethenny Frankel had a miscarriage on *Bethenny Ever After*. In *Ice Loves Coco*, Coco was diagnosed with seriously high blood pressure when she was seeing doctors to talk about pursuing pregnancy. She and Ice-T then had to put their baby-making plans on hold. Giuliana Rancic, the E! news anchor, and her husband, Bill, have been candid about their quest to have a child, both on their reality show, *Giuliana and Bill*, and in their public appearances. She was pursuing IVF when breast cancer was discovered. The couple then froze embryos prior to her treatment and ultimately had a baby through a gestational surrogate in 2012. On *Keeping Up with the Kardashians*, the viewer got to see Khloé Kardashian visiting a fertility clinic as she struggled to have a child with her husband, basketball star Lamar Odom. Khloé's sister Kim later announced that she would pursue IVF if she didn't have a baby by the age of forty—but a year later, she was pregnant by her boyfriend, the rapper Kanye West.[28]

While we can debate the benefits of having reality stars as role models for people struggling with infertility, I suggest it is good to have these issues in the public eye. What's most important is that the information given be accurate and responsible. For instance, while it's great that Kim Kardashian speaks up about potentially pursuing IVF, forty years old is too late to start. As I discovered, your chances of a live birth through IVF at that age are not much better than your chances of a live birth without it.

In March 2013, Sofia Vergara, the TV star on the hit sitcom *Modern Family*, revealed that she was freezing her eggs at the age of forty.[29] While I respected her decision and admired her honesty, I couldn't help but think about my doctor's warning that freezing eggs is not advisable at that age. One of the numerous stories I read about Vergara's plan pointed out that reality by presenting hard statistics about pregnancy at advanced maternal age. The digital news site, VOXXI, which targets Hispanic American readers, included facts about how women at the age of forty have only a 10 percent chance of getting pregnant over the course of a year and a 28 percent chance of a successful IVF pregnancy. The piece also mentioned the suspicion that many stars in their forties and even fifties (like Jennifer Lopez, Mariah Carey, and Holly Hunter) might have used ARTs, even though they haven't disclosed this possible scenario. Conversely, it commended stars who have been honest, like Celine Dion, who went through six rounds of IVF before getting pregnant with twins at the age of forty-two, and Brooke Shields, who also went through six rounds before having a daughter at the age of thirty-eight.[30]

Giuliana Rancic has done a great deal to educate the public by talking about how she was blindsided by her lack of fertility knowledge. On chasing her career instead of pursuing a family life, she said, "Everybody was patting me on the back. No one ever told me, 'Oh, by the way, your eggs change when you reach a certain age.' I didn't think 35 was old! So when the doctor said, 'It's not as easy as you thought it would be,' it was a real blow. Because I felt so young."[31]

Aisha Tyler, a cohost of *The Talk*, revealed her struggles with infertility during a weeklong series of "Big Secrets" on the show during September 2013. Her cohosts (including Sara Gilbert, also the executive producer, who came to fame playing Roseanne Barr's daughter on *Roseanne*) had no idea she had pursued IVF two years before with her husband of twenty-one years. Tyler, forty-two, said, "I'm old. In baby years, that's too old to be trying to get pregnant." Eventually she and her husband felt compelled to abandon treatment: "After going through the procedures and spending a lot of money . . . the doctor said, 'Look, based on what we're seeing here, I just don't think this is going to happen for you.'" However, she hasn't given up on her dream of having a child and spoke about the possibility of adopting after recovering from her painful experience. She said, "I feel like this is such a fresh wound that I want to let it heal for a while before I think about what we could do."[32]

Some public figures take honesty a step further by lending their names to causes that increase fertility awareness. In 2011, *Redbook* magazine launched a video series, "The Truth about Trying," in which celebrities like Sherri Shepherd of the TV talk show *The View* shared their stories. Fox News anchor Alisyn Camerota, after struggling to become pregnant from the age of thirty-five and dealing with multiple IVF attempts and miscarriages, became a volunteer for RESOLVE, the national infertility association.[33]

In addition to celebrities in their real lives, we've seen characters on television and in films dealing with their choices to have children or not. In a February 2013 interview in *Salon*, Marlo Thomas talked about the impact of her show *That Girl* in the 1970s. "I think the most important thing . . . is that everybody thought this was a revolutionary show: A girl doesn't want to be married, a girl who wants to get a job, a girl who doesn't want to live at home, who wants to live on her own, have her own apartment . . . we were a gigantic hit and it's because she was not really a revolutionary figure, she was a fait accompli, she was in every home in America. Every home in America had a 'That Girl' in it."[34]

Thomas cited other shows that also galvanized modern portrayals of women on TV: "*Kate & Allie* was a big jump, to have two single women be mothers, that was pretty interesting. And the next one after that I thought was a good jump was *Roseanne*, as an angry mother who kicked her kids around, that was really interesting. And the payoff, I think, is *Murphy Brown*, the woman who's an alcoholic, has a baby out of wedlock, screams at her staff."[35]

Dan Quayle, George H. W. Bush's vice president, publicly chided *Murphy Brown*, which aired from 1988 to 1998: "It doesn't help matters when prime-time TV has *Murphy Brown*, a character who supposedly epitomizes today's intelligent, highly paid professional woman, mocking the importance of fathers by bearing a child alone and calling it just another 'lifestyle choice.'"[36] Later, on *Friends*, one of the most popular television sitcoms of its time during its run from 1994 to 2004, Jennifer Aniston's character Rachel had a child out of wedlock. Feminist author Amy Richards appeared on the *O'Reilly Factor* to discuss what message this show was sending to teenage girls.[37] About that experience Richards told me, "My main point was that teen girls idolized Jennifer Aniston who was married to Brad Pitt (as she was at the time) and very likely to have a baby under much more conventional standards. That said, 'Rachel' having a child out of wedlock would likely send an unrealistic message—that single parenting was easy. I know from my own upbringing [being raised by a single mother] that it's possible (and wonderful)—and yet I also know that it was hard—and harder when you are more marginalized. When I said 'I am a product of single parenting and don't know my father,' O'Reilly said, 'I'm sorry.' I said, 'I'm not.'"[38]

It's important to note that after Aniston and Pitt split, the tabloids became equally obsessed with the fertility of both. In Aniston's case, there has been constant speculation about whether she will ever have a kid—and maybe she has frozen her eggs? With Pitt, it has been the expansion of his brood with Angelina Jolie—both the kids they have naturally and the ones they adopt.

TV critic Alessandra Stanley has written that although fertility, single motherhood, and other women's issues have long been explored in films and television, what is different now is the age at which some of these mothers are first having or considering having babies of their own. For instance, Tina Fey's character on her TV show *30 Rock* contemplated having a baby alone in her early forties (by the end of the show's run, she got married and adopted twins).

On February 15, 2012, a few days after my first tumor was discovered, I was watching "The Spanish Teacher" episode of *Glee*, the musical comedy series about a high school glee club. The show opened with fifty-something cheerleading coach Sue Sylvester talking to a group of high school boys and soliciting them to donate sperm for her. The glee club coach, Mr. Schuester, scolded her about this, saying he never saw her as "the mothering type." She responded by saying that, like many other women who had chosen career over family, she'd decided to go in a different direction while she still had time, explaining that she had frozen her eggs in the late '70s. Mr. Schuester looked at her incredulously and pointed out that she couldn't have frozen her eggs because that technology wasn't even available then.[39]

Later, we see Becky, a cheerleader with Down syndrome, injecting Sue with fertility drugs, and then, lo and behold, Sue is pregnant by the end of the episode. Although the misinformation—she couldn't have frozen her eggs in the '70s and thus couldn't be pregnant in her fifties with her own eggs—was astonishing, the fact that the subject of egg freezing and older mothers had become worthy of satire on mainstream television was remarkable.

A more realistic slant on fertility panic occurred on the sitcom *New Girl*. A November 2012 episode, appropriately called "Eggs," depicted how the main character Jess and her friend Cece, both around thirty years old, decide to have their ovarian reserve tested after hearing from a pregnant friend that 90 percent of a woman's eggs are gone by the time she is thirty. Although the women are around the same age, Jess discovered she had tons of eggs, while Cece found out she didn't. Entertainment writer Megan Angelo remarked in *Glamour* that she "could hardly make out the jokes in *New Girl* last night over the deafening rhythms . . . of a zillion ticking biological clocks."[40] But she praised the show: "*New Girl* did a beautiful job, I think, of condensing a typical response to this sobering stat. Jess was shocked, then alarmed, then determined to solve the problem by being informed. Meanwhile, it was the determinedly Zen Cece who ended up having her world rocked by the reports."

While on an international flight, I came across another example of a humorous but responsible fertility-related story. *Vicky Donor*, a Bollywood film about childless couples seeking sperm donors, was part of the in-flight entertainment library. The film had done big box office when it came out in India in April 2012.[41] After its release, according to Indian sperm bank reports, inquiries from potential sperm donors went up by as much as thirty calls per day.[42] In addition, more couples struggling with infertility came forward to ask about sperm donation. As Dr. Anirudh Singh, of the Dr. Singh Test Tube Baby Centre in the city of Meerut, said to India's *Economic Times*, "The social stigma on such issues is gradually diminishing."[43]

Normalizing these conversations in popular culture is a big step toward increasing public debate and awareness. Take, for example, what happened with menopause. It used to be taboo until books like *The Secret Passage* by Gail Sheehy came out on the subject and celebrities (like Lauren Hutton when she appeared on *Oprah*) talked about their experiences. Katie Couric, speaking about her experience with menopause, has said, "I think emotionally and psychologically it's weird to feel like, *Gosh, my childbearing years are over.* And of course they've been over for a long time, but still, they're *officially* over now. It's kind of a head trip, to tell you the truth." She recognized that her willingness to talk publicly helps other women: "I'd like to help women get the latest information; it's one of those things people don't talk about, and doctors don't have time to really work with women. . . . I mean, let's *talk* about this stuff."[44]

Incorporating menopause into storylines on television and in films also helped to bring the subject out into the open. In 1974, the television show *Maude* broke ground when the main character accused her husband of having male menopause and talked about the symptoms of menopause. But seeing menopause on screen was still uncommon in the years that followed. Kate Valk, a theater actress in her fifties, told me, "I wish there had been more tropes in literature and cinema that dealt with menopause and its effect on women in terms of identity and societal power. The only thing I remember seeing was Ellen Burstyn's character in *Atlantic City* [1980] cutting her hair short and taking all her clothing to the beach and burning them in a huge bonfire."[45]

Over the past fifteen years, more examples of menopause in films and television have popped up. In a 2001 episode of the British sitcom *Absolutely Fabulous*, the main characters Patsy and Edina attended a meeting of Menopause Anonymous. In a 2002 episode of *That '70s Show*, the character Kitty thought she was pregnant because her periods had stopped, until her mother, played by Betty White, explained that she was actually going through menopause. In the 2010 film *Sex and the City 2*, the character Samantha started having hot flashes and night sweats as she went through menopause.[46]

The same needs to happen with fertility issues. According to a 2010 *SELF* magazine survey, "More than half of the patients included in the survey reported that it was easier to tell people they didn't intend to build a family rather than share their troubles."[47] When celebrities talk publicly about having a miscarriage or undergoing IVF and when fertility-related stories appear on TV and in film, we can capitalize on those moments and start connecting the dots.

A friend of mine who was a television executive for many years said part of the problem in what gets covered and what doesn't is "there's not enough dialogue from and between women leaders in a male-driven media and communications society." Another friend, Laura Dawn, the creative director formerly of MoveOn.org, said part of the problem with the media's representation of these issues is "because we live in a deeply misogynistic country with a political party that literally tries at every turn to devalue women."[48]

Jennifer Siebel Newsom's 2012 documentary *Miss Representation* examined the subjugation of women through the mass media. She argued that "women are aspiring to do great things in leadership, yet the glass ceiling is still there because of the way media depict women. It influences our culture and dictates our gender norms and values."[49] Change on a broad scale usually happens incrementally and can take generations to become entrenched. But the results can be resoundingly clear. For example, three female-fronted films broke the top ten in 2012: *Brave*, *The Hunger Games*, and *Snow White and the Huntsman*. In the eleven years before that in the twenty-first century, only two female-fronted films had made the end-of-year top ten lists: *My Big Fat Greek Wedding* in 2002 and *Mamma Mia* in 2008.[50] Looking ahead, Gamechanger Films (founded in 2013 by producers Julie Parker Benello, Dan Cogan, Geralyn Dreyfous, and Wendy Ettinger) intends to fund only women-helmed narrative feature films.

On television, a wave of trailblazing women from Roseanne Barr to Ellen DeGeneres to Tina Fey have transformed the world of comedy. In Tina Fey's memoir, *Bossypants*, she described a scene in the *Saturday Night Live* writers' room when Amy Poehler was new to the show. "Amy was in the middle of some such nonsense with Seth Meyers across the table, and she did something vulgar as a joke. I can't remember what it was exactly, except it was dirty and loud and 'unladylike.'" Jimmy Fallon told her to stop. She turned to him and said, "I don't fucking care if you like it," and went back to doing what she was doing. Fey explained, "With that exchange, a cosmic shift took place. Amy made it clear that she wasn't there to be cute. She wasn't there to play wives and girlfriends in the boys' scenes. She was there to do what she wanted to do and she did not fucking care if you like it. . . . I think of this whenever someone says to me, 'Jerry Lewis says women aren't funny,' or 'Christopher Hitchens says women aren't funny. . . . Do you have anything to say to that?' Yes. We don't fucking care if you like it."[51]

Speaking of Jimmy Fallon, he and his wife, Hollywood producer Nancy Juvonen, made headline news in August 2013 for talking on the *Today* show about struggling with infertility for many years before having a baby through a surrogate. Sarah Elizabeth Richards, the author of *Motherhood, Rescheduled*, wrote in *Time* magazine, "Fallon's openness came as a surprise, considering that most celebrities have been notoriously mum on the subject." She pointed out that "Hollywood stars having baby-making troubles haven't received much public sympathy, amid criticism of being able to 'buy' their way out of fertility problems with expensive medical help that many Americans can't afford." I second Richards's statement that "we should applaud Fallon—along with his wife and other high-profile women willing to share their stories—for going public with facts so many would prefer to keep hidden."[52]

Openness on these issues is growing as more women break through in comedy and on TV. Recent hits like *Girls* and *New Girl* have female creators, writers, and stars. As Lena Dunham, the force behind *Girls* has said, female friendship is "the true romance of the show."[53] When women run the show, women's stories are more likely to be told. Take, for example, the fertility test episode I cited above from *New Girl* (which is helmed by Liz Meriwether). On *Girls*, Dunham's character took an HPV test. As Alyssa Rosenberg, who writes about culture and television for *Slate*'s "XX Factor" blog, remarked, "It's great when a show can both educate viewers and find drama in the actual details of women's lives."[54]

A goal for our collective future should be to chip away at demeaning or misleading images of women and fertility in popular culture. While Octomom and the teenaged moms of *16 and Pregnant* might be entertaining, these stories do not advance the science, policies, and healthcare affecting women who struggle to have children. Moreover, they do not inform young people about the myriad problems—societal, economic, and otherwise—that arise when you do what these people are doing on TV. When stars aren't forthcoming about how they got pregnant, they unwittingly dupe women into thinking they might be able to get pregnant without assistance, too, even though other stars are forthcoming about their fertility struggles. Women might choose to go with the fantasy in their goals for motherhood.

Celebrities and the media are not required to educate the public, but they should recognize when they do more harm than good. Kids today grow up much faster than ever before and have access to information instantaneously. They can ask any question they want and get an answer from a computer—even though it might not be the right answer. They don't have to ask a parent, teacher, or peer. Also, they can get entertainment anywhere they want on their smartphones and tablets. They don't have to be at home or in a classroom to watch TV. Because of these conditions, the media could do more to present stories that are honest—and thus influence viewers toward making better decisions about their own fertility and parenting futures.

CHAPTER 7
THE ROLLER COASTER

*A*ll *I know is that my plans to have a baby are on hold.*

Two days after a growth was detected near my ovaries and my IVF cycle was halted, I had an appointment with Dr. Souter. I was happy to hear her familiar accent that I hadn't yet placed. Maybe Eastern European? South American? *One day I'll ask her.* In the waiting room it was all men, which was unusual. *This must be a popular day for semen analyses.*

A nurse escorted me to the ultrasound room after confirming my name and date of birth. I took off my pants and settled onto the examining table. Dr. Souter entered and began the scan. Sometimes ultrasounds look like murky lava lamps. Globs of fluid and tissue undulating. But today the cyst was clear, obscuring my right ovary. Dr. Souter told the nurse it was about 4 cm, and the nurse took notes.

Dr. Souter asked me to get dressed and meet her in her office. I focused on what I was told to do and avoided making any leaps in my brain to what could happen. I got dressed and walked to her office.

She wanted another blood test and a pelvic ultrasound. She said there was definitely stuff in the cyst and that it was probably a functional cyst. I asked her to explain. There are different types of functional cysts, like endometrioma (a benign, estrogen-dependent cyst) and hemorrhagic cysts (a sac filled with blood from a ruptured blood vessel). She said I could have ovulated when I was on the Pill a few weeks before I began the cycle, and then blood could have collected inside the cyst. This would be a good scenario, she said. Then the cyst might go away on its own within six weeks, and I could get back onto a cycle. She said the size of the cyst indicated it hadn't just happened; it had been growing for at least a few weeks. But she wouldn't know until the test results came in. I asked her, "What's the worst it could be?" Dr. Souter is a very honest person; I knew she would give me a straight answer. She looked slightly startled by my question and, knocking on the wood of her desk, said, "We hope not . . . but we test for malignancy." I thought she was going to say that.

She asked if I had been feeling anything. "What could I be feeling? I don't know. I'm South Asian. I eat curry and spicy food. I get bloated; I get gas." She told me that if I felt an acute pain it could indicate a torsion (rotation of the ovary), and I should not bend or lift weights. She asked if I had any more questions. I didn't. She stood up, and so did I. She walked me across the hall to Pam in the nurse's office. Before she left, she said, "Tanya, I am very sorry. I can only imagine how disappointing this must have been on Sunday." That small acknowledgment of what I was going through lightened my mood. I smiled and said, "Whitney Houston had died, so I was distracted." She said, "Well, I'm glad you had something to distract you."

The earliest appointment I could get for the pelvic ultrasound was eight days away. I went home and waited. It was Valentine's Day, February 14. I hadn't realized that before. What a coincidence. Instead of being with my husband celebrating adding a child to our family, I was far away from him, thinking, *Not only might I not have a baby, I might find out I'm going to die.*

This convergence and conflict between the holiday fantasy and my personal reality brought back memories of my father. He had found out he was going to die on Christmas Eve, 1992. I was visiting from college, and we were on our way to a friend's party. I was driving, and my father was in the passenger seat. Suddenly, he put his hand to his chest and had trouble breathing. We thought he was exaggerating, but he said, "Take me to the hospital." The doctor said he was fine, but my father, also a doctor, asked for more tests. The next day he got the results. There was a tumor on his lungs. The day after that he had a biopsy. Two days after that we got the news. He had lung cancer. The week after that, the day after New Year's, one lung was removed.

Of all the memories left behind from those last two years with my father, the last week of his life is the most vivid. My mother called to say that Daddy was in the hospital but that I didn't need to come all the way from New York to Long Beach, California. Nonetheless, I had a feeling that I should go.

I went straight from the Los Angeles airport to the hospital. Random brown people, other Sri Lankans, were milling around in the hall by my father's room. He was in a special ward for people who were on their last legs. A black girl with sickle-cell anemia was moaning in a room at the top of the hall. She was only fourteen years old. Nobody was visiting her today. Next door was a man in the last stages of AIDS. My mother said he'd been in and out of the ward for the past year. He would walk accompanied by his portable IV stand and smoke cigarettes in the garden. He had a big smile, and his teeth took over his emaciated face. In another room, I could make out a tiny white-haired woman with her eyes closed. Walking down the hall to my father's room was like rowing across the River Styx. My father looked like death kept alive, with his skinny frame, bald head, and tubes up his nose and around his arms.

Two days after I arrived, he died. I had relieved my mother from her bedside vigil while she went home to shower. Fifteen minutes after she left, he stopped breathing. I didn't notice at first. I was reading *People* magazine to give me something to do, something that wouldn't take any brainpower. I realized I wasn't hearing his deep phlegmy breaths. I walked to his bed and leaned in. His chest wasn't moving; I looked at his eyes. They opened for a second. I tried to read them then. Blank. And his mouth, which was open before for him to breathe, opened wider. Mucus gurgled in his throat. He died like a balloon dies. His body made a quick and slight move forward. Then he was gone.

My father was only fifty-three. There's a saying that originated in China and is attributed to Confucius: At thirty, you can stand on your own two feet. At forty, you have no more confusion. At fifty, you know your fate.

On the morning of February 22, 2012, I had a pelvic ultrasound. I had gotten used to the wand, but this time it moved around more and deeper, and it stayed in a lot longer than usual. The female technician had a pleasant demeanor and smiled a lot, which helped my mood. After fifteen minutes, she said she had enough images and that the results would be available that afternoon.

Around 2 p.m., I grew impatient and left a message for Nurse Pam. She called me back around 5, with a voice that was both heavy and trying to be light. Dr. Souter did want me to have an MRI. She said it might be a fibroid, a broad ligament fibroid. I asked her what that was. It's a growth from the lining of the musculature of the uterus. Unless it causes a problem with the uterus, they won't touch it. The good news was that it wasn't a polyp, which they would have to take out. If it wasn't a fibroid, it might still be a hemorrhagic cyst, but the MRI would tell them more.

Dr. Souter called me that evening a little before 7 p.m. She reiterated what Pam had told me—that this could be a broad ligament fibroid. She also said that it was not in the uterus and that it was moving. When she saw it, it was on the left, but the pelvic ultrasound showed it on the right. I asked her if anything caused it. She said it could be genetic. None of the dozen or so ultrasounds I'd had over the past few months had shown it. If it was what she thought it could be, it wouldn't interfere with my ability to conceive because it was separate from the ovaries.

The next morning, I scheduled the MRI. The first available appointment was Wednesday, February 29 at 10:15 p.m. A day that happens only once every four years. I had never had such a late medical appointment, but maybe I could be half-asleep during the MRI. I had had one before, after an accident during a show I was in. It wasn't a big deal, but I remember having to maintain a Zen-like calm.

The night of the MRI, it was snowing and raining at the same time, so I drove instead of taking public transportation. "I'm here for an MRI." A guard pointed me down a long corridor toward the Founders Building, "Take a left at the café." I ended up in a cramped section of the hospital where the MRI waiting room was located. For such a big hospital, this room was tiny. *Why are hospitals so ugly?*

The receptionist asked for my name and date of birth. She gave me pants, a top, and a robe and told me to put my things in one of the old metal lockers. I changed in a small cubicle with a door and walls that didn't go all the way to the ceiling. I took a seat and read an old issue of *People* with "Murder at the Palace" on the cover; the body of a dead teenager had been found at the Queen of England's estate. I had read this at the Fertility Center last month. I should have brought a book.

A bald light-brown man came to get me. He looked at my chart and said, "Has anyone told you you don't look forty?" "Yes." As he led me through double doors to a room resembling a '70s-era space research lab, he remarked again about how I didn't look forty. He asked if I'd had an MRI before. "Yes." I was ready for this, but then he brought over an IV, and I flinched. I didn't have one for my last MRI, I told him. "What was your last MRI for?" "They were looking at my head." He said you don't need an IV for an MRI of the head.

I was poked with a needle for the umpteenth time. "You don't like needles, huh?" I said no, even though I should have been used to it by now. This time, it really hurt. The needle was thicker than the usual needles.

Another male technician, who was white and balding and wore a wedding ring, was in the room. They led me into the MRI chamber and instructed me to lie down on a plastic bed. They rested a plastic cage-like object on my pelvis. I felt like Jodie Foster's character—a scientist attempting to make contact with extraterrestrial life—in the movie *Contact* as they slid me into the machine. *I am not a good candidate to be an astronaut.* It's not that I felt claustrophobic, a common reaction to an MRI machine. I just wanted it to be over. Every time I thought I was zoning out, a scary noise surrounded me. It was the worst avant-garde electronic music compilation I had ever heard. *And does it have to be so loud?* After forty-five minutes, I was released. I went home with my head buzzing with awful sounds.

The next day, around noon I saw the familiar "blocked" caller ID on my phone. It was Pam with the results of my MRI. I'd heard this heavy-light tone from her before. She said I might have a tumor of the adrenal gland. She said I needed to do a workup with an endocrinologist. It's not a gynecological problem, and they wanted me to see my primary care doctor as soon as possible.

She said, "I don't want you to worry." It was probably benign, but I could be at risk for other issues like high blood pressure. I asked her if this would affect my ability to be pregnant. She said they wouldn't know until they knew exactly what it was, but who knows; it could be an underlying reason for what had happened with the past pregnancies. I asked her where I could look up information about what I might have, and she said I would find information online. She said she'd make sure Dr. Souter called me because she knew I must be anxious, and, again, she didn't want me to worry. After I hung up, I searched "adrenal gland tumor" and realized that Google was not my friend.

According to *Wikipedia*, "an adrenal incidentaloma is an adrenal tumor found by coincidence without clinical symptoms or suspicion. It is one of the more common unexpected findings revealed by computed tomography (CT), magnetic resonance imaging (MRI), or ultrasonography. . . . Tumors under 3 cm are generally considered benign and are only treated if there are grounds for a diagnosis of Cushing's syndrome [a disorder associated with high levels of cortisol] or pheochromocytoma [an adrenal tumor]."[1] My tumor was over 4 cm.

Then Dr. Souter called. She told me that I might need a biopsy, but before that they needed to make sure it was not a pheochromocytoma. She said the tumor was not gynecological in origin. It wasn't in the uterus or ovaries. It moved around. They couldn't tell if it was toward the back (retroperitoneal) or inside the belly (peritoneal). She said I needed to see an endocrinologist. We needed to make sure it didn't secrete hormones. If it wasn't a pheochromocytoma and the biopsy showed it was benign, then we could proceed with the IVF cycle. She asked if I had any questions. I didn't.

That night was a weird night. It snowed more than I'd seen all winter. I went to see a play where, instead of watching, I replayed in my head the sequence of events that had led to this night, going all the way back to when Jay and I first met, our marriage in Sri Lanka, buying a home together, my three miscarriages, and the beginning of fertility treatment.

At 1:50 p.m. on Friday, March 2, I saw Dr. Shapiro at the university clinic. I had prepared questions:

What is the difference between a cyst, fibroid, and tumor?
Is the tumor the object they thought was a cyst in the initial ultrasound?
Where is it?
What causes it?
Will any changes in lifestyle help it? Stress? Diet?
Does my feeling thirsty a lot have anything to do with it?
I feel a slight pain on the side of my belly. Is that related?

I saved these questions until I heard what Dr. Shapiro had to say. She said the localization of the mass was not clear. She said that although it hadn't been detected before, at 4.5 cm—bigger than I thought Dr. Souter said it was—it hadn't just appeared. Most tumors like that were within the adrenal gland, but some were separate, like mine. She said I hadn't had any symptoms, like palpitations and sweating, but she didn't want to stick a needle into one of those tumors. It was filled with substances that could cause my blood pressure to go very high. I asked her what the substances were. She said it was full of metanephrines, which cause headaches and other problems. Two ways to look for them were either in the blood or the urine. Usually people came in with symptoms, but my case was different. The object was actually seen, so I needed to do both tests. During my MRI, I had been pumped with a contrast substance through the IV so that might have tainted the results and given a false positive. But in any case, I needed to see an endocrinologist at Massachusetts General.

She also said that these tumors were rare.

I'd been writing in my little green journal from Sri Lanka the whole time. She asked if I had any questions. "Could this have had anything to do with my miscarriages?" She said they wouldn't know until they knew exactly what it was, but if it was what they thought it might be, I could imagine the effect of that stuff being released by the tumor.

I was calm, but I felt like I had been hit by a truck. The two sensations collided inside me. I felt frozen, yet I was able to get up.

She sent me down to the lab to have my blood drawn and to pick up the 24-hour urine-collection kit. As a needle was stuck into me yet again, I said to myself, *I am tired of giving blood.* I was exhausted. I was spent.

The next morning, I spoke via Skype to my husband in Hong Kong. He asked me about the doctor's appointment. I told him I was seeing an endocrinologist on Tuesday, and only after that I would know. I told him that it had nothing to do with my fertility treatments and it's a miracle it was discovered. Jay said, "So it was a happy accident." "Well . . . I wouldn't call it a happy accident. We don't know." He told me about his rehearsals, but I was distracted. Then he said he was going to look into coming back two days early, and I perked up. We told each other "I love you" and hung up.

I had been distracted because I wanted to know more about pheochromocytoma, this intimidating word, and looked it up again online. The tumor could be nothing. It could also mean death.

A number of the links I found were to cancer sections on websites, like those of the Mayo Clinic and the National Institutes of Health, even though it was made clear that most of these tumors were benign. *Wikipedia* was the top search result, so I clicked on it first. Some of the symptoms are elevated blood pressure, headaches, and palpitations, as I had already been told. But at the top of the list was "skin sensations." My skin had been feeling strange lately, tingly and often itchy. I had been thinking that it was the dry winter air. Maybe it wasn't.

"A pheochromocytoma can be fatal. . . . Tumors may grow very large, but most are smaller than 10 cm," according to this online source. Mine was 4.5 cm, so it was like most. "About 11.1 percent of adrenal cases are malignant, but this rises to 30 percent for extra-adrenal cases." I knew that mine was not in the adrenal gland but outside it. "The diagnosis can be established by measuring catecholamines and metanephrines in plasma (blood) or through a 24-hour urine collection." I was doing both tests.

They most often occur during "young-adult to mid-adult life." I was in the latter age group. It is "rare." It "often goes undiagnosed until autopsy," according to *Wikipedia. So people don't find out they have one before it kills them?*

Surgery is "the treatment of first choice," but there is "the potential for catastrophic intra- and postoperative complications." I knew I'd be in good hands at Massachusetts General. People who have it experience "excessive fluid loss in the urine." Yes, I had noticed this for the past year or more. I went to the bathroom a lot, and I couldn't drink enough water. I had assumed this was because I had a low and small bladder.

The condition was seen in only two to eight people per million. Pheochromocytomas were mentioned on the TV show *ER* a few times as an extremely rare diagnosis.

I was scared, and then I became sad as I read that the British actress Katrin Cartlidge died from one at the age of forty-one. I was almost forty-one. And I was sometimes an actress. I loved Katrin Cartlidge in the Mike Leigh movies. *Would I end up like her?*

I finished reading the *Wikipedia* entry and surfed to other sites. One listed vision disturbance as a symptom. Six years ago I had developed central serous chorioretinopathy (a leaking of fluid into the retina) while performing in New Zealand. All of a sudden I had trouble doing simple tasks like grasping a cup or walking down stairs. The world became 2-D. When I got back to the United States, I went to an eye specialist who asked, "How did you get this?" It's uncommon and usually found in older people. I had no idea how I had gotten it. I just wanted to get rid of it. I cut down my stress levels, went out less, and slept more. I also wore an eye patch for about seven months. It went away on its own.

Another site said that if the diagnosis of pheochromocytoma is over-looked, the consequences could be disastrous, even fatal. But if found, it can be cured. As I read this, I became catatonic. I didn't know what to tell people, if anything. All my efforts at discussing my health openly after the miscarriages were now eclipsed by this new development. I might have a life-threatening condition, which could have prevented me from becoming a mother in the first place.

In many respects, I had played things safe. I didn't take helicopter rides. I wouldn't get on cruise ships. I liked to drive—but as little as possible. I knew the odds of the helicopter or ship or car crashing were low, but I preferred to be safe than sorry.

What am I supposed to do now? Maybe I should go ahead and take a cruise.

I couldn't tell Jay right away. He was in Hong Kong for another two weeks. He couldn't do anything from there. He had to finish his show. My mother was visiting my brother in New York. I was supposed to go there the next week. *Should I go? She knew I'd been going through the IVF process and that it had been delayed, but how could I tell her why?*

I felt stuck. I couldn't say I was sick. I couldn't say I was dying. I couldn't say I was unhappy. I was catatonic. I didn't know where to go. I decided to postpone making decisions until my head was less full. It was 11:50 p.m. I was tired. I wanted to go to sleep.

I thought about what I shouldn't have thought about, which was that I might have cancer. If that were the case and I had to go through treatment, it could take a while. At that point, even if I were given the all-clear, I might not be able to have my own child. This was a truly cruel turn of events.

I didn't know where this train was going anymore. I thought the issue was whether I was going to have a child or not. But even if I didn't want to have a child and wanted to get off the train, I couldn't. I had to keep going and find out if there was anything else wrong with me. I thought of all the things I had done in my life to tempt the fates of health: eating breakfast cereal and McDonalds all the time as a child, developing bulimia in high school, smoking in college. It didn't matter how healthy I was now; the damage could have been done. But all those things had no relevance to me now. I saw my whole future not working out before me, but I wasn't ready to go.

I thought that, as the roller coaster of medical appointments was bound to continue, I would try to emulate my father. Thinking back to the time when he was sick, I appreciated more the resoluteness with which he went to his appointments. Sometimes I went with my mother to pick him up from chemotherapy. I thought about the insanity of knowing you are dying but having to do things as if you're living. All those moments you experience, not knowing they might be your last.

As part of the testing ordered by Dr. Shapiro, I had to spend much of the weekend peeing into a plastic bowl that sat on top of the toilet seat and pouring the urine into an orange jug that I kept in the fridge. There was a sticker on the jug that said "POISON." *Is urine poison?* I remembered hearing as a child about a politician in Sri Lanka who used to drink his own pee. The last few days I had sensed a slight pain toward the middle right of my torso. I wondered if it was the tumor making its presence known or if it was my imagination.

That Monday, March 6, I dropped off the 24-hour urine sample at the clinic and took the subway to my appointment with Dr. Christopher Cutie, a urologist at Massachusetts General. The waiting room at the Endocrinology Center was radically different from that of the Fertility Center. Both were sterile, but the Fertility Center felt new and rich while the Endocrinology Center felt shabby and poor. The seats were crammed closer together, and the carpet looked worn.

I walked into Dr. Cutie's office wearing a John Lennon T-shirt, which I had gotten from Forever 21. I was amassing a small collection of John Lennon T-shirts, one of which—my favorite—showed him and Yoko Ono in bed holding white flowers for peace. I felt stronger and cooler when I wore them. Dr. Cutie looked not much older than me, somewhere in his forties. I thought I saw him glance at my shirt.

He said the doctors suspected it was a pheochromocytoma because of its unusual location. There was something about the way he looked at me that seemed concerned, but he could have just been gentle by nature. He described the tests they would need to do, but I told him Dr. Shapiro had already ordered the blood work and urine sample. He said that I had done all I needed to do for now.

My appointment with Dr. Cutie went quickly, and I rushed to get the next train to New York. I was supposed to be on the 1:40 p.m. regional train, but I paid the difference to get on the more expensive Acela. I wanted to get out as fast as possible.

Being in Cambridge away from most of my friends had made it easy to hold in what I'd been going through. Now that I was going to New York, I would have to face people. Faking it is not in my vocabulary, even though I am a performer. I alternated between wanting to be very private and wanting to share the news about my unexpected health adventure. All I knew for sure was that I needed to be with people. I was happy reading books, taking baths, sleeping—as I had been doing in Cambridge. But I wanted to see friends, to have someone outside of myself to connect with.

When I hit my forties, I had started to look back more. I felt the weight of all the stuff I'd amassed—the experiences, the memories, the people. I could understand more why people dropped out and became hermits. The brain can only hold so much.

In those days after seeing Dr. Cutie, I found myself overwhelmed by anything beautiful—turns of phrase, sunlight, ideas, and people. Now, everything beautiful felt like something I might not see in the future. I had to hold onto them in the present.

During the week I was in New York, my brother and his fiancée had their engagement party. I decided not to tell anyone what was going on, so that we could all just have fun. My brother had made his famous horse-radish vodka. He had lived in Russia for a time and while there learned how to infuse vodkas. For my own engagement party with Jay, he had made these vodkas in flavors of cardamom, cucumber, and my favorite, horse-radish. The night of my brother's party, though, I felt like I couldn't drink too much. *Who knows how alcohol might interact with whatever it is I have?*

A few days after I arrived in New York, Dr. Cutie's office called saying they needed to do a biopsy. Jay was coming back from Hong Kong on March 17, so I scheduled the procedure for March 19.

When Jay got home, I was the happiest girl in the world. It was torture having been apart for that long a stretch. For the first time ever, we had broken our rule of seeing each other at least every three weeks. His first night back, we went out for dinner to our favorite Mexican restaurant and cuddled in bed. It was the kind of night I loved most with him.

The next night was the night before my biopsy. I took a bath in lavender salts and listened to a meditation podcast. I never used to meditate, but a few months earlier, a friend had turned me on to the Chopra Center's 21-Day Meditation Challenge. "I am Deepak Chopra and welcome to the Mind-Body Odyssey. . . . Here's one thing to remember: your mind, your body, your consciousness, which is your spirit, and your social interactions, your personal relationships, your environment, how you deal with your environment, and your biology are all inextricably woven into a single process. This is an integrated process. . . . When you experience negative or toxic emotions, such as fear, greed, anger, hostility or doubt, then of course that creates stress and then that creates damage to your body. Through meditation you can actually reverse the effects of this toxic experience of life. . . ."[2]

The biopsy was a straightforward experience. I laid down in a contraption that provided an image of the area where the doctor would insert a fine needle below my belly button and draw out a sample. The doctor conducting the biopsy, Owen O'Connor, who had a thick Irish accent, referred to the mass as a "lesion." He said he hoped that I would get good results. I hoped that since it was two days after St. Patrick's Day, which was taken very seriously in Boston, the luck of the Irish would rub off on me.

For my birthday the next day, Jay took me for dinner to Craigie on Main, one of our go-to restaurants for special occasions. I felt completely in the moment with him. As we walked home, he said, "We both have a scary history with these sorts of things." I knew exactly what that meant. His sister's death at the age of twelve, and my father's at fifty-three.

As we continued our walk home, holding hands, I imagined what it would be like to tell people I had cancer, even though I hadn't been told that I had it. For an instant, I was assuming the worst.

The day after, I called Dr. Cutie's office to see when I might get the results. Probably next Wednesday. I left a message for Nurse Pam at Dr. Souter's office. "I had a biopsy on Monday and should be getting the results later next week. I was wondering, because it doesn't look like this situation is going to resolve any time soon, should I think about freezing my eggs or is it too late for that?"

I got a call back from a nurse who was covering Pam's calls while she was on vacation. She said, "None of the nurses here could really advise you about freezing your eggs, so I'm going to have someone call you to set up an appointment to talk to Dr. Souter. I'm looking at your notes. Sorry you are having to deal with this. I hope the results of your biopsy are good. That must have been uncomfortable." Yes, it was. "And your birthday is the same day as mine. First day of spring."

I could live forever or I could die tomorrow, I felt at that time. But any of us could say that. I resolved that if I knew my odds of living changed, I would throw a party where people could talk to each other. I did sometimes think about the possibility that my tumor was malignant. When I did, I imagined how it might affect my life. I felt an overwhelming responsibility for the experiences of my husband and mother. I will never forget my mother saying over my father's dead body, "God is wicked."

In the days of waiting between appointments and results, I avidly read the news. An unemployed man, Matt Green, was walking every block in all five boroughs of New York City over the course of two years. President Obama chimed in on the shooting in Florida of an unarmed black youth, Trayvon Martin, by a self-appointed neighborhood watchman, George Zimmerman. More women than men supported Rick Santorum for president.

I watched a documentary about the making of the first Plastic Ono Band album. More John Lennon. I don't know why exactly I'd grown so attracted to him and his music recently. Maybe it was the way he stuck to his beliefs, spoke his mind, let himself dig deep inside to learn more about himself. After the film, I listened to John Lennon songs, like "Isolation" and "Hold On."

That weekend Jay left town, this time for Norway, where he was directing another show. On March 26, I had to go to New York to work on a photo shoot with the artist Carrie Mae Weems. After I boarded the train, I thought about my biopsy results, which had not yet come in. Even though I had been told it might take until Wednesday, two days from then, I decided to call Dr. Cutie's office. *If the results are bad, I can hurry off the train.* His assistant answered the phone. "Hi, I had the biopsy last week." "Okay." "I was wondering if the results had come in." "What's your medical record number?" I could feel her typing in the numbers and looking at her screen. "Okay. I'll give the message to Dr. Cutie and have him call you." *Does that mean she has the results? She must be seeing something on her screen, or she would have said they hadn't come in yet.*

A few hours later, still on the train, I saw Dr. Shapiro's number on my caller ID. I answered the phone. Her words stunned me: "The cells in the mass are a GIST tumor. It's not normal but it's not always malignant. Usually they are in the stomach. You should meet with Sam Yoon, a surgeon in the oncology department. Because of size, these are often observed over time. Often you don't do anything about them but they do cause problems. Usually a patient has symptoms but with you, we're in a space where it's not causing problems."

Dr. Cutie's assistant had known when I spoke to her earlier. I felt the irony of being almost in New York when I received the news. If I had found out last Friday or even that morning, I could have changed my plans.

My brother's wedding was in a week. I made a few on-the-spot decisions: *I won't tell my brother and his fiancée until after the wedding. I also won't tell my mother. I don't want to burden them with the knowledge as they get ready for the happiest day of their lives, and I don't want them to think I'm making a noble gesture by being at their wedding.*

Before the train arrived in New York, I called Dr. Yoon's office, per Dr. Shapiro's request. The receptionist asked, "What is your diagnosis?" "GIST." She told me he only had office hours on Thursdays and made an appointment for me on April 12 at 3:45 p.m., Yawkey Center, third floor, 3B. I knew the third floor was where a cancer department was. I remembered a man I saw with a bandana wrapped around his head who had gotten off on the third floor before I went up to the Fertility Center on the tenth floor.

I started to fixate on this GIST. *The tumor might have had something to do with my miscarriages, so my age was not the reason. But because I started trying to have a kid so late, the delay now caused by my tumor might result in it being too late for me to have my own kid.*

That night I called my childhood friend, Uma, another Sri Lankan who had become a GI specialist in San Francisco. First thing she said was, "How did you get that?" She said no one ever talked about GISTs ten to twelve years ago. Usually they were seen in the stomach. Usually they came with pain or blood. When she encountered them in her patients, she sent them right away to an oncological surgeon. Almost all GISTs are taken out. It's caused by a genetic mutation. It's not familial; it doesn't run in the family. If it's in the pelvis, it could have mechanically impinged on the uterus. Removing it could be a good thing. She ended by saying she was going to e-mail a GI friend at Massachusetts General because she thought I should speak to a specialist in addition to the surgeon.

The next day I went to a meeting with Carrie Mae Weems to prepare for the photo shoot, and I didn't want to focus on anything else. She talked about wanting to explore how women victimize themselves and what men and women think about when they look at each other. She wanted to re-create Magritte's painting *The Impossible*, which depicts a man painting a nude woman into being, and subvert it with two women in the scene. In Magritte's original, the painter is applying his brush to her partially formed arm. We had someone to play the painter, but Carrie needed someone to pose as the woman. I volunteered. I didn't know then that this would become the last shot of my torso unscarred.

But in that moment, it started to sweep over me—the feeling that what I had might change my life and not just be temporary. The burden of telling people made me sadder than the experience of the thing. It sounded worse than it felt.

But I also felt calm. In those days after I got the news, I felt tears come to my eyes every so often, though I suppressed them for the most part, especially in the presence of others. I felt incredibly focused. I hear some people are like that when they find out they have cancer. Instead of freaking out, they acquire an aura of peace.

I thought, *My life is becoming a movie.* And perhaps, *infertility saved my life.*

The scrutiny of the fertility treatment led to the discovery of an illness that would have otherwise taken years to reveal itself. But it's also frightening that with modern medical technology we know more about what is wrong with us before we feel like there is something wrong. Now I wouldn't be able to plan more than a few weeks into the future because I didn't know what the doctors were going to tell me. Every week had seemed to bring a different set of revelations and tasks.

Regardless, I felt very much the same. My mind was occupied. The diagnosis was abstract to me. I felt healthier than ever. *Accept the things you cannot change.*

Per my friend Uma's suggestion, I made an appointment with a Dr. David Harmon, an oncologist, for Tuesday, April 3, at 10 a.m. Jay would be in town, thank goodness, because he was coming from Norway—which I was amused to read online had the best research on GIST—for a few days to attend my brother's wedding.

The Cancer Center was vast. It was busy. I saw people of all ages, though most of them were very old. Some were sipping Creamy Vanilla Smoothies of barium sulfate, preparing themselves for scans. I noticed the poster above the receptionist: "Cancer in the Family: Living with Uncertainty." My name was called, and Jay and I were led to an examination room. There were DVDs on the counter: "Preparing for Chemotherapy." I took one because I was curious.

Dr. Harmon entered. He seemed a kindly older man with a temperate voice. He said my GIST had a low mitotic rate (at which the cells were dividing), but it was malignant. That was the word I didn't want to hear, the one that Dr. Souter had said I should hope not to hear.

Dr. Harmon continued. These things were rare and needed to be treated. He said they stage them and assess the risk. "We estimate the risk of recurrence after surgery. The risk for you is intermediate based on the biopsy. You have a very good chance of being cured. The main thing is surgery. Dr. Yoon'll do right by you." I asked, "Do I definitely have a GIST?" He replied, "We don't mince words about this sort of thing." I asked, "What would have happened if it hadn't been found now?" He said, "You would have gotten very sick." At the end of the appointment, Dr. Harmon arranged for me to have a CT scan of my torso, which he advised so we could be sure there wasn't anything else going on in my body.

Afterward, I asked Jay, "How did I get this?" He responded, "It's a genetic mutation. You got it because you were born. You are now in the murky world of cancer research centers. But when you walk into the hospital, you give yourself over to the process. You kind of hibernate. It makes you an awesome patient. You put your faith in the system. You do your research. You are prepared."

That night I decided to tell a few people whom I could trust not to tell anyone else. I needed to let it out, so I wrote to three friends.

Hi, F, G, Z.

I got the results of my biopsy last week and yesterday saw a specialist so now I have more information.

I like the doctor and feel like I'm in the right city and hospital to get treatment. I gotta have a CT scan on Sunday and see another doctor next Thursday and then schedule surgery. It's all mucho complicated, but I have faith in the process.

If you want to know more about this strange condition, here's what I've referred to about it.

http://www.cancer.org/Cancer/GastrointestinalStromalTumorGIST/ DetailedGuide/gastrointestinal-stromal-tumor-what-is-gist

Sorry I don't have better news. I am in very good spirits though. Keeping my mind occupied and seizing the day.

xoxo

T

When I started acting in theater, I taught myself to cry by thinking of others crying. And I could stop myself from crying by not thinking about others crying. Maybe I could use that technique to get me through the next little while. The worst part about my life then was thinking about telling others. The sound of it was worse than the experience of it. It sucked being the one who would make others worry.

In New York the next day, I took a walk in Prospect Park with my aunt who had traveled from Sri Lanka for my brother's wedding. In the past, I had always been candid with her. We talked about the family, her business, Sri Lanka. We talked about her daughter—my younger cousin whose wedding Jay and I had attended the year before. I sensed her hesitation to talk about my cousin's pregnancy—the baby was due in June. The truth is I felt no disappointment about my not having had the first child among my generation, and my mother didn't badger me as much about having a child now that she knew about my three miscarriages. My aunt told me she was sorry for what I'd been through. I told her about my hopes for IVF. But I didn't tell her about the GIST. On the subway back, I thought about how hard it was for me to be in New York with my family and where so many people knew me so well. In Cambridge, it was easier to keep secrets. Later that day, I had a meeting with a director, who is also a good friend, to discuss her film project. I told her my news and could see her tearing up. She said, "I'm a worrier." I said, "I'm not, so follow my lead."

The hard part about having so many amazing friends and family in my life was that I was not ready to go. I was going to fight as much as I could. Be positive. Be happy. I actually needed not to talk about the GIST. I needed to be distracted. Love hurts.

After I left my friend and got on the subway, I heard a voice above me and looked up. I wasn't listening to the words, just the sound. I looked around. Nothing remarkable was happening, but having my eyes open and full of other people helped me stop thinking about myself.

That evening, at a friend's house in Tribeca, I looked out the window at a deep-blue sky. There was a massive American flag waving in the wind on top of a building a few blocks away. The flag reminded me of 9/11. A melancholy overtook me. These days I saw beauty in everything around me. I had a visceral connection to the material world. I wanted to hold onto everything. *I have cancer.*

My brother's wedding was a beautiful and intimate affair with thirty of their closest friends and family. I made an impromptu toast in which I praised my new sister-in-law for giving my brother and me more motivation to spend time with each other. I knew my brother felt that way about Jay, too. We loved to double-date. I told the crowd that if my brother hadn't married his wife, I would have married her, a statement that made everyone cheer. No one could tell what I was hiding. Except Jay, and I felt his worry, but we had a great time anyway and stayed out until 2 a.m., hanging out after the dinner with the younger members of the wedding party at a bar in Brooklyn.

Easter Sunday, back in Cambridge, I went with Jay to the hospital for the CT scan of my torso that Dr. Harmon had ordered. I asked at the main building reception how to get to Blake, second floor. The woman behind the counter looked like the Church Lady character from *Saturday Night Live*. She smiled so widely. She pulled out a little piece of paper and checked off Blake from the list of buildings. "Cat scan?" she asked, guessing what I was there for. "The cool thing is when you get off the elevator, it's right across."

As I checked in on the second floor around 9:30 a.m., the receptionist passed me a Creamy Vanilla Smoothie of barium sulfate suspension. One of the questions I had to answer on the health history form was "Have you fallen in the last 3 months?" Jay said out loud, "In love." At 10:08 a.m., they gave me a second smoothie. I sucked the straw expecting the familiar flavor of vanilla, but it was berry and tasted horrible.

The worst part of the CT scan was when the nurse stuck the IV needle into my hand. Needles always hurt me, because, I thought, I have small veins. But she did a great job, and the sting only lasted for a few seconds. The scan itself was done in a minute. As I left the room, I could see the technicians behind a window looking at the screen. I knew they had an image of my insides on their monitors. I tried to read their faces, but I couldn't. I could tell they weren't smiling though.

The next day, Jay had to return to Norway to get back to his rehearsals. As I waited for the results of the CT scan, my greatest fear was that I would be told the cancer had spread. Maybe the occasional and slight tingling I had in my chest or breast was a tumor. I spent the rest of the day in a daze that my life in this world might be shorter than I thought. I worried a lot about my husband.

I did some online research on GIST. I joined the Life Raft Group newsletter for people living with GIST. Now I was part of this community.

I also did research on my doctors, Dr. Harmon and Dr. Yoon, mostly by looking at their pages on the hospital website.

The day after that, I called Dr. Harmon's office because it had now been two days since the CT scan. The receptionist said she would have Dr. Harmon call me with the results. Her tone reminded me of the tone I'd heard in Dr. Cutie's assistant's voice. *She knows*, I thought. Later that afternoon, Dr. Harmon called. He said that he'd seen what he expected to see, a mass in the abdomen. There was no spread to the liver. There were a few tiny nodules in the chest that would need follow-up in three months. But in the middle of the chest, there was something to look at. "Do you have any chest pressure or cough?" he asked. "No." I asked him what it could be. He responded, "Benign tumors are usually in the chest. Germ-cell tumor, lymphoma, and thymoma." I didn't know what these words meant. He said, "It's unusual to pick up these things. It might need a biopsy. I'm going to speak to the chest doctor and find out what he wants to do." I said, "Okay, so I'll wait for your call?" He said, "Yes, I'll call you after I speak to him."

I felt the blood rush out of my body. I felt cold. I started shivering. I tried to concentrate, but it was hard. I had another tumor. "In the chest" sounded bad. My head hurt for an hour until I couldn't take it. I called Dr. Harmon's office again. He called me back quickly. I asked him if the growth was in my lung. "I hope you understand I'm nervous about this sort of thing because my father died of lung cancer." He said it was in the mediastinum in front of the heart. "How big is it?" "It's a few centimeters." "Do I need to get it evaluated before I have surgery for the GIST?" "That shouldn't matter." "Is it unrelated to the GIST or could it have caused it?" "More likely not."

While I was on the phone with him, I looked online for info about germ-cell tumors. One connection with my health history was early entry into puberty. I was eight when I hit mine.

I said to Dr. Harmon, "I'm just nervous because the plot keeps getting thicker." He said, "This is another plot twist, but it should have a good outcome."

I told him, "I look on the Internet and I get concerned about the GIST having been biopsied and reseeding. Am I wrong?" He said, "Sometimes the Internet doesn't tell you what you need to know." I asked, "Is it that a lot of people if they had a CT scan would find a growth that needed to be evaluated?" "No, but some."

I called my friend Uma again to get her advice on how to approach my next doctor's appointment. She said to ask if the tumor could be removed laparoscopically because that would reduce pelvic adhesion and have less of an impact on fertility. What is the recovery time? How long will I be in the hospital? Any restrictions or limitations after? Impact on fertility? I took notes as she rattled off questions. She said it was a good thing it had been found because of IVF and before I had started the hormones. I asked her, "Is it because they were looking harder at me that they found this? Wouldn't you find something wrong with a lot of people if you scanned them?" She responded, "A lot of people have CTs but don't have 5-cm masses in their abdomen." Then she reiterated what she had said in our first call about how GIST, though rare, is more common today: "When I was a fellow, no one even talked about GISTs. Are there more out there or are they being diagnosed more?"

I told her that another mass had been found in my chest. I could feel her get a lump in her throat. She said I would need to see a pulmonologist, who would probably want a biopsy. I told her Dr. Harmon had already arranged for me to see a thoracic surgeon, Dr. John Wain, whom I would see the same day I saw Dr. Sam Yoon.

That night and for many days thereafter, I cried. I cried myself to sleep. I woke up feeling like I was in a bad dream. I thought about a world without me in it, and I was sad, inconsolably so. I imagined my friends growing old without me. I imagined my husband alone.

On April 12, around 11:15 a.m., I heard what sounded like stones falling outside my window. I looked out, and there was a big hail storm, in the middle of April. This was a very strange day. I had to walk to the subway while the hail still came down. Cherry blossoms on Inman Street were falling from the trees. Cherry blossoms in a hail storm. In Japan after the 2011 tsunami, the cherry blossom season—a long-revered ritual—was bittersweet, a sign of what endured despite the sadness and a reminder that there was some beauty that remained.

In the thoracic surgery waiting room, two men in their sixties or seventies were seated across from each other, one with his wife to his right, the other with his wife to his left. One wife said, "He operated on my mother. He saved her life." The man opposite said, "He operated on me last year," as he gave a thumbs up. "My wife worked here, so she knows he's the best." They were all talking about Dr. Wain, my surgeon.

Another man sleeping in his chair at the other end of the room was called for an appointment. He woke up and bounced down the hall, clutching two helium balloons. One balloon said, "Thank you for all you did." The other said, "Nurses are the greatest."

During my appointment, Dr. Wain showed me a 3-D movie of my chest cavity. I loved peering at the insides of my body. I loved the way the bones and the organs looked. What an incredible machine. But he pointed out a blob that he said "isn't supposed to be there." He said it could be a thymoma, which was usually benign and could wait to be removed. Or it might have spread from the GIST. Or it could be a lymphoma, which would be treated with chemo or radiation. If it had spread from the GIST, it would be removed or treated. It's a localized process, if you have surgery, and it's successful.

I asked him how big it was. He said it was 40 mm by 27 mm, or 4 cm by 2.7 cm.

I looked at him, stunned. I started to utter, "How . . ." and he completed my question, "How did you get this? Well, these could be genetic changes that couldn't be avoided." He said there were 1- to 2-mm spots in the lungs, but those were probably nothing. I asked him how long I had had the growth. He said if it's a thymoma, it could be about four years; if a lymphoma, then six months. I would have a needle biopsy and follow-up CT scans. If it's a lymphoma, the recurrence rate is 45 to 50 percent all the way to 75 percent.

After this appointment, I went to the sarcoma waiting room for my appointment with Dr. Yoon. A friend joined me to keep me company, which was comforting especially after the stress I felt upon speaking with Dr. Wain. Although the doctor had a kind manner, I was scared and found it hard to focus.

After an hour and fifteen minutes, the waiting room was empty, and my name was finally called. A nurse named Donna brought me and my friend to the examination room. Dr. Yoon was much younger than I thought he'd be, probably about my age. He explained about the tumor and GIST. The CT scan had taken images in what looked like slices of a loaf of bread. GISTs arise from the bowel, the Cajal interstitial cells that serve as the pacemaker in the gastrointestinal tract. There are about 5,000 to 6,000 cases a year, compared with breast cancer, of which there are 170,000 a year. They are usually in the stomach or small bowel. They can be benign or malignant. There are three main factors. Number 1 is the mitotic (cell division) rate. Under fifty high-powered fields, less than five out of fifty, is considered low; five to ten is intermediate. With my biopsy, there were no mitoses in all fifty fields. (Very good!) Number 2 is size. If it is less than 5 centimeters, it's considered low-risk. Mine was just pushing it at 4.7. The third factor is location. He said mine was probably at the small bowel.

Dr. Yoon said Sloan-Kettering Hospital has the largest database of GISTs and went to their website to check out the nomogram (a two-dimensional diagram) with me. The recurrence rate for mine was 86 percent in two years and 74 percent in five years, but that estimate was based on zero to four mitoses. I have zero. GIST has become one of the most studied tumors.

He said he would remove the GIST laparoscopically, making a five-centimeter incision. There are four port sites—near the belly or in the abdomen. He would inflate my abdomen, make an incision below my belly button, remove the GIST, then staple the ends of my small bowel together. The surgery would last two and a half hours; I would be in the hospital for about three days and could expect to recover in about three weeks. The pathology report would come back one week after the surgery and would show whether all of the tumor had been removed. The risks of the surgery would be bleeding, infection, and bowel connection leak.

He had answered all my questions from Uma without my having to ask them. I felt like I would be in very good hands and went home.

Around 7 p.m. that evening, my phone rang. It was Dr. Yoon, who had bumped into Dr. Wain at a sarcoma conference after my appointment, and they had spoken about my case. He said I should call Dr. Wain to discuss my surgery because it was more involved than he thought. While Dr. Yoon's surgery would be relatively simple, Dr. Wain couldn't do his removal of the thymoma laparoscopically, so he would have to cut through my chest bones.

I sent an e-mail to Jay:

I'm sorry I have such health dramas and that you have to witness them. What to do. I love you!

To which he responded:

Don't be sorry about anything. I LOVE YOU

I spoke to Dr. Wain the next day, and he confirmed what Dr. Yoon said. I was to have a sternotomy, which is the same type of opening of the chest that is done for heart surgery. I asked him if there was any urgency to get the surgery done because I wanted to wait for my husband to return in May. He said I absolutely could wait.

While I waited, there was a lot of cancer in the news. Warren Buffett announced he had stage 1 prostate cancer. He sounded like me when he said that, regardless, he felt "healthier than ever." Ryan O'Neal also announced he had prostate cancer. Barry Gibb was in a coma from his cancer.

I have a vast network of friends and colleagues with whom I stay in touch via an occasional e-mail blast. I let them know what I'm working on and what I'm excited about. Rarely is the news personal, but I decided to use this format to tell everyone once and for all what was going on. I was getting tired of telling people one by one. Also, I needed people to send me good energy and think about me. On April 18, I sent this note, with the subject header "From Tanya re: April news health and art."

Hello.

I hope you are very well and enjoying April.

What I'm about to say will be a shock to almost everyone, and I decided to tell people this way for a few reasons. 1) I would rather you heard it from me than someone else. 2) Some of you might have information that could help. 3) My story could help someone else.

Recently I was diagnosed with GIST cancer, which is rare and related to a genetic mutation. Nothing causes it; nothing can prevent it. I have it because I was born.

A few months ago, I said I was taking a break. The reason was that after three miscarriages, I had decided to pursue IVF. In February, after beginning the first cycle, a growth was seen on a routine ultrasound. IVF was halted until further assessment, and I went through a bunch of tests (an MRI, biopsy, CT scan etc.).

There turned out to be tumors in two locations; they might be related to each other or of different origins. One is about 5 cm and the other is 4 cm, but the mitotic rate of the one already biopsied is low (which is great). The first step is surgery to resect them. After they are evaluated, I will know if I need follow-up therapy. I'll have about a week in the hospital and a month of recovery. My prognosis is good. It might have been years before I experienced symptoms. Thinking positively, my trying so hard to have a kid might have saved my life.

I feel—and think I look—healthier than ever, so my condition is abstract to me. When I first heard the diagnosis, I asked the doctor if he were sure, to which he replied, wryly, "We don't mince words about this sort of thing."

The best medicine is to be distracted and occupied, and creatively I have never been more satisfied. A friend recently emailed me a poster that said: The EARTH without ART is just EH.

I love my life. I love what I do. I love my home, husband, family, friends, doctors (especially their names—Sam Yoon and John Wain), insurance, and Mass General. So don't feel sorry for me, not that you were going to. It's important to remember that cancer is a big catch-all phrase for cells behaving badly. It takes many different forms and has a range of repercussions. Right now for me it's one day at a time and seize the day, but I'm looking forward to life after I recover.

Please don't feel like you have to write anything back. I just wanted you to know what was going on. Some of you have been on my email list for as long as twenty years, and some of you I met recently. Thank you all for your support. And thank you as always for reading!

All best,

Tanya

I didn't mention where the second tumor was, i.e., near my heart, or what it might be, because I thought that would be too worrying and that it would be better to wait until I knew for sure what it was.

I got dozens of e-mails back—the most extraordinary stories of people who had dealt with or knew someone who had dealt with cancer, suggestions for what I could do, alternative therapies, dietary changes, names of shamans, and beautiful words of support. These messages all gave me hope.

My second biopsy on the tumor near my heart was scheduled for May 1. Jay took a few days off from rehearsals in Norway and flew back to be with me. At the hospital, as the doctor explained the procedure to us, Jay joked, "The fastest way to Tanya's heart is through her chest." I was happy he was there. Everything was much better when he was there. Unfortunately, he had to leave that night.

At home, I was scared to take my clothes off because I didn't want to see the wound on my chest. By the third day, I started getting itchy. I scratched the right side of my torso, and my hands discovered electrode receivers still stuck there. I found another one by my neck. On the fourth day, when I finally got up the courage to remove the dressing on the wound and take a shower, I thought the bruise wasn't so bad, but it was odd. It looked like a vampire had tried to bite me but missed the neck and landed above my left breast. I also found another electrode receiver. Then I took the longest, hottest shower ever.

Adam Yauch of the Beastie Boys died that day, from a cancerous tumor on his parotid gland. He had been a Buddhist, didn't drink or smoke. I searched for obituaries about him. He was forty-seven, only six years older than me.

After I read about him, I sobbed and sobbed. I thought I should accept that my time on earth might be shorter than I had anticipated.

Looking back at those two weeks before my surgery is hard. Jay was in Norway. I had told him to finish the show, that there'd be plenty for him to do to support me around my surgery and thereafter. I kind of enjoyed the quiet in Cambridge. I could just focus on myself. Of course, there were moments when I felt utterly despondent. Many times I considered the possibility that something might go wrong and that those moments before my surgery would be my last moments. During a pre-surgery appointment, the nurse had asked if I had prepared my will and health proxy. She suggested I should. I read an essay by author Bruce Feiler in the *New York Times* about "last words." He wrote, "Last words have an almost mystical significance in both Eastern and Western cultures, in part because they hold out the possibility of revealing a deep insight or lifting a veil on the meaning of life. . . . The odds are so 'vanishingly small' that you'll know when you're in a final conversation, you should avoid any possibility of regret by initiating interactions earlier. This includes what kind of medical interventions the person might want as well as what that person meant to you."[3]

Even though I knew my odds were very good and that I was at one of the best hospitals in the world, I thought about death. I wanted to make sure that my loved ones didn't worry about me. I also wanted to make sure that if anything happened to me, they wouldn't have a mess to clean up. I remembered how hard it was sorting through everything after my father passed away. I decided to be proactive and prepared a document with all my account numbers, passwords, etc. I printed out three copies of this and my will and placed them in envelopes with the words "In Case of Untimely Death" on them. I planned to put these envelopes in different locations so that they would be more likely to be found. I listened to Whitney Houston for the first time since that week she died, when my tumor had first been detected. And I cried and cried and cried. It hit me that I was facing mortality at a relatively young age and how twisted it was that until just a few weeks before I had been on a journey to bring a new life into this world. I had gone from extending my legacy to maybe being the end of the line. I was tired and went to bed.

The next day, wanting to shake the malaise of the night before, I decided that I must have a party in New York before my surgery, so I could see people, just in case. A friend helped me find a location, and my brother offered to foot some of the bill. I sent out an invitation for an "Under the Knife Party."

One night after Jay returned from Norway, a few days before my surgery, as we sat at our dining table, the air between us was calm. I told him I wanted to talk to him about the instructions I had prepared in case anything went wrong, about my will and health proxy. I told him clearly and directly. These were things I had prepared just in case, but I assured him that everything would be fine. However, I felt him tighten up. I felt fear. *No, Jay, everything has to turn out okay. It will.*

With Jay, I was where I wanted to be. *I love this man so much. We've done so much together. We've been through so much together. Our love is strong and true.* Before I married Jay, my mother had asked, "Can you look at him every day?" I could, every day, many times a day.

A few hours before the party began on May 12, I had trouble breathing. I felt like I was preparing for the last supper. I called a doctor friend who said I was probably just anxious. He said he would take me through some breathing exercises. "Push back your shoulder blades then drop them down. Arch your head and neck slightly back. Wait a minute, taking the same shallow breaths. Then try and take a deeper breath. Don't wear yourself out." I started crying as he talked to me. I felt weak. He said I shouldn't feel bad if I didn't make it to the party. People would understand. But I was determined to go.

I wore a vintage sequined, black and gold, one-shoulder Oleg Cassini dress with a plunging neckline. This would be the last time people would see my cleavage without a scar running down my chest. Dozens of friends turned up, some I hadn't seen in a long time. Many brought presents: stones they said had healing properties, books of poetry by E. E. Cummings and Rumi, nice-smelling soaps. Some people cried. Some people cried a lot. One friend said, "You're such a good person," as he sobbed. I heard from a friend that Jay had teared up a few times, too. I was overwhelmed by the love in the room but very glad I had gone through with the party.

The next morning, we all drove back to Cambridge. My brother was with us because I had asked him to come and keep Jay company during my surgery. That night we ate a fancy meal at Craigie on Main.

We woke up around 4:30 a.m. I took a quick hot shower then put on sweatpants and a new John Lennon long-sleeved T-shirt. I didn't put in my contacts, usually the first thing I do in the morning. Jay drove our car. My brother was in the backseat. I put on an upbeat face. The day was here.

At the hospital, after I had been checked in and examined, Jay and my brother came into the room. I took a good look at them. My brother left the room, and I held Jay's hand. "I love you." "I love you."

The last thing I remember was being on a gurney in a hallway with the anesthesiologist's hand on my shoulder. I felt like a child, vulnerable and worried. I had an IV in my hand. *It stings*, I told him. He looked at me with gentle concern and said it would stop being uncomfortable soon.

This was it, time for me to go under.

CHAPTER 8

THE GLOBAL LANDSCAPE OF INFERTILITY

When I began the IVF process, I didn't think much about its cost. I was lucky to be in a state (Massachusetts) with generous insurance coverage for the treatment. When the process was derailed and I was stuck with thousands of dollars of unusable fertility drugs, it hit me how much more disappointing it would have been if I'd had to pay for these drugs myself. I began to think about the exorbitant price tag of bringing a baby into this world through assisted reproductive technologies (ARTs) and wondered how women in other places coped. In the United States, for example, with only fifteen states providing some form of insurance coverage for fertility treatments, many couples simply cannot afford treatment and consequently suffer.

Having a child is a costly venture no matter how you do it. According to the US Department of Agriculture, a parent can expect to spend about $235,000 on a child's first seventeen years.[1] When you factor in infertility, the cost of treatment can make childbearing even less feasible. The United States has the highest average price of IVF treatment in the world, and the woman's age adds another layer of complexity and expense, as the odds of a successful live birth decline. Despite these deterrents, many women want to exhaust all possibilities for achieving their dreams, regardless of their age.

About 130 million babies are added annually to the world's population, and in 2012, the seven billionth person was born somewhere on the planet. While presenting a vast array of statistics, I explore the questions: How do fertility rates in different countries impact the world's ecological balance? What is the global landscape of infertility and ARTs? How do the costs and regulations of treatment vary from region to region? How much economic support do governments provide? And what are the creative and at times unorthodox ways that people attempt to fund their treatments? While this chapter could turn into a book of its own about the class, race, and cultural discrepancies that have emerged with regard to infertility and parenthood, my intent is to offer a glimpse into the complexity of the global situation.

Around 97 percent of the world's population lives in countries where the fertility rate is falling.[2] This can indicate progress in women's status, economics, and family planning. In countries with overpopulation and resource problems, declining fertility rates are positive outcomes. For example, between 1960 and 2009, Mexico's fertility rate fell from 7.3 children born per woman to 2.4. During the same time period, India's fertility rate dropped from 6 to 2.5, despite it being one of the most populous nations in the world and having the highest predicted population growth through 2015.[3] Africa continues to have high fertility rates (between 6 and 7 in countries like Uganda and Somalia), and the average woman in Africa can expect to have five children compared with 1.7 in East Asia. However, despite having twenty-nine of the world's thirty-one high-fertility countries (the other two are Afghanistan and Timor-Leste), fertility rates in Africa are expected to fall to 3 by 2030 and possibly below 2.5 by 2050, due to the rapid economic growth of the past fifteen years.[4] According to an article in the *Economist* in 2009, "An emergent African middle class is taking out mortgages and moving into newly built flats—and two children is what they want."[5]

When the fertility rate falls below 2.1, the replacement rate (of people being born versus those dying) can cause an imbalance between the young and old generations, resulting in concerns about whether there are enough people to take care of the aging population and enough new workers to keep the economy going. According to a 2012 United Nations report, approximately 48 percent of the world's population lives in low-fertility countries. For example, America's fertility rate is around 1.93, and continental Europe has an overall fertility rate of 1.5 (with every European country except Iceland considered a low-fertility country). In Germany, the fertility rate has been around 1.4 for forty years.[6] Thailand's is 1.66, and in Japan, where in 2010 one in three women in her thirties and one in five in her forties were single, the rate is an alarming 1.3.[7] Despite many women in Japan undergoing ARTs (311,000 cycles in 2011 alone—almost double the number of procedures done in the United States), according to the *Wall Street Journal*, in 2012 "the Japanese bought more adult diapers than diapers for babies."[8] Of the 222 nations ranked in the US Central Intelligence Agency's *World Factbook*, Singapore has the lowest fertility rate: 1.15.[9]

By 2030, more than a third of the population in a number of countries, such as Japan and Korea, will be over sixty-five years old, and in Singapore, the ratio of people of working age to senior citizens—sometimes referred to as the "dependency ratio"—will plummet from its current 6.3:1 to 2:1. In China, where the fertility rate is 1.54—largely because of the country's one-child policy—by 2040, the number of people older than sixty could more than double to 411 million; today it is around 171 million.[10] In America, the dependency ratio will double by 2050 to thirty-five retirees for every 100 workers.[11]

As the 2012 UN report explained, persons aged 60 or over comprise the fastest-growing segment of the world's population, and that segment is expected to increase by 45 percent by 2050. In 1950, in the more developed areas of the world, the number of people under the age of fifteen was more than double the number of people over the age of sixty (27 percent of the total population versus 12 percent). By 2013, the proportion was almost flipped, with older persons in the more developed areas comprising 23 percent of the population versus younger persons at 16 percent. In 2050, that number is projected to be 32 percent versus 16 percent, and around the world in general, seniors are expected to outnumber children for the first time in history.[12]

Researchers have estimated that by the year 2070, Earth's population will reach nine billion people and then start to decrease. At current fertility rates, by 2100, Western Europe's population could fall from 460 million to 350 million; Russia's and China's populations could be half of what they are now; and Japan's population will be less than half.[13] According to a 2008 report from the Austria-based International Institute for Applied Systems Analysis, if the world stabilizes at a fertility rate of 1.5 (like continental Europe already has), by the year 2200, the total global population could be less than half its current level; by 2300, it could top out at one billion (down from today's seven billion). As a January 2013 article in *Slate* explained, "On the bright side, the long-dreaded resource shortage may turn out not to be a problem at all. On the not-so-bright side, the demographic shift toward more retirees and fewer workers could throw the rest of the world into the kind of interminable economic stagnation that Japan is experiencing right now."[14]

Considering these population forecasts, the issue of fertility rates around the world is pressing, but not cut-and-dried. While keeping fertility rates down in some regions represents the success of education and modernization, in others it is a threat to the ecological balance. And advanced maternal age and the accessibility of fertility treatments influence fertility rates around the world.

In the United States, the average age of women having their first births rose about four years between 1970 and 2006, from age twenty-one to twenty-five. Although there is a wide variety between states—with twenty-eight being the average age of a new mother in Massachusetts compared with 22.9 in Mississippi—the average age did increase over time in all states, e.g., by over five years in the District of Columbia, New Hampshire, and Massachusetts, and by over two years in New Mexico, Mississippi, and Oklahoma.[15] The rate of first births for women in their thirties and forties has quadrupled since the 1970s, while it has dropped by a third for women in their twenties.[16]

According to a Pew study on "The New Demography of American Motherhood," teens had more births overall (13 percent) than women aged thirty-five and over (9 percent) in 1990; by 2008, that statistic had completely switched, with 14 percent of births overall to women aged thirty-five and over and 10 percent to teens. Despite this reversal, the total number of births remained fairly stable—4.2 million in 1990 and 4.3 million in 2008—and in fact, the number rose every year between 2003 and 2007.[17] Then birth rates began to fall with the onset of the recession. From 2007 to 2011, there was a 9 percent decline in the overall fertility rate, and the drop was greatest among young Hispanic women ages twenty to twenty-four—with the rate down by a third. 2012 was the first time in five years in which the rate remained stable.[18] However, even during the recession, the rate among women between the ages of forty and forty-four was the only one not to experience a decline, rising 6 percent between 2007 and 2009.[19]

In Canada, according to the Society of Obstetricians and Gynecologists of Canada, the average age of Canadian women giving birth rose from twenty-seven to almost thirty over two decades beginning in 1987, and the number of women thirty-five and older having their first child rose from 4 percent in 1987 to 11 percent in 2005.[20] Looking at Europe, the United

Kingdom is tied with Germany for the highest average maternal age of thirty at first birth. In France, Greece, the Netherlands, Luxembourg, Switzerland, Spain, and Italy, the average age ranges from 28.5 to 29.9, and in Scandinavian countries, it's around twenty-eight.[21] In poorer countries of Eastern Europe and Latin America, the average age is much lower, for example, 24.5 in Latvia and around twenty-one in Mexico, but in Ukraine, one in seven women becomes a mother after forty, and one in five after age thirty-five.[22]

Despite having the highest average maternal age, the United Kingdom has had a baby boom, with births going up every year for a decade. In 2011, the number of babies born in England and Wales was 22 percent higher than the total in 2001. This growth has been attributed to immigration and to thousands of older women deciding to have children before their window of fertility disappears. Over a decade, the number of mothers aged thirty-five to thirty-nine increased by 51 percent, and those mothers aged forty and older increased by 61 percent.[23]

A British woman, Carole Hobson, went to a clinic in Mumbai to have twins through IVF at the age of fifty-eight. Hobson, a single mother, used donor eggs from a twenty-four-year-old Indian woman and the sperm of a six-foot-tall Scandinavian man. The British writer and filmmaker Naomi Gryn wrote an essay for the *Guardian* about why she chose to have a baby at the age of fifty-one through egg donation with her partner, Pete, who is eight years younger. She spent much of her thirties recovering from a near-fatal car crash, met the love of her life when she was forty-two, and subsequently suffered two miscarriages and four failed IVF cycles. Many of the comments on her article were vicious. One person, who posted under the name "flowergrrl," wrote, "This makes me physically ill. I'm sorry but it is the height of selfishness (yes, selfishness) for a 50+ woman (or even a 50+ man) to have a child. Do you think you're going to live forever?"[24] (I actually know Naomi's brother, David, and she and I have other friends in common. They say she couldn't be happier to be a mother and has more energy than ever.)

In Singapore, which as stated earlier has the lowest fertility rate in the world (1.15), the government has taken extreme measures to encourage childbearing. According to its 2010 census, among the thirty to thirty-four age group, 43 percent of men and 31 percent of women were not married. To counter this trend, the government has sponsored matchmaking and fertility-boosting campaigns. It also gave out bonuses of up to S\$4,000 (around US\$3,223) for each of the first two babies, and S\$6,000 (around US\$4,835) for the third and fourth; and offered matching grants for deposits made into a Child Development Account. Despite these measures, in response to a TV panel survey question, "Can Singaporeans be persuaded to have more children?" 74 percent said no.[25] Meanwhile, in Quebec, where the average age of a woman having her first birth is 28.2, the government announced in 2009 that it would cover up to three fertility treatments per woman who can't afford them in an effort to boost birth rates.[26]

While researching for this book, I asked friends of different ages around the country "to what factors (e.g., social, governmental, economic) do you attribute why women today are having kids so late?" The answers included "the feminist revolution," "wanting careers, enjoying life," and "shortage of decent men." However, the majority cited economics as a reason to delay. Laura Dawn, a Brooklyn-based creative director who had her first child at age forty-three, said, "As artists, my husband and I were forced to travel for work all the time and both had to work constantly, so without affordable childcare options, we just said 'no way.' We frequently thought about moving to France just for the free healthcare/childcare and educational opportunities."[27]

The conflict between home and career can also be a deterrent to pursuing motherhood, especially when considering the statistics on domestic task sharing. Despite evolving gender dynamics, women still bear the bulk of parenting and domestic chores. Most US households are dual-income (in 2011, only 16 percent of households contained a breadwinner husband and a stay-at-home wife), and the number of men who left the workforce to raise children doubled in a decade to 176,000.[28] In fact, according to a 2007 survey by CareerBuilder.com, 38 percent of working dads said they would take a pay cut to spend more time with their kids.[29]

However, according to the *Atlantic*, women are 30 percent more likely to do chores at home than men.[30] In a *New York* magazine article about feminists who choose to stay at home, Lisa Miller wrote, "Despite their stated position, men still do far less housework than their spouses. In 2011, only 19 percent spent any time during the average day cleaning or doing laundry; among couples with kids younger than 6, men spent just 26 minutes a day doing what the Bureau of Labor Statistics calls 'physical care,' which is to say bathing, feeding, or dressing children. (Women did more than twice as much.)"[31]

A study by the *American Sociological Review* showed that women do 48.3 hours of multitasking per week compared with 38.9 for men, with working mothers multitasking more than two-fifths of the time compared with one-third for men.[32] Also, the stigma of interrupting and possibly forfeiting a career to have a child still looms large among women. As Dina Bakst, a founder and president of A Better Balance: The Work and Family Legal Center in New York City, argued in a 2012 op-ed for the *New York Times*, "Thousands of pregnant women are pushed out of jobs that they are perfectly capable of performing—either put on unpaid leave or simply fired—when they request an accommodation to help maintain a healthy pregnancy."[33] As reported in *Time* magazine, "Married women with kids who lost their jobs between 2007 and 2009 had a 31 percent lower chance of finding a new job than married fathers with kids," while "single women who weren't moms had a 29 percent greater chance than single men without kids of finding a new job."[34] These economic and work/life balance issues have an indelible impact on whether women in the United States can view having children as part of their futures.

The disincentive to have children exists in other countries as well. According to recent research from the Organisation for Economic Co-operation and Development (OECD), women without children in countries such as Ireland, Australia, Luxembourg, and the Netherlands generally receive higher wages than men.[35] In the United Kingdom, because of involuntary and age-related infertility, 30 percent of university graduate women are projected to be childless by the age of forty-five.[36] As Suzanne Moore, a columnist for the *Guardian*, wrote, "I am not at all surprised, though, that more women are choosing to remain child-free as it is obvious there is less and less support. As childcare costs soar and two wages are needed to support a family, some kind of reproductive strike happens."[37]

According to a *Marie Claire* survey in the United Kingdom, almost one in three respondents said they had delayed motherhood for their careers, and three-quarters of respondents in their twenties and thirties said that their work "is either very important or the single most important thing in their lives."[38] Many women, however, do not delay motherhood by choice. More than half of women responding to a poll on MumPoll.com said they would like to have children but can't afford them.[39] In addition, according to a 2012 Modern Motherhood Report for *Red* magazine in the United Kingdom, which surveyed 3,000 women between the ages of twenty-eight and forty-five, 54 percent described themselves as "emotionally infertile," meaning they wanted to have children but hadn't found a partner or their partner didn't want to have children.[40]

I have noticed this attitude among my friends who are able to have children but haven't because they say they are not in the right place or with the right person in their lives. I personally feel that if they really want to be mothers, nothing would prevent them from that goal. I have a few friends who went to a sperm bank when they hit their late thirties and are very happy single mothers. One of them, Jenny Laden, had her daughter in New York City then moved to Pennsylvania, where she is the director of environmental art at the Schuylkill Center for Environment Education. I asked Jenny about how she made her decision to be a single mom. She explained,

> At thirty-three I decided to give myself until thirty-six to find the love of my life. During that time I seriously considered the alternative—to have a child on my own. I got curious about what else I might do to have a child if I hadn't found a partner I loved and wanted to commit to by age thirty-six. I also spent that time mourning the loss of things happening like the hetero-normative fantasy I'd unconsciously bought into—of falling in love, getting married and making kids together. But the reality is that my own parents were divorced, my father was gay, and died from AIDS. One of my communities was a world of gay parents and kids, and I met all these amazing parents with their amazing kids and they all were parenting outside that box. And I thought, "Well who am I not to be open to another way to make a family?"[41]

To me, Jenny and other single mothers by choice I encountered were pioneers. I didn't have the courage or determination to do what they did, but they opened my eyes to the fact that women had options. Today, it is still a big leap to do what they did.

However, for many people around the world, having a biological child is not a choice they can make for themselves; their bodies don't cooperate. Infertility affects approximately 10 percent of couples worldwide. In 2012 in China, according to the China Population Association, 12.5 percent of people of childbearing age were diagnosed with infertility, compared with only 3 percent twenty years ago.[42] In Nigeria, although it has a high fertility rate of 5.7, infertility has been on the rise, with 20 percent of cases in gynecology clinics being fertility-related.[43] Nepal, which had its first test-tube baby born in 2005, also shows 20 percent of couples have fertility-related issues.[44] In India, 15 to 20 percent of couples experience infertility.[45] Some of this infertility can be attributed to environmental factors— pesticides, cigarettes, and other pollutants that impact fertility—and some of it to age-related factors.

Around 5 million babies have been born worldwide through IVF since the first was born in 1978 in the United Kingdom. Every year, approximately 1.5 million ART treatments resulting in 350,000 babies occur. The United States and Japan are the most active countries for ART use, but more than a third of the cycles happen in Europe.[46] In many European countries, like Finland, ARTs account for as much as 4 percent of live births.[47] Around 3 percent of babies born in Belgium, Slovenia, Denmark, the Netherlands, and Sweden are conceived through ARTs. The number is also around 3 percent in Australia.[48] In the United States, that number is around 1 percent.[49] In the United Kingdom, where the number is around 2 percent, the number of cycles for women in their forties increased by more than 500 percent over two decades since 1992.[50] Israel is one of the most robust countries for IVF, with 4.1 percent of births resulting from treatment, up from 2.5 percent in 1997; and in just over a decade between 2001 and 2011, the number of IVF cycles per year nearly doubled.[51]

Until recently, Costa Rica was the only country where IVF was banned (it had been legal between 1995 and 2000). In 2012, the Inter-American Court of Human Rights ruled that "by prohibiting IVF, Costa Rica has 'violated the rights to private and family life, to personal integrity . . . to sexual health, to enjoy the benefits of scientific and technological progress, and the principle of non-discrimination.'"[52] The court ordered the ban lifted and also directed that the Costa Rican government compensate those affected by the ban between 2000 and 2012.

According to Dr. Anna Pia Ferraretti, chairperson of the European Society of Human Reproduction and Embryology's IVF Monitoring Consortium, the global demand for ARTs is estimated to be at least 1,500 cycles per million population per year. Many countries in Europe surpass that average, such as Denmark, Belgium, the Czech Republic, Slovenia, Sweden, Finland, and Norway, while other countries show much lower numbers, such as Austria, Germany, Italy, and the United Kingdom.[53]

In the city of Beijing, China, alone, 5,000 babies are born each year through IVF. Zheng Mengzhu, the country's first IVF baby, was born in 1988 to a thirty-nine-year-old mother. She is now twenty-five and working in the gynecology center of Peking University Third Hospital—a touching continuum of giving back to the world that helped create her.[54]

Every year in the United States, about 1.2 million women seek fertility treatment, and about 150,000 cycles of IVF occur (which is just the tip of the iceberg of those that could occur, since many people cannot afford treatment due to poor insurance coverage).[55] During an IVF cycle, ovulation is suppressed, eggs are retrieved and fertilized in the lab, and then embryos are transferred back into the uterus. According to the Centers for Disease Control and Prevention (CDC), the national average is 2,361 ART procedures per 1 million women of reproductive age, with four states (Massachusetts, New York, New Jersey, and Connecticut) and the District of Columbia doubling that average, and three states at one and a half times the average (Maryland, Illinois, and Delaware).[56] Not surprisingly, all these states, except Delaware, have some form of mandated insurance coverage for fertility treatments.

Liza Mundy, in her book on how ARTs are changing the world, *Everything Conceivable*, noted that the pioneering funders who drove the development of ARTs were women. In fact, the first IVF clinic in the United States, the Jones Institute for Reproductive Medicine in Virginia, was seed-funded in the late 1970s by a woman who had a child through a drug regimen devised by Dr. Georgeanna Jones. Also, the IVF project of Dr. Robert Edwards and Dr. Patrick Steptoe—who had delivered that first IVF baby, Louise Brown, in 1978 in the United Kingdom—was partially underwritten by a California woman.[57]

Since then, ARTs have ballooned into a robust business, valued at around $4 billion per year in the United States alone, and around $770 million in the United Kingdom.[58] Many of the companies that make the drugs and medical devices for ARTs can each generate billions of dollars a year in revenue. Pharmaceutical giant Merck increased its fertility drug revenue by 6.1 percent in 2011 to about $936.5 million (Europe accounted for nearly half their sales, with double-digit growth rates in Asia, Africa, and Latin America).[59]

Where you live or seek treatment has a major impact on what you pay and what obstacles you face. As a result, there are geographic differences in terms of the dilemmas inherent to IVF, surrogacy, adoption, egg and sperm donation, and gender selection.

The United States has the highest costs in the world for fertility treatments, largely because of a lack of government and insurance support for underwriting and regulating the costs. Pricing is left to private institutions, and most IVF clinics charge between $10,000 and $20,000 per treatment.[60] Because multiple rounds are often necessary, the price for a single pregnancy can be in excess of $40,000.[61] Mini-IVF can help reduce costs because the procedure requires fewer fertility drugs and results in the retrieval of fewer eggs, but regular IVF is the more frequent choice. According to *Newsweek*, the average cost per IVF treatment in 2010 was around $13,775 in the United States, $8,740 in Canada, $4,012 in Japan, and $3,109 in Belgium.[62] In parts of the Middle East that have robust fertility treatment centers, such as Jordan and the United Arab Emirates, a cycle costs around $4,000. In China, where there is often a waiting list for treatment because of high demand, the average cost for an ART procedure is around $6,000 to $7,000.[63]

Aside from the cost of the IVF cycle alone, the American Society for Reproductive Medicine (ASRM) has reported that medications for IVF can cost between $3,000 and $5,000 on average per fresh cycle in the United States.[64] Using an egg donor can cost an additional $12,000 to $15,000.[65] For those who want a biological child but cannot carry the child themselves, gestational surrogacy can cost from $70,000 up to over six figures.[66] Those who struggle with infertility have to pay a lot more to pursue having a child than those who don't.

Peggy Orenstein movingly captured her journey through fertility treatments in her 2007 book, *Waiting for Daisy*. After a failed donor egg cycle, Orenstein attempted to contact the clinic again, only to be told that she would have to fork out an additional $13,000, beyond the $16,000 she'd already spent, to try another donor cycle. She wrote,

> I felt like the high roller whose new friends disappeared when his stake was gone. The caring brochures, the chummy smiles, the warm affect of the clinic "team" seemed abruptly stripped away, revealing nothing more

than a cold-blooded business. We had wanted so desperately to believe that we had ignored the sales pitch in the compassion, the coercion in the photographs of babies and sunflowers. But I finally got it—these guys may have been doctors, but I was also a consumer. I was undergoing a procedure, but I was also making a deal—and they were making a buck.[67]

Some medical practices do, however, take a humane approach and have stepped up to ease the financial burden. For example, in 2010, Fertility Partnership in St. Louis, Missouri, discounted its pricing to $7,500 for a standard course of treatment.[68] Also in 2010, a clinic in Davis, California, advertised "Pregnancy for $9,800 or your money back."[69] Shady Grove Fertility Center, which has multiple branches in Maryland, Pennsylvania, Virginia, and Washington, DC, also has a money-back guarantee. You pay a higher fee up front, and if you do not have a successful pregnancy after a certain amount of cycles, you get a significant amount of your deposit back.[70]

In the United Kingdom in March 2012, reproductive surgery pioneer Lord Winston accused fertility clinics of "exploitation" when it came to treatment pricing.[71] The National Institute for Health and Clinical Excellence (NICE) guidelines, which have been in place since 2004, state that women who are aged twenty-three to thirty-nine or who have been infertile for at least three years should be covered for up to three cycles of IVF, but the National Infertility Awareness Campaign found that women were being denied treatment based on the stricter policies of Primary Care Trusts, which were allowed to regulate themselves.[72] In a landmark case that made headlines in the United Kingdom at the end of 2012, a couple, referred to as Mr. and Mrs. K in legal documents, sued Health Secretary Jeremy Hunt for age discrimination after they were denied treatment at the NHS Berkshire Primary Care Trust (PCT) because the woman was considered to be too old at thirty-seven.[73]

Israel has the most liberal policies for ARTs. All women up to the age of forty-five can have free and unlimited IVF procedures for up to two live births.[74] As a result, Israelis are the highest per capita users of IVF in the world. Vered Letai-Sever, a thirty-two-year-old who had a son after eight IVF treatments, said to the *New York Times*, "There is something deeply humane about this policy, this idea that people have the right to be parents."[75] In 2012, the health ministry began to consider measures to increase coverage for up to three kids and to consider limiting funds to women over forty-three who tried repeatedly for a first child.[76] Nonetheless, Israel's encouragement of and financial support for women pursuing IVF results in a more benevolent system in which women of varied means can become mothers. In addition, Israel was the first country in the world to legalize surrogate-mother agreements.

Israel also allows posthumous reproduction, which has been officially recognized through guidelines issued in 2003. This allows a dead man's wife or partner to use his sperm as long as he doesn't leave explicit instructions to the contrary. Vardit Ravitsky, an Israeli-born assistant professor in the bioethics programs at the University of Montreal, commented on Israel's position, "Where we are with reproductive technologies is a result of the fact that we have refused to accept infertility as a fact."[77] In a 2011 article in the *Jewish World News*, he spoke of cases where grandparents have attempted to give themselves grandchildren using the sperm of their dead children. Ravitsky said, "I remember really being struck by an elderly father who lost his son in the army who spoke before the committee with tears in his eyes and talked about what it would mean to him to have grandchildren, and the grief he had about the fact that at the time his son died, the technique wasn't there to extract sperm. I remember thinking we should think outside the box here. It's too simple to just say no."[78]

Although other countries might not have the liberal policies of Israel, they have developed their own ways of addressing cost issues. In the United Arab Emirates, about 7,000 couples per year seek IVF treatment and pay out-of-pocket expenses of more than $5,000 per cycle. In 2012, the Emirates Family Network joined together with the Dubai Gynecology and Fertility Centre and the National Bank of Abu Dhabi to provide loans for IVF financing.[79] Meanwhile, in Nigeria, Nordica Fertility Centre—after ten years in business and 1,090 babies born—offered free treatment to twenty-five needy couples in 2012.[80]

Elsewhere, prospective parents are given no financial support. In Poland, where there is no law on IVF but the conservative Law and Justice (PiS) Party has tried to submit bills to ban it, couples have to pay for treatment themselves.[81] In Ireland as well, treatments are available mostly to private patients who pay out-of-pocket. An article in the Irish newspaper the *Herald* reported that Irish couples are increasingly visiting the Czech Republic, where treatment is half the price.[82]

Against the backdrop of wide price fluctuation in fertility treatments, many people seek medical care away from home, with many Americans and Europeans in particular traveling to countries like South Africa, Argentina, and India. Fertility tourism has become a thriving outgrowth of the infertility business. A 2010 study by the European Society of Human Reproduction and Embryology (ESHRE) estimated that the number of cross-border IVF cycles was as high as 24,000 to 30,000 cycles per year.[83]

No country has benefited more from fertility tourism than India, where there are more than 1,000 registered and unregistered fertility clinics across the country. Dr. Anjali Malpani, who runs an infertility clinic in the city of Colaba with her husband, said 60 percent of her clients are from foreign countries. Many of these patients are aged thirty-eight and above and have tried IVF before. Dr. Malpani said, "They insist on us implanting more than three embryos per cycle to improve their chances of pregnancy—a procedure that is banned in many foreign countries." Although fertility clinics in India are unregulated, Dr. Hrishikesh Pai, head of the IVF department at Lilavati Hospital in the major city of Mumbai, argued that fertility tourism makes a lot of sense: "Why shouldn't they come to us? We have the latest equipment and a level of skill unmatched by doctors in any other country. I have an embryoscope, the first in Asia, which I use to observe embryos without exposing them to the laboratory air and select only the healthy ones. I have freezing containers to preserve the embryos for the next treatment cycle. I do around 1,000 embryo implants in a year."[84]

In addition to standard IVF services, surrogacy—which was legalized in India in 2002 in an effort to boost medical tourism—has become an estimated $2.3 billion business, according to an article in *Mother Jones*.[85] However, India's Home Ministry issued a memo in 2012 to Indian missions abroad that "gay couples, single men and women, non-married couples and couples from countries where surrogacy is illegal be prohibited from hiring a commercial surrogate in India."[86] Despite the discriminatory restrictions, an estimated 25,000 couples per year visit India for surrogacy services, resulting in more than 2,000 births in 2011.[87] Akanksha Infertility Clinic, the most successful surrogate childbirth business in the city of Anand, charges about $15,000 to $20,000 for the process, compared with $50,000 to $100,000 in the United States. The surrogates themselves make between $5,000 and $6,000. This practice has attracted much criticism, including from a professor in the city of Chandigarh, who told Al Jazeera, "Earlier, men and women were made bonded laborers but now even wombs are being made to do bonded labor . . . the way women are dragged into this profession" is exploitative.[88] Despite a rapidly growing middle class, India is still beset by social and economic conditions that are obstacles to women's advancement. India has been rated the worst country for women among all of the G-20 countries (which represent the major economies of the world). In this climate, women desperate to make money can be vulnerable to being lured into surrogacy.

Instead of or after exhausting options for fertility treatments and surrogacy, some decide on adoption as their route to parenthood. However, adoption services can also be expensive, costing up to $50,000 or more for American parents wishing to adopt from other countries. In addition, as with cross-border surrogacy, international adoption can be fraught with ethical and political issues. The Hague Adoption Convention on the Protection of Children and Cooperation in Respect of Inter-Country Adoption was signed by the United States in 1994 and entered into force in April 2008.[89] Seventy-five countries are parties to the convention, which calls for a central authority to regulate adoptions within a country and aims to prevent the abduction and sale of children, but numerous disturbing developments have nonetheless arisen from the exchange of children across borders. For instance, China is a party to the convention, and as the *New York Times* reported in 2011, according to the State Department, between 1999 and 2010, 64,043 Chinese children were adopted by parents in the United States—more than any other country. However, many of those children might have been adopted illegally, even kidnapped to be sold.[90]

Another popular point-of-adoption for Americans is Russia, which is not a party to the Hague Adoption Convention. But Russia became off-limits in December 2012 when President Vladimir Putin banned the adoption of Russian children by Americans. Prior to the ban, Americans had adopted more than 60,000 children from Russia since 1991, when the Soviet Union collapsed. But there had been public outrage over a few cases of Americans abusing their adopted kids, and Putin's action was seen as retaliation for US sanctions against Russian officials suspected of human rights abuses.[91] After the ban, about 200 to 250 parents already in the adoption process were left in limbo.[92] Putin later compromised and grand-fathered in the adoptions already approved by the courts, but that didn't help the people who hadn't gotten final approval.

The purchasing of eggs internationally, like surrogacy and adoption, has become another outgrowth of the global infertility industry, especially as egg-freezing technologies improve. From the Nordica Fertility Centre in Nigeria to the Sher Institute in America, egg freezing has been on the rise around the world as an insurance policy against infertility. In the United States, where egg freezing is considered elective (not medically necessary), the cost can be upward of $15,000 for a cycle that retrieves ten to fifteen eggs. A 2012 article in the *New York Times* explored how potential grandparents are footing the bills for their children to freeze their eggs. One doctor said that about three-quarters of his one hundred recent egg-freezing patients had parents who paid all or part of the bill.[93] Frozen Egg Bank in California, where the cost is typically $9,257 excluding egg storage and fertility drugs, has offered a holiday special price of $4,900.[94]

For cancer patients seeking to preserve their fertility (as opposed to those who are freezing for nonmedical reasons), there are many ways to find financial support. For example, the organization Fertile Action, which collaborates with Mindy Berkson, the Chicago-based infertility consultant, has a network of egg-freezing doctors in twelve states who offer discounts for cancer patients.[95] Fertile Action also offers cash grants, which cancer patients can apply for online. In order to be considered, people have to submit a letter to their future child along with other supporting materials.[96] The Sher Institute, with locations around the country including Dallas, Las Vegas, and St. Louis, freezes the eggs of cancer patients for free.[97]

In Canada, clinics charge between $3,500 and $5,850 for egg freezing, excluding the cost of drugs.[98] In the United Kingdom, the cost at London clinics is typically between $6,000 and $8,000.[99] Although only twelve babies have been born from frozen eggs in a decade in the United Kingdom, the number of women who freeze their eggs has grown by five times in that same period. In Israel, egg freezing is not only covered by the government but is also considered to be preventive medicine. Rabbis have been known to recommend that any single woman over age thirty-two should freeze her eggs.[100]

There is also a growing market in frozen donor eggs, which can cost thousands of dollars less than fresh ones. For example, coordinating with a donor for a fresh egg can cost between $25,000 and $38,000 per cycle and can require three to twelve months of coordination, as opposed to $18,000 for a frozen egg cycle completed in as little as one to two months using eggs from companies such as Donor Egg Bank USA. According to a 2012 CNN report, "In the not-too-distant future, nearly all donor eggs will be bought frozen online instead of fresh locally."[101]

Egg and sperm donation are bustling businesses, and the United States is the largest exporter of human sperm, with tens of thousands of vials going to more than sixty countries. A 2012 article in *Time* noted a few trends: fair-haired donors are preferred, even in South America, Africa, and Asia, while Israel requires that the imported sperm not be Jewish.[102] (This latter requirement is in place because by prohibiting a Jewish sperm donor, the government is lowering the likelihood of certain genetic issues that can result from combining the genetic material of two Jewish people. Tay-Sachs disease, for instance, a rare autosomal recessive genetic disorder, is a serious threat among Orthodox Jews who tend to partner with others within their community.)[103]

In the United States, a college-age man can make as much as $12,000 per year for twice-weekly sperm donations. There have been numerous articles about the lack of regulation of the sperm bank industry. As Debora L. Spar, president of Barnard University and author of *The Baby Business: How Money, Science, and Politics Drive the Commerce of Conception*, told the *New York Times*, "We have more rules that go into place when you buy a used car than when you buy sperm."[104] One woman discovered that her child was one of 150 children born from the same donor's sperm.[105]

With regard to egg donation, the ASRM recommends that women donating an egg receive up to $5,000 in compensation, and anything over $10,000 is inappropriate. However, without direct oversight, women with desirable characteristics (like being an athletic Harvard grad) could potentially earn more. Abroad, egg-donation services can cost anywhere from a few hundred dollars to $10,000. In the United Kingdom, the Human Tissue Act prohibits the sale of eggs and sperm per se, but the donor is paid for her labor. For example, in the United Kingdom, the fee is currently capped at about $390, but the agency in charge of that cap is pushing to raise it to closer to $1,200 in order to increase the number of donations.[106] In Spain, the fee is $1,350 (donors are anonymous and unpaid but get "travel expenses" of about €1,000).[107]

Donation companies can act like brokerages, specializing in eggs from countries where the costs and regulations are more amenable. Dr. Ilya Barr, a fertility specialist from Israel, established GlobalART in the late 1990s in Romania to work with egg donors there to obtain eggs for clinics in various countries. Some clinics have established ties with foreign clinics in countries like Cyprus and Ukraine, where it's also easier and cheaper to get eggs.

Gender selection is another complicated world within the fertility industry—with an estimated 4,000 to 6,000 procedures done per year. According to *Slate*, the service, which is carried out during preimplantation genetic diagnosis (PGD) at a cost of about $18,000, brings in revenues of at least $100 million a year.[108] PGD was designed in the early 1990s to screen for birth defects and diseases. The United States is one of the few countries to allow it to be used for gender selection. Other countries such as Canada, the United Kingdom, and Australia made it illegal to use gender selection for nonmedical reasons. One Australian medical tourism company, Global Health Travel, said it sent 106 couples for "family balancing," or gender selection, services to a Thai clinic in 2012, up from 72 couples in 2011. These couples paid at least $15,000 for the service.[109]

In some countries, gender selection can be used to disastrous results. There are 163 million infant girls "missing" from the world's population due to sex-selective abortions in the last thirty years, and up to 12 million of those girls have been aborted in India.[110] In Uttar Pradesh, India's most populous state with almost 200 million people, men outnumber women by nearly 10 million. Mohammad Asif, director of program implementation with Plan India (an NGO dedicated to improving the lives of underprivileged children), said that he expected this imbalance to end soon: "Before, women's work was either at home or on the farm. With globalization, girls are now picking up jobs in banking, manufacturing and hi-tech. This is creating a lot of buzz in the family to start considering girls."[111] In China, another country reputed to have an alarming number of sex-selective abortions, the ratio of men to women is 121 to 100. Gender selection is an ethical problem that needs more international oversight—without it, this procedure is inherently ripe for transforming into eugenics run amok.

The eugenics debate has been applied to various aspects of the ART industry, even by those within it. At a lecture for the Society for Reproduction and Fertility (SRF) in Edinburgh, Scotland, Lord Winston cautioned, "We may find that people will want to modify their children, enhance their intelligence, their strength and their beauty and all the other so-called desirable characteristics. That is going to become an increasing risk as a market. That will be a form of eugenics which will actually have all sorts of serious implications for developed societies."[112]

Andrew Solomon, in his book *Far From the Tree*, about family and identity, wrote of a case where a lesbian couple electively had a deaf baby by getting a fifth-generation deaf friend to donate sperm. Solomon pointed out that no one would be up in arms about a straight deaf couple naturally having children who would most likely be deaf, and he had a fascinating take on how this case relates to the general debate over trait selection:

> Designer babies aren't going anywhere; they will undoubtedly become increasingly common as technology advances. The very phrase *designer babies* is pejorative, but not so long ago *test-tube babies* was used with disdain, before IVF became standard operating procedure for an aging middle class. In 2006, nearly half the PGD clinics surveyed by the Genetics and Public Policy Center at John Hopkins University offered a gender selection service. . . . The Fertility Institutes in Los Angeles declared that they were planning to help couples select for gender, hair color, and eye color, though such a salvo ensued that they suspended the program. Such choices are inevitably the future. How different are they from standard protocols for sperm and egg donors, which screen donors for undesirable hereditary traits and provide information on physical attractiveness, coloring, height, weight, and college entrance scores? Most people are attracted to others with desirable traits; our very impulse toward sexual congress is a subjective screening process.[113]

*   *   *

In the following section, I explore the issue of governmental support in different countries for fertility treatments and present some interesting methods people have developed to take funding into their own hands.

Around the world, while some parents struggle to have children, other parents are abandoning the ones they do have. A large number of people have found themselves in a situation where they can't afford to raise children. In a heartbreaking indication of the impact of the economic crisis, a kindergarten teacher in Athens, Greece, found a note with one of her students a few weeks before Christmas that said, "I will not be coming to pick up Anna today because I cannot afford to look after her. Please take good care of her. Sorry. Her mother."[114] In addition, babies left at churches and other centers hit all-time highs in 2011 in countries like Greece (1,200) and Italy (750). Italy, despite being Europe's third-largest economy, has the highest percentage of child poverty of all twenty-five European countries.[115] Eleven countries (Austria, Belgium, the Czech Republic, Germany, Hungary, Italy, Latvia, Lithuania, Poland, Portugal, and Slovakia) out of twenty-seven in the European Union permit baby hatches for people to leave their children. (A baby hatch can be a door or flap, usually found in a hospital or social center, with a bed and sensor that sends an alert when a baby has been left inside.) Some countries give the parents ninety days to change their minds and get their baby back.[116]

More government support for medical expenses is needed across the board. In a study of fertility policies of twenty-three countries in Europe from 2007 on, Dr. Mark Connolly of the University of Groningen in the Netherlands found that the highest ratings for reimbursement were in Belgium, France, and Slovenia. These as well as Italy, Montenegro, and Portugal all had higher levels of funding than the United Kingdom, which was third from the bottom—above Russia and Ireland—in terms of reimbursement.

Despite being the birthplace of IVF, the United Kingdom lags far behind some of these countries in terms of cycles per year per million people. For example, in Belgium, the number is over 2,500 compared with over 800 in the United Kingdom.[117] When Dr. Connolly spoke in 2012 at the annual conference of ESHRE in Istanbul, he said British clinics were "feeble" in providing treatment.[118] Although 13,000 babies are born in the United Kingdom every year through IVF and ICSI, that number could be three times higher if not for restrictive public health–funding policies.

The fertility policy study cited a 2009 review, which showed that although the United States had the largest number of ART cycles overall, the United States—like the United Kingdom—had among the lowest utilization rates of ART treatment for a developed country. At the time, there were 373 non-donor cycles (in which the couple's own egg and sperm were used) per year per million people compared with 1,574 in Australia and 1,465 in Scandinavia.

In the United States some form of insurance coverage for fertility treatments is mandated in only fifteen states: Arkansas, California, Connecticut, Hawaii, Illinois, Louisiana, Maryland, Massachusetts, Montana, New

Jersey, New York, Ohio, Rhode Island, Texas, and West Virginia. However, the extent of that coverage varies from state to state. For example, some states (like Arkansas) require two years of an inability to conceive, and others (like Massachusetts) require one year; some (like Rhode Island and Connecticut) cap coverage at age forty, and others (like New York) at age forty-four. And some states (like Texas) require that the sperm used be only from the patient's spouse.[119]

Adding to the quagmire is the fact that women tend to pay more for health insurance than men. Only fourteen states, such as California, New Jersey, and New York, have made attempts to ban or limit gender rating, and according to a report from the National Women's Law Center, in states that have not banned it, more than 90 percent of the bestselling health plans charge women about 31 percent more than men of the same age. According to an article covering the report in the *New York Times*, "Insurers said they charged women more than men because claims showed that women ages nineteen to fifty-five tended to use more health care services. They are more likely to visit doctors, to get regular checkups, to take prescription drugs and to have certain chronic illnesses."[120]

Some estimates, such as those presented in the September 2007 issue of *Fertility and Sterility*, assert that adding IVF coverage would increase insurance premiums by as little as $10 to $120 per year.[121] Despite the fact that a 2006 survey of 900 companies by Mercer Consulting (a human resources and benefits consulting firm) found that over 90 percent had no increase in healthcare costs when they provided infertility coverage, only 20 percent covered IVF, and about 37 percent covered drug therapy for infertility.[122]

A 2010 *SELF* magazine story on infertility claimed that "part of the problem is that the insurance industry considers infertility akin to cosmetic surgery; having a child is deemed by many insurers to be something men and women would like, but it's not necessary for their health."[123] Also, without widespread coverage, infertility disproportionately affects those with less financial resources. As science writer Liza Mundy has explained, "The poor are more likely to be affected by infertility because they are less likely to have been able to deal with illnesses and underlying conditions that can result in it and because they aren't able to afford the treatments to address it."[124]

Moreover, poor coverage results in poorer health outcomes. A study published in the *New England Journal of Medicine* in 2002 found that the percentage of high-order pregnancies (those with three or more fetuses) was greater in states without mandatory coverage, and multiples are higher risk.[125] In 2011, Dr. Pasquale Patrizio of the Yale Fertility Center also conducted a study, which confirmed this finding.[126] Without coverage, patients are more likely to transfer more embryos in one cycle with the hope that this will increase their chances of having at least one of them succeed. They want to avoid paying for multiple cycles.

In his foreword for the book *Budgeting for Infertility*, the late Dr. Sam Thatcher, who was based at the Center for Applied Reproductive Science in Johnson City, Tennessee, denounced the financial obstacles caused by uneven insurance coverage for fertility treatments. He wrote, "Denying a pregnancy to a patient with Polycystic Ovary Syndrome (PCOS) and ovulatory infertility is as unjust as denying insulin to a diabetic. To not assist fertilization for a man with a low sperm count is as wrong as not intervening in a cardiac arrest."[127] However, doctors themselves, as the book pointed out, are split on the insurance issue. For example, Dr. Thatcher said, "If physicians really care about patients, then he or she also really cares about the financial well-being of patients as a stressor." But reproductive endocrinologist Mark Perloe said, "Mandated coverage would simply mean that we would do a greater volume of IVF, but we would have to limit the relationships we have with patients because we have to pay the bills."[128] (I find Dr. Perloe's opinion offensive that if insurance coverage for people's medical treatment results in more people seeking medical treatment, he would have to limit his relationships with his patients. I understand that a private medical practice is a business. My father had one, a psychiatry practice. But he made sure that alongside his paying patients, he served those who needed his help but couldn't pay for it themselves. He especially liked working with the immigrant refugee community in Long Beach, California, where we lived.)

Members of Congress have recognized the inequalities in access to fertility treatments and have stepped up to remedy them. Senator Kirsten Gillibrand (D-NY) introduced the Family Act of 2011 to the Senate in May 2011, and Representative John Lewis (D-GA) introduced it to the House of Representatives in November 2011. The act would provide for a maximum lifetime tax credit of $13,360 to families who must use IVF, similar to the $13,000 tax credit offered to those who adopt.[129] It would be available to "taxpayers with an adjusted gross income of less than $182,500 and phases out for those whose incomes reach $222,520." Representative Lewis's home state of Georgia does not have mandated coverage but is where he said almost 200,000 people were dealing with diagnosed infertility. Representative Lewis argued, "Without this credit, access to all the advances of modern medicine and the ability to bear children . . . becomes, for average Americans, a luxury defined by the size of their wallets or the digits in their zip code."[130] Unfortunately, the act died in the 112th Congress and will have to be reintroduced.

Increased coverage and government support through a tax credit are necessary for a better reproductive future in this country. Until measures like the Family Act become law, many people throughout most of America will not be able to afford having children. One friend told me about a couple she knows who maxed out their credit cards for multiple rounds of IVF—which sadly didn't prove successful. Their monthly bill became a horrific reminder of what they hadn't achieved. Nowadays, credit card debt, along with home equity loans, which have often paid for fertility treatments, are not as easily used because of the poor economy. Instead, fertility-focused lenders have emerged to fill the gap. The *Wall Street Journal* reported that fertility-related loans totaled as much as $4 billion in 2012 alone. According to Doug Weiss, senior vice president of IntegraMed America, Inc., a fertility clinic operator based in Purchase, New York, fertility finance is "pretty much a recession-proof business, since the biological clock doesn't stop."[131] Also, interest rates can run as high as 22 percent (compared to the average credit card rate of around 17 percent).

Dr. Nancy Snyderman of the *Today* show researched dozens of fertility-focused lenders and found that many of them enjoy a robust business. As one lender, Jules Segal of Capex MD, said, "At present we're funding about a million dollars of loans a month. We're on a very steep growth curve and we're looking to fund about $15 million in loans in 2012."[132] Snyderman also discovered that some go so far as to give doctors "kickbacks or a stake in the company in exchange for sending customers their way."[133] Covering Snyderman's report for *Slate*, Cassie Murdoch wrote, "In theory, they're just like any other loan company—except that they're dealing with a population of borrowers who are often far more emotionally vulnerable than your average home buyer, and many of these lenders seem totally comfortable taking advantage of that fact."[134]

As mentioned earlier in this chapter, in 2012, the National Bank of

Abu Dhabi in the United Arab Emirates partnered with the Emirates Family Network to provide the financial resources to make treatment feasible. The bank offered loans to couples pursuing IVF, while the network counseled them on the health and emotional issues. The interest rates were far more amenable than those found in the United States: 6.49 percent—but the loans had to be repaid within a year.[135]

Some clinics have started to hold contests for fertility treatments. In this way, they boost their publicity while seeming to provide a service to needy families. In the United Kingdom, South East Fertility Clinic in Tunbridge Wells offered five couples the chance to win £1,000 off IVF treatment and a free consultation.[136] In the United States, during National Infertility Awareness Week 2012, Long Island IVF launched an annual "Extreme Family-Building Makeover" contest, through which the winner would receive a MicroIVF cycle.[137] Contestants were asked to submit "the most emotional or entertaining essays and homemade amateur video." The announcement said, "Make us laugh with you or cry with you. Tell your story straight from the heart."[138]

An October 20, 2012, article in the *New York Times* pointed out that ethicists are concerned about these giveaways and how they trivialize the process. Authorities in the United Kingdom and Australia have condemned them and even proposed banning them, but others feel that it opens up the playing field to those who might not be able to afford IVF. The ASRM has said it has "no problem with it." In a June 20, 2012, article in *Time* magazine, Samantha Pfeifer, chair of the ASRM's practice committee, said, "It's a publicity maneuver. What makes it weird is that you're creating a life, and that puts it into a different category. But if you think of it as a medical procedure you have to pay cash for, you could think of it as giving away a free car. We need a car, but we can't afford it—let's go for it."[139]

Those who don't have the chance of winning an IVF prize can fundraise on their own, especially through social media and online platforms. For example, Giveforward.com is a website for medical-expense fundraising. It takes 7 percent of your donations, which are not tax-deductible.[140] Brandi and Shelton Koskie from Kansas set up a website, BabyOrBust. com, in 2006 and raised $20,000 in two years. They went on to have a daughter, Paisley, through IVF.[141] After trying for three years and spending about $40,000 on IVF with donor eggs, Todd and Ula Nelkins from Texas planned to auction off their rare football card (worth up to $20,000) in

2012 for their IVF treatments.[142] As Todd told the *Washington Post*, "I would love to keep the card, but I would rather have a kid. It's a wonderful card. You daydream that maybe 30, 40 years from now, our son or daughter will find out where the card is and what happened to it."[143]

Sometimes the publicity about fertility fundraising can be positive; it can create a sense of community around the issue. On a Saturday in June 2012, people gathered in Illinois for the first annual Race for the Family "to raise funds for families undergoing infertility treatment or pursuing domestic adoption."[144] When Liza Mundy wrote in the *Washington Post* about people who couldn't afford fertility treatments, some readers sent in checks to support specific people mentioned in the article.[145]

With the increasing costs of raising a child, whether to have one at all has become an overwhelmingly economic issue. When you factor in infertility rates, the price tag is even harder to surmount. There are people working to change the paradigm. For example, Dr. William Ombelet, a professor of obstetrics and gynecology at the Institute of Fertility Technology in Genk, Belgium, has been conducting studies of an IVF method that would cost only $300 by using less expensive materials (like keeping the embryos alive with a culture made of citric acid mixed with sodium bicarbonate). As of this writing, twelve babies have been born with this cheaper treatment.[146] But for now, as I have attempted to show, the infertility industry is a business in which the consumer is vulnerable. The global demand for IVF and other ARTs has exploded over the past few decades. Fertility tourism is booming and has fostered a brave new world of practices and technologies, but against this backdrop, a dark side of exploitation has emerged.

Because of the increasing globalization of the infertility industry, government and medical institutions must join together to increase intercountry research and oversight. In the same way that there is a Hague Adoption Convention with seventy-five countries as parties, there could be a Global Convention on ARTs. Policies on pricing and practice in every country could be more deeply scrutinized while preserving the noble aim of having children accessible to and safe for all.

CHAPTER 9
FRIENDS WITH KIDS AND FRIENDS WITHOUT

I started this book with the idea that every woman has a story to tell about miscarriage or infertility, her own or her friend's. Every woman also has a story to tell about motherhood—about whether she has kids or whether she doesn't, and whether having kids was by choice or out of her hands. My friends and women I meet seem to fit into categories: mothers, want-to-be-mothers, never-want-to-be-mothers, will-be-mothers, never-will-be-mothers, almost-were-mothers, and more.

Once I was at a party where there were a couple of women I had known for more than twenty-five years. One had given up her career as a lawyer to raise two kids. Another also had two kids but continued to work as a lawyer at one of the top firms in the United States. The one who had stopped working talked about how she enjoyed being able to focus on tasks like overseeing the renovations of her house. The other woman said that her husband's flexible hours as a professor made it possible for her to focus more on her job because her husband was such an active parent. But she said that she often felt the tug-of-war between career and motherhood, and that sometimes she felt like she failed at both. As I listened to their revelations, I confess I had to check my inner judgment of the woman who wasn't working. Why couldn't she work and be a mom, too? How does she hold her own against her husband if she's dependent on him to pay the bills? I had to remind myself that happiness is important and that, as another friend put it, "one-size-fits-all" does not apply to women's choices about these matters.

Another night, I was having dinner at Hecho en Dumbo, a Mexican restaurant on the Bowery in Manhattan, with two of my closest friends. They're a few years older than me, both in their forties, and both have toddlers a few months apart. Within a few minutes, one of them started talking about something cute her kid did recently, and the other joined in with something cute that *her* kid did recently, and soon they were talking only to each other about their kids, and I was tuning out. I had nothing to contribute to the conversation, and, to be honest, I wasn't interested in it. Whenever I'm alone with one of them, it doesn't feel so bad because then we are sharing directly with each other, but the dynamic is different when there are three of us and I am the only one not having the same life experiences.

A few days after that dinner, I saw Maureen Angelos, a cofounder of the Five Lesbian Brothers theater company. Maureen, or "Moe," as her friends call her, is in her fifties, doesn't have kids, and earns a living as a scenic painter in addition to her work in theater. I asked her how she felt around groups of women when they talk only about their kids. Moe said, "Many of the women I work with are straight and married and have kids and they do talk about them a lot. I ask after the kids and do my best to engage in the conversations, but there comes the realization that it is not how my life is oriented. So I get kind of quiet, I guess. I feel anything from on the margin of the discussion to bored to exasperated when it seems it is all they can sometimes talk about."[1] Moe said she always loved kids, but when she came out at the age of twenty-two, becoming a parent was not really a natural inclination for a lesbian. Most of her gay friends with kids actually had them before coming out—when they were in straight relationships.

Now, of course, the winds have changed with regard to queer parenting. Many are having kids through surrogates, sperm donors, and adoption. But in Moe's generation, this trend had not yet emerged.

For me, as time goes by and the possibility that I might not have my own biological child increases, I grow more aware of the differences between various categories of friends: basically, those who have children and those who don't. It's hard for those with kids not to talk about them a lot, and it's hard for me to hang out with them and not be able to contribute to the "child" conversation. When I am with women around my age who don't have children, I am also sometimes preoccupied, wondering what sacrifices and disappointments they might not be acknowledging about being childless.

To help me explore these ideas, I developed a questionnaire and distributed it to thirty friends of various ages and life stages. In addition, I asked them to forward my questions to their own friends. The quotes used in this chapter are excerpted from their responses and in-person conversations. I also collected articles and studies to contextualize my observations within the larger framework of women's choices about motherhood and the effect of those choices on peer dynamics. Globally, women are judged by where they are in the motherhood spectrum, yet more women are choosing to be childfree.

One night at a group dinner, I was seated next to a thirty-six-year-old woman who ran a think tank in Canada and whom I was meeting for the first time. I told her I was working on a book about motherhood and feminism, and she started to tell me her story. In her twenties, when she had to choose whether to work on a political campaign or to focus on her personal life, she decided that she was not going to have a family. I revealed to her that I hadn't wanted to have a family until I was in my late thirties, when I met the man I married. She said that she had been seeing someone for eighteen months and that the two of them hadn't talked about having kids, but she did have a friend who was forty-five years old and her friend told her recently that she just started to feel the ache for the children she didn't have.

For some women, the aspiration to be a mother is crystal-clear to them from a young age. For example, Gabriela Poma Traynor, a forty-three-year-old based in Cambridge, Massachusetts, and originally from El Salvador, has three kids between the ages of eight and thirteen. She told me, "I always assumed I would have kids because that is what women did. I come from a very traditional Latin background in that sense, and even though I was treated as a peer by the men in my family (I had an American education after all), at one point they sat me down and told me I had to settle down, get married and have kids!" But she added that her choice was not immediately clear: "I mainly felt confused about having or not having kids. One day it would be: I want six kids! Another day, I'd think: there is no way I'm having kids, I won't ever be free."[2] Ultimately, she got pregnant while she was in graduate school at Stanford University and ended up not pursuing her doctorate degree, although she still hopes to return to academia.

Some friends, especially those who don't have the financial resources to hire domestic help, spoke about the disruption caused by their kids, but it was hard to get them to speak on the record about their negative impressions. In his book about family and identity, *Far from the Tree*, Andrew Solomon described this resistance: "Parents willing to be interviewed are a self-selecting group; those who are bitter are less likely to tell their stories than those who have found value in their experience and want to help others in similar circumstances to do the same. No one loves without reservation, however, and everyone would be better off if we could destigmatize parental ambivalence."[3]

Although these friends of mine love being moms and wouldn't exchange having children for anything, they wish there had been another path, one that hadn't forced them to put aside their personal ambitions. They hoped that once their kids were old enough, they would be able to do more for themselves—one wanted to open a design store, another wanted to complete an advanced degree, etc.—but now they worry that they have taken too much time out to get back into the game. As Solomon wrote about a woman named Bunny Harvey who "intended to be a painter who had a child and ended up as a mother who also paints," "it's a classic feminist bind: she could have had a richer career if she hadn't been a mother, and might have been a better mother if she hadn't had a career."[4]

In a controversial 2010 piece for *New York* magazine titled "All Joy and No Fun: Why Parents Hate Parenting," contributor Jennifer Senior cited many reports of parents, especially mothers, who love their kids but hate their lives. As she explained, "A few generations ago, people weren't stopping to contemplate whether having a child would make them happy. Having children was simply what you did. And we are lucky, today, to have choices about these matters." Of the numerous studies on the subject, she said the one most often cited is from 2004 by Daniel Kahneman, the Nobel Prize–winning behavioral economist. He had surveyed 909 working Texas women and "found that childcare ranked sixteenth in pleasurability out of nineteen activities."[5]

For some of my friends, having a child was either never a goal or stopped being one at a certain point. Mary Kaye Schilling, a journalist and editor in her fifties, had had a miscarriage when she was in her thirties and then decided that she didn't want to have kids.[6] Elaine Chen, a Manhattan-based forty-five-year-old marketing executive, said, "I always thought I would have kids because it never seemed to be an option not to have them. Growing up in the suburbs in the 1970s to 1980s, I met very few adults who did not have children." As she got older, her perspective shifted. "In today's society if you have children you are expected to put them first and sacrifice a lot of your own ambitions and identity. I spent a lot of time in my thirties thinking about whether having children was what I wanted and decided that I would be fine without them; when I see how tired and stressed many of the mothers I know are, I feel very comfortable with the decision I made."[7] Jenny Davidson, a forty-two-year-old author and tenured professor at Columbia, said, "I never did! I looked at my mother and saw a life of self-sacrifice and domestic drudgery. I wanted nothing to do with either!" When Jenny was between the ages of ten and thirteen, she babysat but was "very glad" once she "was old enough to work as a temp in an office instead."[8]

In her book *How to Be a Woman*, Caitlin Moran wrote that "the inference of the word 'childless' is negative: one of lack, and loss. . . . We make women feel that their narrative has ground to a halt in their thirties if they don't 'finish things' properly and have children."[9] However, I found among my childless friends that many of them had chosen that path and were happy, even relieved to have avoided motherhood. A 2010 Pew Research Center study on childlessness showed that in 2008 there were equal numbers of women aged forty to forty-four who were childless by choice (6 percent) versus unable to have them. Commenting on the study, Amy Pienta, a researcher at the University of Michigan, told the *Huffington Post*, "Childless women are as happy as women who had children at typical ages. They are not any more depressed; their psychological well-being is just as high."[10]

Katie Gard, a freelance writer and photographer, explained in a March 2013 piece for the *Huffington Post* that she has embraced a woman's right to choose by being "the woman who has the guilt-free ability to join her co-workers for a cocktail after a rough day. The woman who has time to work out in the morning. The woman who can cook an amazing, stress-free meal and enjoy eating it with her significant other at 8:00 p.m." Despite having been married for seven years, Gard did not feel the urge to bear children. But, she wrote, "when it comes to the pressures society—especially other women—especially my *mother*—places on me to get pregnant, sometimes it seems like not getting pregnant during wedlock is far worse than getting pregnant outside of wedlock."[11]

In some studies, childless women are actually depicted as happier than mothers. For example, the *Wall Street Journal* presented research showing that "if you take two people who are identical in every way except for childbearing status, the parent will be on average about six percentage points less likely to be 'very happy' than the nonparent."[12] According to a 1988 General Social Survey, 39 percent of interviewees didn't think people without children "lead empty lives"; by 2002, that figure had grown to 59 percent.[13]

Furthermore, not having kids of your own doesn't mean you don't have kids in your life. After the childlessness study was released, Pew Research Center analyst D'Vera Cohn commented on National Public Radio, "You can be taking care of nieces and nephews in informal adoptive situations or just making sure you're looking out for them."[14] Kate Valk, a theater artist in her fifties who chose not to have kids but is a godmother, said, "The role of 'auntie' is always welcome in any household."[15] Also, there are many paths to being a caregiver. Mary Kaye explained that she is "as much of a nurturer as any parents" she knows, "and there are ample opportunities to do that in your life: co-workers, friends, family, lovers. You don't have to have a child to do that."[16]

Supreme Court Justice Sonia Sotomayor has spoken publicly about her regret that she didn't bear or adopt children. But, as she described in her memoir, *My Beloved World*, she has many kids around her because she has more godchildren than anyone she knows.[17] In 2009, around the time she was confirmed for the Supreme Court, CNN ran a story in pictures about her life. One of those pictures depicted her hugging her niece, with a caption that read, "Sotomayor divorced in 1983 and has no children of her own but enjoys the company of her nieces and nephews and godchildren."[18]

As I engaged more with my friends about their choices regarding motherhood, I was amazed to learn how many of them who don't have kids did at one point face the possibility of becoming a mother. I had assumed that some of these women chose not to have children because they were so career-minded—like a friend who is a high-powered television executive and another one who is a well-traveled journalist. But I discovered, through the questionnaire or conversations, that they had actually tried to have a child, and it was only after it didn't work out—because of a miscarriage or failed IVF—that they changed course.

Among these friends, there was great variety in their current positions toward kids. Some felt good about avoiding motherhood, like Mary Kaye, who told me, "I was relieved after I had the miscarriage. I had never wanted children (I had one abortion before that), and kind of got seduced into it by my boyfriend at the time. And I've never regretted not having children since. I'm not one of those people who love every baby they see."[19]

Other friends, however, continued to consider motherhood a possibility, even though they couldn't have their own biological child. Natalie Dean, a forty-year-old teacher, made several attempts to have a child and is now pursuing adoption. She said, "As a child I always imagined I would have children. I also begged my parents to have a younger sibling for me (they never did). I wanted to take care of and play with kids both my own age and much younger than me. I started babysitting neighborhood kids at the age of nine."[20]

Some friends described adoption as *the* way they would like to become mothers. For instance, Jennie Boddy, a forty-eight-year-old publicist, often thinks about it. She said, "My sister is autistic, and I thought it would be wonderful to adopt a special needs kid, perhaps a Down syndrome kid that needs a home. I just adore those kids."[21] Moe Angelos explained, "I have never felt the biological pull to produce offspring. I always thought if I was ever with a partner who really really wanted kids, we could adopt, because of course there are many children in this world already."[22]

Like Natalie, I am sad about not having had a child. There is no silver lining yet, although we know that we can still be mothers one day, most likely through adoption. But where we are now is that we've gone through years of trying, and it feels unfair that we don't have kids while others who also delayed motherhood do. Natalie happens to be my neighbor in Cambridge. Not only do we share this experience; we live on either side of the same wall.

I don't resent my friends who've "succeeded" at motherhood, but my childlessness distinguishes me from them. In an essay for the UK *Daily Mail*, Samantha Brick, a journalist and producer who had been trying to have a baby for five years since the age of thirty-seven, wrote, "Fertility envy has severed decades-old friendships. Among women of a child-bearing age, it is the biggest divider."[23] It can be as uncomfortable for the women with kids as for the women without. Laura Dawn, a forty-three-year-old former creative and cultural director of MoveOn.org, who had a miscarriage before a successful pregnancy, said, "I have friends who have had multiple miscarriages, and I got pregnant very easily, so I feel a slight sense of guilt over that as well."[24]

For many women, having a child is associated with feelings of fulfill-ment. Mary Kaye depicted it as a cultural issue: "I do think America is about achievement, and if a woman perceives her inability to become pregnant as a failure, she might feel ashamed about it."[25] Amy Richards, the feminist author and mother of two boys, told me, "We wrongly attri-bute so much value to children in terms of giving women an identity."[26] Laura said that before she had a baby, "If I had a quarter for every woman that had cornered me and asked a thousand, none-of-her-business ques-tions about why I hadn't had kids yet. . . ."[27]

Women of my generation delayed motherhood because it seemed like the logical and even prescribed thing to do. We looked at our mothers and our mothers' friends and thought they had made too many sacrifices with regard to their personal ambitions. Many of my friends expressed that they delayed motherhood because it seemed an obstacle to self-fulfillment or enjoyment. Natalie said, "As a child who grew up in the seventies there were many moms who were younger than my mom, and most of them stayed at home or worked part-time at jobs that didn't earn them much money. Under these circumstances, how do women survive if their marriage fails?"[28]

She added that many women of our generation in particular spent at least ten years "working very hard *not* to get pregnant" and then didn't think it would take longer than six months to make a baby. Natalie's words resonated strongly for me. Many of us matured earlier than women of previous generations did, and we had sex for many years before wanting to have kids. We associated sex with what was for us, at the time, the *freedom* to have sex. It took us longer to associate it with childbearing.

The word "motherhood" arouses conflicting emotions. Betty Friedan made this case in *The Feminine Mystique* in the early 1960s, a time during which 60 percent of women entering college didn't graduate. She wrote, "Despite the fact that many of these women had achieved the domestic life they'd wished for—a home in the suburbs complete with modern appli-ances, children, and a bread-winning husband—they were miserable. It was a 'silent problem.'"[29]

The concepts of motherhood and domesticity continue to push buttons today. Around the 2012 Olympics, Procter & Gamble, the multinational manufacturer, launched an ad campaign showing different moms cheering on their Olympic-hopeful children. The slogan was "The hardest job in the world is the best job in the world. Thank you, Mom. P&G—Proud Sponsor of Moms." Reacting to the ad, *Salon* staff writer Mary Elizabeth Williams said it was "freaking annoying." She explained, "'There is no tougher job than being a mom' takes 'the formerly quotidian institution known as parenthood' and shoehorns it into the realm of 'professional status.' It turns motherhood into a title, creating a false equivalency between child rearing and every other calling in the world."[30]

However, according to a February 2013 article in the *Atlantic*, 71 percent of Americans think motherhood is more challenging today than it was twenty or thirty years ago.[31] With more women in the workforce, working mothers are forced to be consummate multitaskers. In her book *Lean In: Women, Work, and the Will to Lead*, Sheryl Sandberg, the COO of Facebook, wrote, "Integrating professional and personal aspirations proved far more challenging than we had imagined. During the same years that our careers demanded maximum time investment, our biology demanded that we have children. Our partners did not share the housework and child rearing, so we found ourselves with two full-time jobs. The workplace did not evolve to give us the flexibility we needed to fulfill our responsibilities at home. We anticipated none of this. We were caught by surprise."[32]

As Caitlin Moran wrote, "Give a new mother a sleeping child for an hour, and she can achieve ten times more than a childless person. 'Multitasking' doesn't come near to the quantum productivity of someone putting in an online grocery order, writing a report, cooking the tea, counseling a weeping friend on the phone, mending a broken vacuum—all within the space of a 3 p.m. nap."[33]

While our decision to delay might have been clear, we didn't anticipate the multiple repercussions. For example, a big issue I'm noticing among my friends is that if they are successful at having one child, having another one becomes a problem. It's almost like an unofficial one-child policy has emerged. By the time some of my friends got around to being ready for another pregnancy, they were too old and decided not to try or had great difficulty and gave up. Laura Dawn had her first baby at forty-three. After leaving MoveOn.org, she founded ART NOT WAR, an artist-run progressive media company. On delaying motherhood, she said, "In retrospect, I just really wish I lived in a country that supported children and mothers, because I would have done this earlier and without so much worry and weight on it. If for some reason (God forbid) anything were to go wrong, I don't think I'd have another chance, and that's a lot of weight to put on both me and the baby."[34] Tina Merrill, who is based in North Carolina and has run a variety of businesses from a doggie hotel to an energy consultancy, had a son at age thirty-five. A few years later, she began to think about having another, but, she said, "as I considered and decided not to have a second child, my age was largely a factor. I was approaching forty by then, and concerned about risks and my general feeling of being old and tired and physically beat up from pregnancy and motherhood already."[35] While Laura and Tina might seem lucky to me because they delayed motherhood and it worked out, they still deal with disappointment.

For others such as myself, it hasn't worked out, and it's devastating. Hilary Grove, who is in her late thirties and a partner at a private equity investment firm, had tried aggressive IVF treatments for more than two years and then had to terminate a pregnancy after five months when she discovered the fetus had a rare chromosomal abnormality. Thereafter, she said, "I found out I have very low egg reserve, so I assume I will never have a healthy child that is not via egg donor or adoption."[36] Natalie said, "I didn't want to have kids until I was in a long-term, committed relationship. I met my husband at age 31, married within two years, and started trying to conceive about two years into our marriage. I prioritized my career, didn't want to have kids as a single mom, and then was unable to get pregnant or maintain a pregnancy."[37]

Despite the rational motivations to delay childbearing, the truth is that many women end up wishing they hadn't delayed so long in order to focus on their careers. Erin Callan, a former CFO of Lehman Brothers, received a lot of attention for her March 10, 2013, opinion piece, "Is There Life after Work?" in the *New York Times*. At the age of forty-seven, she had been trying IVF for several years. "My boundaries slipped away until work was all that was left. Sometimes young women tell me they admire what I've done. As they see it, I worked hard for 20 years and can now spend the next 20 focused on other things. But that is not balance. I do not wish that for anyone."[38] In a University of California, San Francisco, study of 107 people who had used IVF to have a child after the age of forty, the majority felt that, although they were more emotionally prepared for parenting, the best time to have kids was actually five to ten years earlier than in their forties.[39]

These opinions seem to be impacting the next generation. Younger women are increasingly choosing to have kids regardless of whether they are married to their partner or whether they have a partner at all. Fewer people are getting married in general, with 51 percent of Americans aged eighteen or older married as of 2010, compared with 72 percent in 1960. Between 2009 and 2010, the number of marriages performed in the United States fell by 5 percent.[40] However, a study by the Centers for Disease Control and Prevention (CDC) showed that the number of unmarried couples who live together and have children has nearly doubled since 2002.[41] As a February 2012 article in the *New York Times* reported, by the mid-1990s a third of Americans were born outside marriage, but that figure has risen to 41 percent, with 53 percent of those children being born to women under thirty.[42]

Single parenthood has radically increased, more than tripling as a share of American households since 1960. For example, the number of single dads has doubled since 1990 to nearly 2.79 million.[43] Gail Taylor, a founder of the surrogacy agency Growing Generations, said to the *New York Times* in 2008 that 24 percent of her clients were single men, both gay and straight—double what it had been in 2005.[44]

As reported in the *Atlantic*, this trend belies notable economic repercussions, which are influenced by the pressures of caring for children as a single parent. Single moms account for one-quarter of US households, while single dads make up for another 6 percent. According to the Pew Center, in 2011, married mothers earned almost four times more than families led by a single mother. Moreover, "80 percent of moms with spouses are employed, but only 60 percent of single mothers are in full-time jobs. . . . Similarly, single dads are less likely to be in full-time jobs (69 percent) than married dads (88 percent)." The data suggest that "the presence or absence of children might be the single biggest factor explaining income differences between single and married mothers. For single and married women without children, the average difference in income in 2012 was $857—almost inconsequential compared to the almost $19,000 difference between single and married mothers." Considering that the United States is the only one of fifteen top countries as reported by the International Labour Organization that "does not mandate paid maternity leave, paid sick leave and does not guarantee paid vacation time," it is not surprising that single parents find it hard to cope.[45]

For a March 2013 essay in the *Atlantic*, Stacia L. Brown wrote about her experience and observations as a single unwed mother. As she noted, "The National Marriage Project reports that 58 percent of first births to lower-middle-class households and 40 percent of all US births are to unwed mothers."[46] She founded an online support and advocacy initiative, Beyond Baby Mamas, for single parents of color. In Brown's opinion, "Unmarried mothers' needs are not one-size-fits-all; meeting them will take more than generalizations. We aren't an epidemic to be stemmed or a crisis to be quelled; we're individuals in need of support from friends, family, and community. With the right system of support, we can certainly thrive."

The February *New York Times* article on the rise of children born out of wedlock started out with the statement "It used to be called illegitimacy. Now it is the new normal."[47] According to a 2011 Pew Research Center study, although nearly a quarter of Americans believe marriage is becoming obsolete, many members of the millennial generation (eighteen- to twenty-nine-year-olds) "believe being a parent is more important than being married."[48]

However, some people do hold onto the ideal of children through marriage. In her polemical book *Marry Him: The Case for Settling for Mr. Good Enough*, Lori Gottlieb asked, "What does it mean to be empowered and also want happily ever after? In other words, if feminism taught us that we don't really need the White Knight, how do we reconcile that with the fact that many of us are women who want a husband and a family?" The chapter following this excerpt is titled "How Feminism Fucked Up My Love Life."[49] She said it's not feminism per se that's the problem but rather the feminist ideals of freedom and choice as applied to dating that inspire women to find themselves and seek a variety of partners before choosing to settle down. When they are finally ready to make that choice, they might find that they've waited too long. As Gottlieb explained, "When it comes to dating, we *don't* have the same opportunities as men, especially as we get older. This might seem obvious, but somehow I thought that I could just have a baby on my own, put my dating life on hold for a year or two, and then get right back in the game."[50]

Seemingly in reaction to stories like those of Gottlieb, many women are choosing to opt out; in fact, the number of stay-at-home moms increased between 2010 and 2011 for the first time since 2008. In a March 2013 article, "The Retro Wife," for *New York* magazine, Lisa Miller wrote about feminists who've made this decision. One named Kelly, aged thirty-three, "calls herself 'a flaming liberal' and a feminist, too." She said, "I want my daughter to be able to do anything she wants. But I also want to say, 'Have a career that you can walk away from at the drop of a hat.'" Women like Kelly tend to be more affluent and live in homes with incomes of $100,000 a year or more. While respectful of Kelly's choice, Miller commiserated that it could be a sign that "feminism has fizzled, its promise only half-fulfilled. . . . American women are better educated than they've ever been, better educated now than men, but they get distracted during their prime earning years by the urge to procreate."[51]

As Miller pointed out, some prominent women like Sheryl Sandberg have spoken up against this trend. In *Lean In*, Sandberg called for women to strive for leadership positions, to not assume that being a leader excludes being a mom, and to not be afraid to ask for what they need to achieve balance in their lives, both at work and at home. Sandberg also recognized the importance of mothers who choose to stay at home. She wrote, "Stay-at-home mothers can make me feel guilty and, at times, intimidate me. There are moments when I feel like they are judging me, and I imagine there are moments when they feel like I am judging them. But when I push past my own feelings of guilt and insecurity, I feel grateful. These parents—mostly mothers—constitute a large amount of the talent that helps sustain our schools, nonprofits, and communities."[52]

Supreme Court Justice Sonia Sotomayor wrote in her memoir about the disapproval she felt in her school as the daughter of a working mother: "The nuns were critical of working mothers, and their disapproval was felt by latchkey kids. The irony of course was that my mother wouldn't have been working such long hours if not to pay for that education she believed was the key to any aspirations for a better life."[53]

One friend I knew growing up in California, Jennifer Braunschweiger, is now the deputy editor of *More* magazine. In her piece for the April 2013 issue about stay-at-home versus working mothers, she described her own childhood: "I was looked after by babysitters until I was nine, when I became a latchkey kid, like many of my fellow Gen Xers. As I was growing up, my mother would tell me, 'Jennifer, when you were born, I couldn't *wait* to get back to work!' She was proud of her career and her financial independence, and because of her, working has never felt like a choice to me. It's a given." After Jennifer got pregnant at age thirty-four, "people in my office kept asking if I would return after maternity leave. . . . Why wouldn't they wonder? Two other women were pregnant the same year I was, and neither came back to her job."[54]

Braunschweiger pointed out that "there is a danger in lumping people together too categorically" and that "the issue is further distorted by socio-economic class."[55] For middle-class and lower-income women, the burdensome cost of daycare can be a factor in staying home. Full-time infant daycare can range from about $4,650 per year in Mississippi to $18,200 in the District of Columbia. In an April 4, 2013, op-ed for the *New York Times*, Lilian V. Faulhaber, an associate professor of law at Boston University, argued that the US tax structure and the absence of subsidized child-care—which exists in countries like France and Sweden—almost incentivizes women, who earn significantly less than their spouses, not to work.[56] Childcare is not considered a business deduction, so parents have to pay for it out of after-tax income.

For many women, working but spending all their earnings on childcare doesn't add up. In her *New York* magazine piece, Miller cited New York University sociologist Kathleen Gerson's research, which "found that, in spite of all the gains young women have made, about a quarter say they would choose a traditional domestic arrangement over the independence that comes with a career, believing not just 'that only a parent can provide an acceptable level of care' but also that 'they are the only parent available for the job.'"

In a provocative cover story for the *New York Times Magazine*, Judith Warner tracked down women who had given up their careers to be mothers in the early 2000s. Some of these women had been featured in a 2003 cover story by Lisa Belkin for the same magazine about the "Opt-Out Revolution." In surveying nearly two dozen women who exemplified this movement, Warner discovered varying degrees of satisfaction, complacence, and frustration. She wrote, "Among the women I spoke with, those who didn't have the highest academic credentials or highest-powered social networks or who hadn't been sufficiently 'strategic' in their volunteering (fund-raising for a Manhattan private school could be a nice segue back into banking; running bake sales for the suburban swim team tended not to be a career-enhancer) or who had divorced, often struggled greatly."[57]

One woman, Sheilah O'Donnel, thought giving up her career at Oracle, the technology company, "was what I had to do to save my marriage." Thereafter, her self-esteem plummeted and her marriage fell apart. Eventually she went back to work, though at a salary that was one-fifth of the $500,000 she earned at her career peak before having children. Now she counsels her friends to keep up their careers. She told her own twelve-year-old daughter, "You just have to be able to at least earn enough so you can support yourself."[58]

Another woman, Kuae Kelch Mattox, gave up her career in editorial at NBC after the birth of her second child, which coincided with her husband's salary in the business side at Sony taking off. Also influencing her decision was the death of her mother, who had passed away after the birth of Kuae's first child; Kuae had heard from her father that her mother, a drama teacher and speech therapist, "had always wished she could have spent more time with her children. She [Kuae] didn't want to die with similar regrets." Warner wrote that Kuae's friends and family were surprised: "As an upper middle-class African-American woman, didn't she have an obligation to climb the career ladder?" She joined Mocha Moms, a support group for stay-at-home mothers of color and became its volunteer president. Kuae did go back to work after thirteen years, as a booker for a women's news show on Arise TV, a global network specializing in stories about people of color—but at a salary that was probably half of what she would have earned had she stayed on track at NBC. After just six weeks, the show was put on indefinite hiatus, and she was out of a job.[59]

Her husband Ted said he sometimes wonders what it would have been like if he had been the one to stay at home: "Maybe call it jealousy. Maybe envy. What could I have been in 12 years of self-discovery? I'll go out on a limb and say: 'I'd like to try it. It looks pretty good to me.'" Ted's comment illustrates how men also struggle with shifting gender roles. As the article reported, according to the Families and Work Institute, men "now report more work-life stress than women do." Ted told Warner, "Men want to say we're more than a paycheck. There has to be something more than going to work for 50 years and dying." Warner concluded, "At a time when fewer families than ever can afford to live on less than two full-time salaries, achieving work-life balance may well be less a gender issue than an economic one."[60]

For the most part, though, it's the mothers who continue to walk the tightrope between home and career. As reported in the *Atlantic* by Jordan Weissmann about the "overhyped rise of stay-at-home dads," while the number of stay-at-home dads did more than double over the last decade and a half, "among all married couples with children under 15, only 0.8 percent include a stay-at-home dad—up from about 0.3 percent in 1994— compared to 23 percent that include a stay-at-home mom."[61]

In 2011, nearly 71 percent of women with children under eighteen worked.[62] Gabri Christa, who had a daughter when she was forty, is an artist who works part-time as the director of performing arts at a consulate. She said, "I am the one telling my female friends to think many times before having kids. I am happy with mine but think it is a tremendous sac- rifice and for an artist really difficult. The frustration about all I can't do is constant, yet I know it is not forever and I am clear what my choices are."[63] Caitlin Moran wrote that when women are asked about having kids, the question is actually "'When are you going to fuck it all up by having kids?' When are you going to blow a four-year chunk, minimum, out of your career—at an age when most people's attractiveness, creativity, and ambi- tion is peaking—by having a baby? . . . When do the holes start appearing in your CV?"[64]

In addition to balancing motherhood and work, how do women balance their social lives in light of the demands of motherhood? How do they manage their friendships with mothers versus non-mothers? Gabriela Poma Traynor, mother of three, explained, "I do know people with kids who just socialize with others that have kids, but I think that is limiting. I have friends I adore: some with kids, some without. I make adjustments: having lunch instead of dinner with someone, for example, or early nights of hanging out. It's usually with girlfriends without kids that I have to do this type of 'arranging.'"[65] Isolde Brielmaier, mother of one, said, "I still spend an equal amount of time with my friends who do not have kids as well as those who do. This was something that I really was committed to when I got pregnant and it also says a lot about my friends who don't have kids."

However, socializing with other friends with kids can make life easier. For example, Gabriela said, "With other friends with kids, the play date will be very convenient because we get time together, and if the kids have friends, they get time together, and we kill two birds with one stone." Tina Merrill pointed out that "it can be great to find friends who have kids the same age, because we can hang out and the kids will entertain each other— it's like free babysitting!"[66] But Tina added that because she has only one child, she finds it easier to juggle figuring out the time she can spend with friends who don't have kids. Caroline Reeves, a Chinese history professor in her fifties who had sons at age thirty-nine and forty-one, said, "We have refused to go the 'our friends are our kids' friends' parents' route. But often, we do try to have weekend guests who have kids because it's just nice to have the kids having fun too, and not bugging us."[67]

In *Flux*, Peggy Orenstein wrote that women "as they age . . . their lives diverge sharply and they can become critical toward those who choose different paths."[68] In *Opting In*, Amy Richards wrote that friendships mutate as this divergence begins: "Friendships for the first time require real work, planning, time, and travel. We may never have given serious consideration to how to grow together as we grow up."[69] She said about her own circumstances: "Once I was a mother, I developed yet another guilt: not wanting to burden my friends with my children, either by talking incessantly about them or asking them to eternally accommodate me, for instance, always coming to my house for dinner or choosing a time convenient to my kids' bedtimes."[70]

For the woman who doesn't have kids, spending time with the friend with kids can be affected by many factors. Hilary Grove said, "I generally care more about if the woman works. If the woman works, I naturally have things to relate to and the conversation tends not to center on kids." But she also recognized "how important it is to have female friends." She added, "Being thirty-seven, I would be a very lonely person if I isolated myself from women who had kids."[71] Jenny Davidson said, "It's easy to spend time with single parent friends who share custody with another parent and have child-free time they like to occupy with adult socializing! I do think some people with young children are insensitive to the chaos/noise effect on those without children—that has more to do with parenting styles, though, than pure child presence."[72] Mary Kaye Schilling felt that "people with children, no matter how much they say they don't fixate on their kids, their lives revolve around them, for obvious reasons. Occasionally you meet someone who still very much wants to preserve their own identity, but it's rare."[73] Elaine Chen said she's "more than happy to spend time with people who have kids," but she has parameters: "1) if they can talk about things other than their kids; and 2) if their children are present, that they are well-behaved."[74]

Moe Angelos described this scenario among her friends with kids: "Until the kids are able to be slightly independent, there is little room for adult space/time when the kids are around, I have found. And that's cool, but I do sometimes miss my adult friends once they have gone over to Kidworld. They come back, once the kids get in school for instance. But there is a period of time early on when to see the parent means a shift from the pre-kids friendship structure—unless the friends are very wealthy and can afford childcare all the time. But I don't know anyone like that."[75] Before Liz Mermin, a London-based filmmaker, had a baby at the age of forty, she said it was decidedly easier to spend time with friends who didn't have kids. In her opinion, "Friends without kids go out more often, stay out later, and don't need to be planned so far in advance. They also drink more."[76] Natalie Dean felt that it was easier because of the following: "One, for scheduling reasons—we don't have to work around nap times, meal times, babysitters. Two, we can have adult conversations and not focus on a child most of the time. Three, after struggling with fertility, multiple attempts at IVF, and years of trying for kids (most of our committed relationship), we found that we often felt empty after spending time with our friends and their children. We've spent countless hours analyzing parenting choices and styles and wondering what we'll be like as parents. This gets tiresome and sad."[77]

The tensions don't exist only between women who have kids and women who don't but also between women who have kids and other women who have kids. In 2012, the American public witnessed "the mom wars" on the campaign trail leading up to the presidential election. A raging debate about moms who work or don't ensued after Democratic political consultant Hilary Rosen said on CNN that presidential candidate Mitt Romney's wife, Ann Romney, who had raised five sons, had "never worked a day in her life." Rosen's statement became a flashpoint for both ends of the political spectrum. The Obamas denounced the comment, and Ann Romney herself chimed in on Fox News. She said her husband had told her, "Ann, your job is more important than mine . . . your job is a forever job that is going to bring forever happiness."[78] (On a side note, Mitt Romney's "forever job" also is to be a parent, but that didn't stop him from having another job as well. On another side note, in a 2013 graduation speech at Southern Virginia University, he said, "Some people could marry but choose to take more time, they say, for themselves. Others plan to wait until they're well into their thirties or forties until they think of getting married. They're going to miss so much of living, I'm afraid. If you meet a person you love, get married. Have a quiver full of kids if you can."[79])

Mary Elizabeth Williams, *Salon* staff writer, called for an end to the mom wars and for women to collaborate on solutions. She wrote, "It's in those moments when a spit-up-stained stay-at-home mom who hasn't washed her hair all week looks across the drive at the polished executive mother heading off on a business trip. It's there when a guilt-wracked, stuck-at-the-job mom sees the Facebook pictures of a mother boasting of her 'magical' summer spent with the kids in the Hamptons. And when they both think, 'That bitch has it easy.' It kicks up ugly, uncomfortable issues of privilege. It perpetuates the fiction that all women have the luxury of choice about motherhood, and that my choice is inherently a threat to yours."[80]

Women with kids also often come to blows with each other over parenting styles. As Amy Richards has written, "Every parenting suggestion or portrayal of motherhood inevitably brings a wave of adverse reactions because the topic of motherhood hits us at our most vulnerable."[81] Frank Bruni, op-ed columnist for the *New York Times*, argued that the parenting style obsession is a distinctly modern phenomenon: "As the Me Generation spawned generations of mini-me's, our rigorous self-fascination expanded to include the whole brood and philosophies about its proper care and feeding."[82]

Two of the most popular recent books on the subject are *Battle Hymn of the Tiger Mother* by Amy Chua and *Bringing Up Bébé* by Pamela Druckerman. They explore the differences in parenting styles in other cultures: Chinese in Chua's case and French in Druckerman's. I personally found the books to be humorous and personal more than judgmental, but many women reacted with vitriol.

Some of Chua's points, though honest, come across as deliberately provocative. For example, "Happiness is not a concept I tend to dwell on. Chinese parenting does not address happiness. . . . But here's the thing. When I look around at all the Western families that fall apart—all the grown sons and daughters who can't stand to be around their parents or don't even talk to them—I have a hard time believing that Western parenting does a better job with happiness."[83] On whether to let her daughter go to a sleepover, she wrote, "Sophia didn't need to be exposed to the worst of Western society, and I wasn't going to let platitudes like 'Children need to explore' or 'They need to make their own mistakes' lead me astray."[84] On playdates: "I refuse to buckle to politically correct Western social

204   THE BIG LIE

norms that are obviously stupid. And not even rooted historically. What are the origins of the Playdate anyway? Do you think our Founding Fathers had Sleepovers? I actually think America's Founding Fathers had Chinese values. . . . Ben Franklin said, 'If thou loveth life, never ever wasteth time.' Thomas Jefferson said, 'I'm a huge believer in luck, and the harder I work the more I have of it.' And Alexander Hamilton said, 'Don't be a whiner.' That's a totally Chinese way of thinking." (Chua's daughter, upon hearing these statements, said to her mother, "I think you may be misquoting.")[85]

The *Wall Street Journal* fomented the fire around Chua's book when it ran an excerpt in January 2011 with the headline "Why Chinese Mothers Are Superior."[86] The excerpt garnered more than 8,000 comments online. On the *Today* show, host Meredith Vieira told Chua that viewers had written in with comments like "She's a monster." When *Bébé* came out a year later, it was also excerpted in the *Wall Street Journal*, with the predictable headline "Why French Parents Are Superior." Druckerman's tone and tactics were less "embattled" than Chua's, and reaction wasn't as strong— the excerpt received just more than 1,000 comments. Still, women jumped on the book's praise of French parenting as almost anti-American, which Druckerman attracted with statements such as this: "When American friends visit our home, the parents usually spend much of the visit refereeing their kids' spats, helping their toddlers do laps around the kitchen island, or getting down on the floor to build LEGO villages. There are always a few rounds of crying and consoling. When French friends visit, however, we grown-ups have coffee and the children play happily by themselves."[87] One commentator, Erika Brown Ekiel, a Silicon Valley–based consultant and former associate editor of *Forbes*, wrote an essay for *Forbes* under the headline "Bringing Up Bebe? No Thanks. I'd Rather Raise a Billionaire."[88] She claimed that France does not have many billionaires, at least no self-made ones, and that America's capitalism and individualism are superior to France's socialism.

Adding to the recent array of controversial parenting books, French philosopher and feminist Elisabeth Badinter came out with the English translation of her book *The Conflict: How Modern Motherhood Undermines the Status of Women* a few months after Druckerman's. Badinter denounced "natural" and attentive mothering (natural childbirth, breast-feeding, cloth-diapering, etc.) as being opposed to feminism and working women. In a piece for the *New York Times*' Motherlode column, KJ Dell'Antonia felt the real "conflict" arises from societal demands and economic realities. Badinter did touch on this, but Dell'Antonia felt she missed the crux of the matter. Dell'Antonia wrote, "We don't, as a society, make it easy for parents of either sex to balance the financial demands of raising children with the physical and emotional demands of being there for them as they grow up. For women on one side of the income divide, the societal pressure is to get to work as soon as possible, and the only way to 'balance' a job and parenting in many fields is to quit when family needs become too intense and find a new job when the pressures have eased."[89]

In a piece for The Stone forum for contemporary philosophers on the *New York Times*' website, Amy Allen, a philosophy professor at Dartmouth College, had a similar reaction as Dell'Antonia and called for greater cooperation between both women and men to identify remedies. Allen wrote, "If 'the conflict' continues to be framed as one between women— between liberal and cultural feminists, or between stay at home mothers and working women, or between affluent professionals and working class women, or between mothers and childless women—it will continue to distract us from what we should really be doing: working together—women *and* men together—to change the cultural, social and economic conditions within [which] these crucial choices are made."[90]

I've witnessed how total strangers can come to blows because one woman feels the other has made a bad parenting choice. While I was in line one day at the register of a Whole Foods in Cambridge, a white woman in maybe her early forties came up to the man behind the counter and said, "Just so you know, there are two kids sleeping in the back of a car, and we're about to call 9-1-1." The man looked at her blankly at first, but then realized he was supposed to react. "Oh, really?" he said before looking equally blankly at his coworker behind him. He got out from behind the counter and obligingly followed the woman outside. A minute later, he returned, shrugging his shoulders as he said to his coworker, "I guess you should page. It's a maroon Prius." A few seconds after the page, a white woman in her late thirties or early forties came to the counter and said, "That's my car." The guy said, "You might want to check on your car, uh. . . ." The woman, looking worried, said, "Why? Did something happen?" He said, "Uh, no, but . . . you might want to go out there."

I had already paid up, so I walked outside, a few steps behind the mother, who looked perfectly normal, more so than her accuser, who was by now standing in front of her own extremely dirty white Chevy Tahoe, just two cars away from the Prius, which was immaculate. The kids inside looked like they were about seven and ten years old. The mother said to the lady, "What's wrong? They were sleeping in the car." And the accuser glared, grunted, got into her car, and drove away.

I was upset by the woman who had alerted the store and threatened to call the police. Maybe the mother didn't have help, and it would have been worse to leave her kids alone at home. She had brought them to a Whole Foods in a safe neighborhood with a small and highly visible parking lot. The kids were keeping each other company and hopefully knew to keep the door locked and not go outside. I used to hang out with my brother in the car all the time when my mother took us on her errands. She had to take us with her because she didn't have any other help.

If the woman in the dirty Chevy had genuinely been concerned about these kids, she could have waited by the car while she told someone to get a store clerk, rather than immediately threatening to call 9-1-1. She could have asked the store clerk to send a page simply to make sure the kids' parent was in the store. When the kids' parent answered the page, the lady could have said, "I'm glad everything's okay. I just wanted to make sure."

Our impressions of parenting styles are intrinsically wrapped up in the conflicting attitudes we have toward the concept of motherhood itself. Instead of assessing what kind of mother someone is, we should be looking at what kind of *person* she is. How much money and support does a particular parent have and how does the availability of those resources impact her decisions? What kind of lifestyle does the parent want, and what kind of lifestyle can the parent afford to have? As Jennifer Braunschweiger explained in her *More* magazine piece about stay-at-home versus working mothers, "Many women on both sides feel bad about what they've had to give up, and it's all too easy to let insecurity turn outward into judgment and accusation. No wonder we're fighting."[91] If women focused more on being generous with and helping each other rather than judging and schooling each other, perhaps we could, as Amy Allen and Mary Elizabeth Williams suggested, develop constructive solutions.

Yet society persists in talking about women as existing somewhere along the motherhood spectrum before acknowledging that having a child can be a choice, and that those who choose to be or who end up child-free are equally as valid as those who don't. Caitlin Moran wrote, "I don't think there's a single lesson that motherhood has to offer that couldn't be learned elsewhere. If you want to know what's in motherhood for you, as a woman, then—in truth—it's nothing you couldn't get from, say, reading the 100 greatest books in human history; learning a foreign language well enough to argue in it; climbing hills; loving recklessly; sitting quietly, alone, in the dawn; drinking whiskey with revolutionaries; learning to do close-hand magic; swimming in a river in winter; growing fox-gloves, peas, and roses; calling your mum. . . ." Her list goes on and on.[92]

Women should talk to each other about their experiences, avoid assumptions about each other's fertility or infertility, be open to differences of opinion, and respect each other's choices. That is something we all can do, whether we are friends with kids or friends without.

CHAPTER 10
THE POWER OF OPTIMISM

I'm still here.

I opened my eyes to faint sunlight shining through the window of my room. "Hello," I said. A nurse peeked in. I asked her, "Where's my husband and brother?" She walked down the hall to get them.

I could see a mess of wires around me, some of them poking through my skin, including an epidural in my back. I saw a chest tube snaking out from the middle of my torso and down the side of the bed. There was blood, stagnant, in the tube. My chest felt heavy, and there was a long gauze dressing starting from the top of it that went all the way down the middle between my breasts. This was where they had cut me open. I was scared to move in case the bones in my chest came out of place.

I saw Jay and Troy approach and gave them the biggest smile. "I made it!"

They sat at the foot of my bed and told me about how the doctors had come to update them regularly about the progress of my surgery. Troy made the shape of a big egg with his hand and said that's what Dr. Yoon told him the GIST looked like. After a few hours, it grew dark outside, and I started to nod off. I told them they could go. I was tired and would try to sleep. They said they'd come back in the morning.

Even though I was high on Dilaudid, an opioid for severe pain, I had trouble staying asleep, so I used a remote control to turn on the television, perched high on the wall facing me. A Celtics basketball game was on. Yeah! I love the Celtics. My father had conditioned me to be a fan. He loved Larry Bird. Daddy was bizarrely superstitious when he watched the games. If he was sitting a certain way and they were winning, he wouldn't move. If they were losing, he would alter his position, sometimes just shifting his weight from one butt cheek to another.

I couldn't move even if I wanted to. My chest felt like it was under a ton of bricks.

I called Jay, who told me that he and Troy were also watching the game. They were at Bukowski's, a bar near our house. I told him, "I'm so happy!" It was true. I felt ecstatically happy—as if from here on out, life would be smooth sailing. The worst was over; the best was yet to come.

The next day, my mother arrived from California. It was hard for her to see me incapacitated, and it was hard for me to have her see me like that. But I knew it was important for us all to be together.

During my five days in the hospital, I was struck by how young I seemed compared to the other patients. On my side of the ward, there was a woman in her sixties with colon cancer, another women in her eighties whose room had been quarantined. I felt lucky because I had many visitors, and arrangement after arrangement of flowers arrived at my room. Nurses would stop by to chat even when they didn't have to check my vitals or give me medications. They said some of the patients didn't treat them well, but that I was "real nice." I was in the ward for people recovering from serious trauma, so it's understandable that the patients would not be at their best. They were scared.

I often thought of my father when I was in the hospital. He had been a doctor and even in his final days treated all the nurses and medical staff very well. He greeted them cheerily; he always thanked them. I took my cue from my memories of him.

Every day a nurse gave me a towel bath, which made me feel like a baby. Also, I could only drink chicken broth or eat gelatin the first two days, until I graduated to soft solids, which consisted of mushy chicken and mashed potatoes. On the second day, a nurse made me get out of bed and take a few steps. It was agony lifting myself up. The bones in my chest felt loose, and the pain was intense when I moved my core even slightly. On the fourth day, a physical therapist taught me how to lessen the pain I felt when I got in and out of bed. She told me to cross my hands over my chest and roll slowly onto my side, then make my feet touch the floor while I simultaneously raised my upper body. On the fifth day, I put on street clothes—a long-sleeved John Lennon T-shirt, sweatpants, and sneakers. Jay took me out in a wheelchair to our car and brought me home.

A week after my surgery, we were invited to a theater awards ceremony in New York. Jay and I agreed that he should go even though I was still too weak. I wouldn't have let him miss the event for anything. I suspected we had been invited because our show might be getting an award. We had worked so hard on the last production, and the stress between us had nearly done us in. This award was recognition that our collaboration had been a triumph. Also, my mother was in town to help out so I would be okay without Jay for the night. A friend who was at the ceremony texted to let me know that when Jay accepted the award for his direction of the show, he dedicated it to me.

Around that time, I missed my twentieth reunion at Harvard. It felt horrible to be so close to my alma mater but unable to attend. I couldn't walk more than a block without getting exhausted. My body was still in shock and was working on rebuilding the bones in my chest. To cheer me up, my mother and Jay hosted a party to which many of my classmates came. I held court in an armchair holding a pillow against my chest. I wore a scoop-neck black eyelet blouse through which you could see the top of the surgical strips crisscross my chest. There was a long scar forming underneath.

A few days later, my mother went back to California, and Jay and I were finally alone—for what felt like the first time in months because he had been away so much before my surgery. Over the next few weeks, he and I became closer than ever. He kept a journal in which he noted when I took my medications, and he made sure I took them at the appointed intervals—there was Colace (a laxative), ibuprofen, and Dilaudid. I started to wean myself off the latter medication after three weeks. I had read it was addictive.

It had been months since I had read a book, and as my head started to be less foggy, I decided to read the newest book on my shelf, *Wild* by Cheryl Strayed, which a friend had given to me. The book was a godsend. Strayed's journey got me out of my head and dreaming again. She had hit rock bottom after her mother died of cancer, her marriage fell apart, and she got hooked on heroin. To find herself, she went alone on a treacherous hike of the Pacific Crest Trail. In an early scene, she stands on the trail and looks around in all directions, weighing her options of what to do next. "There was only one, I knew. There was always only one. To keep walking."[1]

I often thought about these words when I felt too tired to lift myself up and take a short walk, which the nurses had urged me to do every day. *Just keep walking. One day it won't be an effort.*

During my recovery, I was totally dependent on Jay—to do the grocery shopping, cook, even bathe me. I couldn't pull, push, lift, or reach without a sharp pain erupting in my chest. Because it hurt to move my arms, Jay soaped me up when I took a shower. As I looked into his eyes, I felt the strongest love, as strong as on our wedding day. When we married in a church in Sri Lanka, we said our vows in front of hundreds of people (mostly my huge extended family). But when we looked deep into each other's eyes, all of a sudden, there was just him and me. I saw so much love in his blue eyes that I cried. A bird in the rafters started chirping as we said, "I do."

In the parable of the missing halves, we are each half a person in search of our other half. *Jay and I are each other's halves. I will spend the rest of my life with him.*

In the nearly six years we had been together, we'd never visited his hometown. Of his family, only his mother had made the long journey to our Sri Lankan wedding, and it had been at least seven years since he himself had gone back to Iowa. We decided that this summer we should make the pilgrimage, and we did so in mid-August after I had recovered enough.

I was excited to visit the Midwest. Iowa seemed exotic to me, like a foreign country. On the drive from the airport to the family farm, where his dad and stepmother lived, I was struck by how expansive the land was, fields and fields for miles. Jay stopped the car to show me the house where his mother, he, and his siblings lived after his parents split. It didn't look like anyone lived there anymore.

The main street was mostly deserted, and a couple of places were shut down. A store named Final Quest stood next to one called Stoner Drugs. It looked like the town in the film *The Last Picture Show.*

We had a peaceful, happy stay at the farm. Jay said it was the best he and his dad had gotten along with each other. We went to an estate auction and an ice cream social at the local church. Everyone we met— both family and strangers—heartily welcomed me, which was reassuring because I had expected to encounter prejudice because of my brown skin and foreign features. But in truth, I felt like I was part of the family.

One day at the house, I scanned photos from Jay's childhood that were in a box his father had saved. There were photos of Jay high-jumping, at his high school graduation, and with his sister. I felt the sadness in the house about the sister who had died from Ewing's sarcoma, for whom Jay had been a bone marrow donor. There were photos of her, smiling with her three brothers. I thought that if Jay and I had a daughter, we would name her after his sister.

For the last two days of our trip, we met up with Jay's mom in Des Moines and stayed at a bed-and-breakfast operated by a couple. The wife was very thin, and her hair was shorn close to her head. At breakfast she revealed to me that she was on chemo. I didn't feel like telling her about my condition, but I realized that I was part of a community of people living with cancer. I had been able to escape chemo for now and hopefully forever. I just had scars on my body, but otherwise I was the same. I hadn't lost a ton of weight and all my hair. In the presence of this woman, I was struck by the difference between our experiences of cancer.

Jay and I left Iowa feeling good about how pleasant our visit had been. We had connected with his family and become even closer with each other. To add to the photos of us with elephants and monkeys in Sri Lanka, we now had photos of us wandering through cornfields.

But when we returned to Cambridge, a horrible situation awaited us. We were about to remount the show for which Jay had won the award. It had been invited to tour in Boston, Poland, and three cities in France. Just two weeks before rehearsals were to begin, one of the actresses pulled out to do a TV show. We had to scramble to replace her, and suddenly what was supposed to be a happy and triumphant occasion became tense. Also, we had to spend a lot of extra time, energy, and money for additional rehearsals to keep the show on track.

After everything we had dealt with in the months before, we were emotionally and mentally wiped out. Around the time of my diagnosis and surgery, we had been audited for two years' worth of taxes. Because of my condition, we got an extension and then spent much of June and July painstakingly assembling our receipts and documentation.

Adding to the headaches over practical affairs, I started to feel a black cloud gathering over me because I didn't know if I was in the clear healthwise. My follow-up appointments were coming up, and although the outlook was positive, I certainly had gotten unpleasant surprises before.

I also got a shock regarding an old college classmate from Athens who had suddenly died. He had stayed with me just recently in July while he was in Boston for doctors' appointments to check his liver, which had been transplanted ten years before. While Jay and I were in Iowa, I heard that he had died while cooking dinner for his two young sons. Some of his clothes were still in our closet because he had planned to return to Cambridge in October for more appointments. I looked at his heavy black garment bag containing a black-tie suit and wondered, *What do you do with a dead man's things?*

The halcyon days of summer we had experienced in Iowa were coming to a clamorously crashing end. Abruptly, it seemed, Jay and I were not enjoying life, which was unfortunate considering how close and kind we had been with each other up until that point. I started to notice more tension in some of our interactions with each other—I thought it would pass after we got through the next little while.

On August 30, 2012, I had a follow-up appointment with Dr. Yoon about my GIST. In the waiting room, I was struck by how devastating cancer is—I could feel it all around me. The staff tried to alleviate the mood by being extra-pleasant and smiling a lot. A petite Asian woman in hospital scrubs wheeled a cart like she was peddling dim sum—but instead she was offering shortbread cookies, apple juice, and peanuts.

Dr. Yoon checked my scars and made sure everything was healing correctly. He told me my prognosis was very good. The chances of recurrence were low, and aside from being monitored every few months, I could go on with life as usual. I felt a huge relief, especially because I had recently read Siddhartha Mukherjee's extraordinary book, *The Emperor of All Maladies: A Biography of Cancer*. He closed the book with a story about a patient with GIST. I was amazed that this condition I had never heard of until I found out I had it was the final moment in a definitive book about cancer.

Mukherjee had written about Germaine, a woman whose GIST was caught too late, only after she started exhibiting symptoms like feeling nauseous and weighted down. As she dealt with the disease, her marriage fell apart, but she developed a closer bond with her brother, who happened to be an oncologist. She said, "Cancer breaks some families and makes some. In my case, it did both."[2] She fought her cancer bravely, researching new medications and signing herself up for the latest trials. Mukherjee described her as always "trying to outwit it." But she died six years after her diagnosis. He said that Germaine "captured something essential about our struggle against cancer: that, to keep pace with this malady, you needed to keep inventing and reinventing, learning and unlearning strategies."[3]

In my case, a complete fluke with the discovery of the tumor during

IVF had likely set me free from having to hustle down the road to avoid cancer's sword.

A few hours after seeing Dr. Yoon, I went to an appointment with Dr. Souter at the Fertility Center. I wanted to go as quickly as possible for what would probably be a last-ditch effort at having my own biological child. Dr. Souter asked how my summer was. "Intense," I said. She responded, "Of course it was." I said, "It's good for the book." She nodded then asked, "What's happening with the book?" I said, "I'm going to write it." She said, "If I remember, you had an excellent title." "The Big Lie." "Yes, exactly."

We got back to talking about my fertility. Dr. Souter said there was no reason I couldn't pursue IVF again, but because it had been a year since my last round of tests, I had to redo most of them for insurance approval. Also, the rules change pretty radically for what insurance covers when you get deeper into your forties. For example, if your FSH (follicle-stimulating hormone) levels are too elevated, you don't get covered.

On September 1, I went in for my day 3 blood work to test my FSH levels. I was having a case of déjà vu. *Here I am again, at the Fertility Center. There is Annie, the nurse I remember with the Irish accent.* She smiled at me, but I couldn't tell if it was because she recognized me. There was the Caribbean-accented phlebotomist who had told me there wouldn't be snow on my birthday. She called my name and drew seven vials of blood. I hadn't given that much blood in about seven months. *I've done this all before. Why am I doing it again? Is it useless? Will anyone tell me if it is?*

An Indian couple walked into the waiting room. I looked around, and everyone looked so old to me.

I couldn't have anticipated how struggling to have a child would result in a hyper-awareness of my surroundings, myself, and my feelings. I guess we spend so much time growing out of childhood and turning outward to fit in, in the world. But as I tried to have a child, I turned inward, and my body ruled my world. I never used to think about the limits of what I could do, but now with the cancer on top of the fertility issues, attending to my body had become a part-time job—one appointment and consideration after another.

While dealing with the multiple miscarriages and pursuing fertility treatment, Jay and I never sought psychological support. Moreover, none of the medical professionals we interacted with even suggested it. In retrospect, I wish we had talked to someone objective. According to a 1993 study on the psychological impact of infertility, many infertile women described it as "the most upsetting experience of their lives." Sixty-three percent rated it as more stressful than divorce, even if they had experienced both.[4] In a study on "life after infertility," which surveyed women who had undergone at least three IVF cycles between 1982 and 1993 with varying degrees of success, one-third of the unsuccessful women reported that infertility had exerted a very negative effect on their marriages.[5] Furthermore, according to a 2010 *SELF* magazine piece on infertility, "Only 5 percent of patients use the psychological support services their clinic offers, despite data showing how helpful they can be."

I'd read studies that couples who go through the arduous process of IVF but don't eventually conceive are more likely to die early. One study analyzed 21,000 Danish couples seeking IVF and found that among the couples who remained childless, the women were four times more likely to die early, while the men were two times more likely to die early. The lead author of the study, Professor Esben Agerbo of Aarhus University, Denmark, said it was important to remember that "association is not causation."[6] However, psychologist Ingrid Collins, commenting on the study for the BBC, hypothesized that "people having IVF tend to be desperate for a child. If they are unsuccessful they may be depressed—it may even be this rather than childlessness that is playing a part [in the incidence of early death]."[7]

When Jay and I went back to the Fertility Center, everything we had gone through the first time played again, but our mood was different the second time. Around my surgery, our optimism and enthusiasm had been tested as we faced my mortality. Now, things at the Fertility Center felt Kafkaesque—disorienting and menacing. Yes, this had been the place that had likely saved my life, but it was also the place that had put fear in our hearts.

A 2009 article in the *Harvard Mental Health Letter* asserted that it's "difficult to know when to stop seeking treatment. Frequently one partner wants to end treatment before another, which can strain the relationship. Most patients need to make the transition gradually, and with great difficulty, from wanting biological children to accepting that they will have to pursue adoption or come to terms with being childless."[8] Moreover, according to studies on gender differences in attitudes toward fertility treatment, women are more likely to initiate treatment than their male partners. Once they have started infertility treatment, women are less willing to stop than men.[9] And the pressure has been known to cause irreparable damage to a relationship. Sarah Elizabeth Richards has written about how some women are even seeking financial support for fertility preservation treatments in their divorce cases.[10]

I asked Jay one night as I made dinner how he felt about being back at the center. He replied, "I don't feel like I really have a choice." I was shocked. I decided not to react. Also, it didn't seem like he was in the right frame of mind to have a conversation. He was focused on his computer, preoccupied with work.

Five years before, Jay and I had gotten engaged, discussing how much we liked kids. We had gone far along this path toward parenthood together. I was determined to see this through, I thought, for *us*.

But in that instant with Jay, I felt a divergence between us.

We spent the next few weeks of September preparing for the show, rehearsing a new actress, and performing at the Institute of Contemporary Art in Boston toward the end of the month. After that, in the first week of October, we went on to Krakow, Poland. The show went off without a hitch, and I was relieved. But I could tell something was not 100 percent right with Jay. He seemed distracted. He felt . . . very serious.

We stayed in Krakow two days later than the rest of our company. Jay had to give a talk at a symposium for artists and academics, and we had dinner with the director of the arts festival. The next day we got in a bit of sightseeing, and everything seemed fine. In the evening, we stopped at a café where Jay had a glass of wine while I had tea because I had come down with a sore throat. I noticed that Jay's energy was directed away from me, almost like he couldn't look me in the eyes. All these weeks that I had been noticing a shift in his behavior, I thought he was simply stressed out and having a delayed reaction to the intensity of the months before, around my surgery and the headaches of the audit, the actress's ill-timed departure, and so on. But in that moment, I felt strongly that the problem might actually be *me*. The realization gripped me like a straitjacket. I broached the subject: "Jay, is there something wrong?"

The rest of the conversation is a blur. I know that he said he had been feeling angry, that he was thinking about times in the past when we had clashed about things related to the show. I told him, "But everything's great now." He said angrily, "Now, now, sure, *now* things are fine."

I started crying but stopped myself because we were in public. I thought, *Okay, now we've gotten this out in the open. We've listened to each other. Everything will be fine. It's been a difficult time, but it will pass.*

After we returned from Krakow, we had another appointment at the Fertility Center, during which we confirmed being green-lighted again for IVF. Dr. Souter greeted me, "You look good. You don't look like you had surgery." She sent us to an examination room while she talked to Cheryl, a nurse, who then called us into her office. Cheryl shook my hand. "Dr. Souter explained to me your story. Wow. Freaky." I smiled and said, "Yeah." Cheryl continued, "So, we're going to get you back on track." I told her that I hoped to start IVF after finishing the next leg of our show's tour at the end of November. She was able to figure out a schedule that would start me on a cycle at the end of December.

I looked at Jay, who seemed overwhelmed, but by what I didn't know. Plus, I wasn't really worried. I had reasons to be optimistic. Jay had told me we would take a vacation after our performances were done. Also, before we left for the last leg of our tour in France, while I was sleeping, he sent me an e-mail:

now it's two. will you wake me at nine?

I love you, blu. A romantic time in paris coming up.

Jay

I thought, *He loves me. He's still calling me by my nickname, "blu." Everything is fine. We've just had a lot going on. Very soon, we'll get to relax and enjoy each other.*

But after we arrived in France in the first week of November, I sensed a worsening. One day in the dressing room, Jay was on Skype with an artistic director in Germany—someone with whom I myself had spent a good amount of time. I waved to him on the computer as I walked by. A few minutes later in the theater, Jay said that this artistic director might be getting a job running another theater and might offer Jay a job. He said, "I'm just going to go . . . and take it." *Whoa. No discussion. No "Hey, Tanya, what do you think of this possibility? Should we move to x place for a while?"*

As the days progressed, Jay seemed to be ignoring me. I felt like he could barely look at me. A guillotine had dropped. Soon, I felt so badly about myself and us that I could barely leave my room, except to turn up for rehearsals and perform. I kept up appearances in front of the company and interacted with the staff at the theaters. In reality, I was shell-shocked from being unable to enjoy the success of our show.

I'm no saint. I know I can be tough and critical. But I also know how strongly I felt about Jay's and my marriage and our devotion to each other. I also felt how much love we always looked at each other with. In addition, after my surgery and our trip to Iowa, we had become closer than ever. I thought, *Sure, we have issues to figure out like most couples, especially ones that work together, but our marriage is solid.*

I tried to talk to Jay a few times about what I was observing, but he was already far away. He felt so shut down, aloof, and angry, and I was too vulnerable and stunned to know how to counter or convince him. Then one night he told me he thought we should separate. I felt a dagger in my heart. The ground vanished beneath my feet. I felt alone on a precipice, and he wasn't there to keep me safe. My angel, my love, my best friend. What had happened? It felt so sudden, although he acted as if I shouldn't be surprised. But how could I have known? Despite the ups and downs we had been experiencing, he had told me we would have a romantic time in Paris. He had told me we would take a vacation after we got back. *Also, we are supposed to start IVF in a few weeks. And wait, I have a follow-up CT scan after we get back. Are you serious? You want to separate from me? I still need you, Jay.*

Still, I thought, *This shall pass. Something has broken, but it will come back together.*

I got through the last show, even though I cried whenever I was alone, in the dressing room before the show and backstage between scenes.

At the after-party, I had a few glasses of wine and confided to a few people that things were over, it seemed, between me and Jay. If I hadn't been tipsy, I probably wouldn't have said anything, but at the same time, I had been holding so much in for so many weeks that I had to let it out. The cat was out of the bag, and word seeped into the company that something was wrong with Tanya and Jay. It felt like the worst dream ever. As we left for the airport, I tried to hold my head up high, but I was dying on the inside. I told Jay before we got on the plane, "Jay, we can work this out." But he could barely look at me. I told him, "It doesn't seem like I have much choice."

What happened to us in the days and months that followed I still don't and may never understand. I was dealing with the emotional whiplash of watching our marriage fall apart so rapidly and abruptly. To go into the rest of our story would turn this into a different book. But I'll tell you about the moment a week after we got back from France when Jay and I actually separated. For the most part, except when I had to be in Boston for the CT scan (which came back clear, no recurrence), Jay and I stayed apart, with him in Cambridge and me in New York. On December 1, 2012, he came to New York for what I had hoped would be a reunion and time for reconciliation, but he hadn't changed his mind. I felt like he wasn't dealing with *me*; he wasn't seeing me for me. I asked him what he wanted to do, and he said he still wanted to separate. I started sobbing. I said over and over, "It hurts so much, Jay. It hurts so much." But I told him that if he wanted to separate, then he should separate, take his things, leave the keys, and go. I said it's not what I want, that I love him, that we still had so much to do, so much to give, but that I didn't feel like it was my call to make.

That night, we slept in the same bed—which felt oddly peaceful and right. But the next morning, I felt shaky and scared, like everything was slipping away. I helped him collect his things, clothes in the drawers and on the shelves, random books. He tried to hug me once, but I recoiled and tears burst out of my eyes. *What had happened to our romantic time in Paris? What had happened to our vacation that should have been happening right now?*

I walked him to the car, and for the first time in weeks, I saw the man whom I had married. He looked gentle, he looked so sweet . . . but yet, he looked lost. We were both lost.

I told him to remember the good times. "There were a lot of nice times," I said. He agreed. I told him that what we needed was stress management, not a separation. He said it's not black and white, that we would check in with each other soon. But he also said, "I don't want to say anything that has a double meaning. And right now everything has a double meaning." "More or less," I said.

A crazy man with a ski cap, anarchist earrings that stretched out his earlobes, and three cigarettes in his mouth walked by. A flock of pigeons lifted from the ground and took flight as Jay and I hugged each other, gingerly.

When Jay settled into the car, I waved. He blew me a kiss. I turned around and walked. I turned around and waved again. He waved back. I turned to my building, held my head up high, and walked toward my apartment.

It was December 2, 2012. *I am struck by how many 2s there are today: 12/2/12. Maybe I'll have twins . . .*

But that was it. He was gone. The love of my life. The father of our future children. *Where do I go now?*

I walked into the bedroom that was stripped of his belongings. I dissolved to the floor and felt like I would sink through it if I didn't grab onto something. I cried so hard that I felt like my eyes were going to fall out of my face. I held my hand to my chest as I heaved with tears—my chest, which had a scar running down the length of it that wasn't there just a few months before. I went to make the bed that he had slept in with me. As I tidied the sheet on his side of the bed, I started crying more. I said to the air, "I love you, Jay. I wish you loved me." I walked to the kitchen. On the dining table was a knife I had used to open a box earlier that day. The knife tempted me to cut into my wrists and make the suffering go away.

After my surgery, a friend sent me a poem, "The Time around Scars," by Michael Ondaatje, a writer who, like me, is from Sri Lanka.[11] The poem tells us how scars mark a time before and after, and it felt especially relevant now that I had my own scars on my body.

Our darkest moments are our most solitary.

Over the next few weeks, to keep myself busy while I hid from the world, I cleaned a different corner of my house every day. I pulled everything out of every drawer and reorganized. In one drawer was a stack of old business cards. At the top was one Jay had given to me the night we met: November 19, 2006. It had an image from a show he had directed at the Norwegian Theatre Academy.

My wardrobe had twos of almost everything: two pairs of sneakers, two black bras, two pairs of rain boots, two wool overcoats. I kept one set of each in Cambridge and the other in New York. That way, I could travel lightly between the two cities. If I wasn't going to be in Cambridge anymore, *what would I do with all the twos?*

After rearranging my drawers, I decided to pull every piece of clothing off my shelves and reorganize them. I put a suitcase and cardboard box on the floor into which I would throw unwanted items. There were so many clothes that didn't fit me properly or that were "too young" for me. I had saved them in case I had a daughter. When I was growing up, I loved pilfering my mother's closet for clothes from the '70s. My daughter could pilfer my clothes from the '80s and '90s. *But for whom was I saving them now?*

During these weeks, I lost a lot of buttons. They fell off my jackets and sweaters. *There, I lost another button today—this time off of a long-sleeved white shirt.* I looked up the significance of buttons and found that they imply the need to find ways to keep certain things together. If you lose a button, or if a button is broken, it means that alternate ways need to be found. Buttons represent the outer self.

Many times in my head I played and replayed my life with Jay. *What drove him away? When will he come back? Will he come back? Were there clues along the way that I had missed? Was it the experience with the Fertility Center? Was it the cancer? Was it our working together?* I don't know if and when these questions might be answered, and Jay's and my story is still being written. But this is where the story has to end for this book.

Cheryl Strayed, the author of *Wild*, the first book I read after my surgery, wrote in her online advice column, *Dear Sugar*: "The best thing you can possibly do with your life is to tackle the motherfucking shit out of love. . . . Let yourself be gutted. Let it open you. Start there. . . . All right is almost always where we eventually land, even if we fuck up entirely along the way."[12]

On Christmas morning, a few weeks after our separation began, I received a text message from a friend: "Merry Xmas Tanya! Let me know how you are. Xxx." I texted back, "Thank you. I'm very sad, but I'll be okay. Please have a great time with your family."

She called immediately.

I said, "I'm sad, and I think he's sad, too. He's still the same person I married. These last few months were awful. He left me no choice. But I miss him." My friend said, "Oh, honey. This softening is good, the remorse. It's better than attack mode. This is more real." She was commenting on the devastation and anger that I had shared with her after Jay first left me. Then she told me about her visit with her family: "We went to my sister's church. It was fabulous. The pastor was fabulous. He gave a sermon about the journey. It's about the journey, no matter how long or hard. Joseph and Mary crossed the desert when she was nine months pregnant. He couldn't leave her alone because they weren't married. She would have been stoned if she were alone. What they didn't know was that the angels were following them, the wise men were tracking the stars. All these things were converging to protect them, but they didn't know that. They just kept going."

Silence as I took this in . . .

Then she said, "I hate to see you go through this. You're a good person, Tanya. I have a feeling though that everything will work out."

I thought a lot about my father during this time. Sometimes I would call out aloud or in my head for him and my grandparents to protect me. The week before my father died, a doctor came to the waiting room where I was sitting with my mother. He whispered to her that my father had told him he was dying. "I'm dying, Doc." Each day after that became a routine. Standing outside his room, sitting by his bedside, watching the monitor for his heartbeat, watching him sleep and breathe—one breath, one long breath, one short breath, one heavy breath, one syncopated breath. Some nights, always at night, he was totally alert. One of those nights, I was alone with him in his room. His mind was melting, and he was far away. But he said to me, "I love you. I'll watch over you. I'll make sure you don't stray."

Shortly after my separation, a friend gave me a book called *When Things Fall Apart* by the Buddhist teacher Pema Chödrön. I learned that Chödrön had gone on her own spiritual quest after her husband announced that he was leaving her and had been having an affair. In the book, she wrote, "Hopelessness means that we no longer have the spirit for holding our trip together. We may still *want* to hold our trip together. We long to have some reliable, comfortable ground under our feet, but we've tried a thousand ways to hide and a thousand ways to tie up all the loose ends, and the ground just keeps moving under us. Trying to get lasting security teaches us a lot, because if we never try to do it, we never notice that it can't be done."[13]

Reading kept my mind occupied in those sad days. Books kept me company when I was most alone. I read a book called *Wave* by a Sri Lankan author, Sonali Deraniyagala. She wrote about losing three generations of her family—her parents, two sons, and husband—in the 2004 tsunami. Everything she lived for was mercilessly ripped away from her in an instant. Lines from her book opened me up to the grief I didn't know how to overcome. She wrote, "How can I sleep? If I sleep now I will forget. I will forget what happened. I will wake believing everything is fine."[14] I had done this. Every morning I woke up thinking that what had happened had been a bad dream.

On February 10, 2013, a few months after Jay left, I forced myself to get out of my house and get some air. I walked up East Broadway on the Lower East Side, and in the distance, I heard drums and gongs. It sounded like Chinese New Year, and I walked toward the noise until I reached a small group gathered at a storefront watching a dragon inside. The Year of the Snake was beginning. A year ago, the Year of the Dragon, I had been about to start IVF.

I started writing this book after my third miscarriage. At the time, I didn't know where my journey would take me. I didn't know I would pursue IVF. I didn't know I would be diagnosed with two types of cancer. I didn't know I would face my own mortality. I didn't know my husband would want to separate.

The year 2012 turned out to be my "rumble strip," the year everything fell apart. It had started out so promising, with the hope that we would finally start a family. But then life happened, and by the end of the year, I felt like my life was over. Instead of completely crumbling, however, I reminded myself to keep breathing, to put one foot in front of the other, to keep moving . . . and I kept writing. *I will share my story so that others don't feel like they're alone. I will share my story so that others can learn from it. I will share my story so that others can avoid my mistakes—and make better decisions about their own futures.*

CHAPTER 11
ACTION ITEMS FOR THE FUTURE

My path had many twists, but every story about delayed motherhood and infertility is unique. I'm not the only woman whose cancer was discovered incidentally through the IVF process. I'm also not the only woman whose relationship was sorely tested while grappling with infertility.

When you enter the world of fertility treatments, what you are willing to do is often miles away from what you thought you'd be willing to do. Where you end up is often completely different from what you anticipated. Although where I am thus far feels devastating, I still have aspirations to become a mother, whether biologically or through other means. And deep down I feel that this dream will be real someday.

Having been through my own experiences, I want to make sure that other women on similar journeys are better prepared and more aware of their options before they begin. I want them to have the basic facts about their fertility at their fingertips and to think about their future fertility before it's too late. I want women to know there are many ways to be a mother, and also that there are many ways to find fulfillment aside from being a mother. I want women to think carefully about why they should or shouldn't pursue motherhood. I want them to be supported more in that pursuit by their partners, families, communities, doctors, insurance providers, and governments.

By nature, I'm an activist. I believe in turning adversity into action. I believe everything we do, no matter how small, can make a difference. Through my struggles to have a child, I learned a lot, and I am hopeful that the ideas I propose will lead to a better reproductive future and better future in general for all women. These ideas are by no means new. Many of them are already being championed in various sectors. They just need to become more widespread and entrenched so that they result in long-lasting changes in individual choices and societal attitudes.

These ideas, which I call Action Items, include

1. Share your stories.
2. Know your fertility.
3. Free yourself from convention.
4. Strategize for your goals.
5. Don't be afraid of feminism.
6. Advocate for a better future.

SHARE YOUR STORIES

When women share their experiences, they help take the shame out of infertility. During my visits to the Fertility Center, everyone in the waiting room barely looked at each other, let alone talked to each other. It was unfortunate that so many of us in the same situation in the same room kept our eyes down as we waited for our names to be called.

A number of women I spoke to for this book did not want their stories or at least their names to be public. This is a personal choice. Infertility is a subjective and individual experience that can often be painful to discuss. Every woman is different. Not everyone wants the world to know what she is going through. But you can talk to a friend or a group of friends. Sharing on an intimate basis is telling your story, too.

You never know when your experience could benefit someone else. The more these stories get out there, the more we will see them in the books and magazines we read and in the movies and television programs we watch. What isn't happening enough now is an intergenerational dialogue on the subject of motherhood and delayed motherhood. At the college level, we have educational programs about reproductive health and well-being, but eighteen-year-olds are let loose on the world without being made aware of the reality of their fertilities and the eventual work/life balance issues that they are sure to encounter.

Some women are taking on the task of informing the next generation in incidental ways. My friend Natalie Dean proactively starts the conversation with her students. She said, "As a graduate school adjunct instructor and a mentor to new teachers, I know many women this age [thirties]. Some of them are married and considering their options; others are not in long-term relationships and are feeling pressure. For those younger women with whom I'm friends, I tell them my story, and I tell them it's not uncommon. I tell them that the only medical reason doctors have found explaining my infertility is that my eggs are 'old.'"[1]

Caroline Reeves, the Chinese historian with two young sons she had at the ages of thirty-nine and forty-one, told me about a recent slipup made by a colleague of hers, but it led to an honest conversation about delayed motherhood:

> I had my women historians of China group over. All *very* smart women, a social networking group of senior and young scholars. One woman, who is finishing her PhD at Yale, came for the first time. She is in the kitchen with me, helping me put out the food, and she says, "I see you have some toys here for young children! Do you have grandchildren?" I nearly swallowed my tongue. Okay, I may be a Chinese History professor in my fifties, but this poor young girl must be soooo out of it if she has no idea that *this is her future* if she is going to procreate—if she thinks she is going to be some hot-shot scholar, she better understand that women in their fifties often have no choice but to be mothers of young children, if they're lucky enough to make time for that *at all*, not *grandmothers*!!!!! Let us just say, she will *not* be making that mistake again. I helped her understand that that was not a good way to put things.[2]

We can also lean on our educators and health professionals to have more honest conversations about these issues. Dr. Arthur Greil, professor of sociology at Alfred University, believes we have come a long way in terms of fertility awareness. He said, "When I started doing research in the mid-eighties, people were unaware of infertility. Many people I interviewed said they hadn't even heard of infertility until they started to try to become pregnant. I think it largely had to do with a culturally based aversion to talking about sex as well as to stigma surrounding infertility."[3] Crystal Wilmhoff, lead clinician at Planned Parenthood Southwest Ohio Region, said, "I do talk about these things—infertility, miscarriage, and delaying motherhood—all the time with patients and with friends and family. I think they are not talked about by people that have not experienced them, but once you have, you are amazed at how many other people have had similar experiences."[4]

As important as it is for women to talk to experts and other women, it is just as vital that women talk to their partners—female and male—and to figure out how best to have these conversations. The problems that erupted in my marriage are an extreme example of the impact infertility can have on a relationship, but there are numerous types of situations out there. One friend who began to pursue IVF said her boyfriend kind of regressed during the process. She said he seemed "overwhelmed" whenever she tried to talk about it. She started to wonder if she was with the right guy. By the time I completed this book, they were still together but hadn't yet gone through with a cycle because he had started saying he was unsure about becoming a parent, at least with her. Another friend had a serious boyfriend with whom she wanted to have children, but he claimed he wasn't ready—he was fifty-five years old! Another friend said her husband avoided going to almost all the fertility clinic appointments with her. She felt like she was totally alone in the endeavor. They ultimately divorced. We need to open up the dialogue about the specific issues men and women face in the dramatically changed landscape of when and how we become parents so there isn't a trail of blood, or at least devastated emotions, when couples cave under pressure.

Infertility is an indelibly existential, exhausting, and often shocking experience. We all need to talk and listen to each other. Don't be scared of the conversation. Be open to each other's feelings. And seek outside help when possible and necessary. We are wired in particular and different ways, and we don't have to face these issues alone.

We can also help break the silence through online networks. Through this medium, women can engage with others on the issues while in the privacy of their homes. Sheryl Sandberg has launched such a community around the issue of women and leadership in conjunction with her book *Lean In*. For those with infertility issues, RESOLVE, the national infertility association, has abundant resources on its website for both in-person and online support groups.[5] Another resource is the Anonymous Us Project, founded by musician and writer Alana S. Newman. The mission, as stated on its website, is to provide "a safety zone for real and honest opinions about reproductive technologies and family fragmentation. We aim to share the experiences of . . . participants in these technologies, while preserving the dignity and privacy for story-tellers and their loved ones."[6] People can anonymously submit their stories about pursuing fertility treatments, being the children of sperm donors, and so on.

Those who have struggled with fertility issues can contribute to the information pool by exchanging their stories. It's not just about having more agency in your own life; it's about recognizing that you are part of a community. Having more stories in the public sphere helps take the shame and secrecy out of infertility. While your privacy is important, your candor can benefit others in profound ways.

KNOW YOUR FERTILITY

It's hard to imagine that women, especially those with a college education, don't know the basics of their own fertilities, but I am constantly amazed by how little women grasp of the reality of their biological clocks. Part of the problem is that they were never taught about the subject in any substantive way. Another part is that, while there is a growing volume of writings on the subject, there is so much mixed messaging in the mass media. Women who see their friends and celebrities getting pregnant in their forties assume they will be like them, too. They don't know, until they try, how improbable getting pregnant and carrying a baby to term can be at that age. Laura Dawn, the creative director who was forty-three when she had her baby, said now she would advise women to wait only until they're around thirty to try to get pregnant. She added, "Don't wait past thirty-five if you can help it."

One of the simpler lessons I took away from my story is that "knowledge is power." As Crystal Wilmhoff of Planned Parenthood explained, "People need to have a fundamental knowledge of how their body works so they are able to make informed choices regarding when and/or how to prevent or enhance their fertility."[7] But because we aren't automatically given information about our fertility, we have to educate ourselves. I don't know if my journey could have been any different, but if I had been more aware of the statistics against me, I might have pursued IVF earlier and more aggressively, possibly at thirty-seven after my first miscarriage instead of at forty. I wouldn't have waited until after three miscarriages for a doctor to tell me to have a fertility workup.

In 2009, the American Fertility Association, based in New York City, came up with a fun and quirky way to get people thinking about these issues. It launched a series of events called "Manicures & Martinis" at the Dashing Diva Nail Salon in Manhattan. A fertility expert was onsite to speak to women in their twenties and thirties. Health advocates criticized the offering of martinis, especially since alcohol can negatively impact fertility, but organic alcohol-free "Fertilitinis" were on the menu as well.[8]

Seek out knowledge about fertility. Don't wait until things go wrong. There are numerous books that can help—some of which I list in the resources section later in this book. Tina Merrill, the COO of a social media technology company, told me, "As a young woman I was primarily concerned with not getting pregnant. I think a better understanding of one's body and cycle is important. I credit the book, *Taking Charge of Your Fertility*, for Sam's quick conception. We had been casually 'trying' by not using contraception for six months with no results. Once I followed the fertility-monitoring program, I conceived on my second cycle. It's very empowering in general to have this deeper understanding of your body."[9]

There are also a lot of great mobile device apps that focus on infertility (like My Mobile Fertility), fertility trackers (like iPeriod), and pregnancy guides (like BabyCenter and Sprout). Search for ones that work for you. Make sure to read the ratings and reviews. I hope more apps will be developed, especially by organizations like RESOLVE and the Guttmacher Institute, both of which have a wealth of resources on these subjects.

In addition, you can ask your doctor to test your fertility. Through bloodwork and ultrasounds, you can have your ovarian reserve and ovaries tested and find out if you have signs of ovarian aging. Insurance typically won't cover an elective fertility checkup, but the tests can be worth the expense because awareness can lead to better choices and better outcomes.

When it comes to fertility treatments, the science can change quickly, so always update your knowledge. For example, when I started writing this book in late 2011, egg freezing was still considered experimental. A year later, it wasn't, and many celebrities, feminists, and even doctors were endorsing it. In a few years, who knows what the landscape will be?

FREE YOURSELF FROM CONVENTION

This book is full of stories from women who tried to set up their lives in a particular order only to discover that neither the timetable nor the outcome was entirely within their control. Gail Sheehy, author of the groundbreaking book on menopause, *The Silent Passage*, also wrote *Passages: Predictable Crises of Adult Life*, about different stages of adulthood. In this latter book she explained, "The Trying Twenties confronts us with the questions of how to take hold in the adult world. . . . [O]ur concentration during the Trying Twenties is on mastering what we feel we are *supposed* to do. The distinction is between the previous transition, the Pulling Up Roots years, when we knew what we *didn't want* to do, and the next transition, into the thirties, which will prod us toward doing what we *want* to do."[10]

She goes on to talk about the many "shoulds" with which some of us grow up, including graduate school, career, marriage, and children, and the impact those "shoulds" have on our approach to making decisions. "One of the terrifying aspects of the twenties is the conviction that the choices we make are irrevocable. If we choose a graduate school or join a firm, get married or don't marry, move to the suburbs or forego travel abroad, decide against children or against a career, we fear in our marrow that we might have to live with that choice forever. It is largely a false fear."[11]

However, we do have a finite amount of time to have a biological child. I've talked about how for much of my twenties I enjoyed my lifestyle and my career and didn't focus on my goal of motherhood. Moreover, I had decided I didn't want to be a single mother. In hindsight, I wished I'd had the courage and determination of my friends who said they weren't going to wait to have everything in place before having a child. I felt that if I bucked certain norms my family would be embarrassed. But in truth, my family would have supported me as long as I was happy and a good person. It was up to me to break free of what I assumed people wanted of me.

I have a friend, a Manhattan-based producer and performer in her early fifties, who I feel truly epitomizes someone who has carved her own way. She said her journey to have a child was a "long and emotionally exhausting process," during which she "was unclear if [she] would actually get to bear a child." She had been in a fourteen-year relationship with a man, and she began to speak with him about having children when she was thirty-two. He ended the relationship when she was thirty-seven. Eventually, she had a daughter at the age of forty-two with a gay male friend who would later become her husband. Initially, she wasn't glad she had waited to have children, but she said, "Once I had the child, I was very pleased to be at this point in my life becoming a mom. Lots of the *sturm* and *drang* of one's twenties and thirties are past, and I was utterly clear that this was what I wanted to be doing. I didn't have the worry that it would overtake my identity ('I used to be an artist, but now everyone just sees me as a mom' sort of thing). I knew who I was and what I wanted." She calls her home now a "commune of a loft" with other adults cohabiting, including a close girlfriend and her daughter. Parenting duties are shared, and everyone has a lot of fun. Another friend who is in her early forties and wants to have children but isn't in a relationship says she has been talking to women she knows in similar situations about going to a sperm bank, moving in together, and jointly raising their children.

Many women think they have to figure out their careers and relationships first. But if you know you want a child, don't make that decision dependent on being established in your career or finding the right partner. Diminish your dependence on tradition; don't let it prevent you from putting yourself boldly forward into a better future that is more in line with your personal vision.

STRATEGIZE FOR YOUR GOALS

For those women who, like me, delayed motherhood then struggled to have a child, we did have options. We chose to prioritize our educations and careers. We also enjoyed our lives without kids, even though many of us wanted eventually to have kids. Basically, we wanted to live by our own timetables without the constraints and responsibilities of motherhood. Victoria Birk Hill went through seven years of fertility treatments and three failed IVF cycles before adopting a daughter. Now she is the managing director of a Michigan-based wellness center called in Harmony and also works with Dr. Carole Kowalczyk of the Michigan Center for Fertility & Women's Health. As she put it, "It is a personal journey, and we are all ready for the responsibility at different times in our life."[12]

Generations of women before mine were told what to do. Then my generation was told to do what we wanted, but we didn't have many role models to emulate. Now there are many role models—women who've dealt with the work/life balance, who've delayed motherhood, who've pursued fertility treatments, who've built families with their lesbian partners or gay male friends. These were new frontiers when I was growing up, but now we have lessons to pass along to the next generation. I have learned the importance of asking questions about what I don't know. Be inquisitive. Be proactive.

No matter how advanced reproductive technologies are, they aren't guaranteed to work. Dr. William Kutteh, director of Fertility Associates of Memphis in Tennessee, said it's important for women to understand before they come to his center that "we can solve some but not all problems."[13] Don't be cynical but be skeptical, and don't be afraid to ask questions. Responsible medical professionals will prepare you with the odds. When egg freezing was being championed in fall 2012, Dr. Eric Widra of Shady Grove Fertility Center cautioned, "This is not a technology that should be used to cure societal ills or societal pressures. We do live in an unfortunately complex society, where women often do have to make these choices. But the reality is, the number one factor in infertility is delayed childbearing."[14]

Be mindful that if you delay, no matter how many precautions you have taken—like freezing your eggs or sticking to a fertility-friendly diet every day—you might not be able to have a biological child. Moreover, there are many factors that impact fertility regardless of age. What holds true for one woman can be very different for another. Ultimately, the most important thing for any individual is to choose happiness—to be a happy and healthy individual, and if you are a parent, to raise happy and healthy children. As much as possible, decisions should be made based on that goal, and you should set goals for yourself that are attainable and adaptable.

Anticipating and figuring out the balance between motherhood and career is a difficult endeavor. Dr. Karina Shreffler, associate professor in Human Development and Family Science at Oklahoma State University, said,

Unfortunately, many professional careers have a period of time where you have to work extra hard to "make it." For example, after medical school, there is a residency period characterized by very long shifts and inflexibility. Some attorneys work to make partner, and professors work to get tenure. If you don't put in long hours, you will not succeed in these professions for which you have worked hard to earn a degree. Unfortunately, the period that you are required to put in all the hours (both in graduate school and as a new professional) overlaps with women's prime child-bearing years. I don't think it's always a case of prioritizing career as much as it is just trying to get your career established so that you can then focus on having children. Of course, sometimes fertility postponed is fertility foregone![15]

Jenny Davidson, a professor at Columbia University, advised,

Think seriously about your vision for your adult life over the long haul. You can choose a few things to prioritize, and if you're lucky you'll achieve a good deal of fulfillment in those few (sometimes, too, success comes in unexpected forms or realms that are not quite what we'd choose but are thoroughly satisfactory replacements for whatever we had imagined). But just as if you want to write novels, you should think very seriously about the costs of entering a demanding career path on some professional track and having children, so if you want to have children you should think about how this fits into the whole picture of other choices before you. Sometimes the desire for one thing or another really will have to take a hit.[16]

Catherine Gund, a filmmaker and cofounder of the Third Wave Foundation, believes we have to start being more creative. She asked,

We know we can pursue school, career and family but what are some new and different ways to combine? How can we enlist more extended family and more of our friends to weave their lives together with us and our children? More and more people are working at least part of the time from home; lots of professions allow for that. And it can be smoothly combined with having kids. Sometimes simplicity is in order, making compromises, but ones that provide the lifestyle you love. I made my office in my house so it's easy to work at night when the kids are sleeping. That way I can be around for them after school. That's what I want. That would make a lot of people crazy, but it makes me happy.[17]

As author Peggy Orenstein has written, "It doesn't help that the world of children continues to be run as if women don't work, or can drop whatever they're doing at a moment's notice."[18] Let your employer know about your goals and the demands on your time. If you are working for someone who does not give you enough leeway to pursue motherhood, then you might not be with the right employer. But ask for what you want before coming to that conclusion. You might be someone who needs a more flexible work schedule. Soon-Young Yoon, the chair of the NGO Committee on the Status of Women in New York, advised, "Hire help even if it costs one's entire salary so that there is no interference with what one wants to do with a career and other projects."[19] As Amy Richards, the feminist author and also a cofounder of the Third Wave Foundation, has written, "There might be a right way for each family, but there's not a single right way for all families."[20]

A number of companies have developed pioneering family-friendly policies. According to an October 20, 2012, article in the *New York Times* on how Silicon Valley is leading the way, "Facebook gives new parents $4,000 in spending money. Stanford School of Medicine is piloting a project to provide doctors with housecleaning and in-home dinner delivery. Genentech offers take-home dinners and helps employees find last-minute baby sitters when a child is too sick to go to school." Facebook also gives employees take-home dinners or their families can eat with them on the campus. In addition, it subsidizes $3,000 per family for childcare and up to $5,000 for adoption expenses.[21]

Along with these measures, the walls of the office should be more permeable in our increasingly mobile and interconnected world. The workplace can be where you need it to be. For some women, that means choosing careers that allow them to work from a home office. For other women, it could mean working out a flexible schedule with their employer. Women should be allowed to work at home or at least work *more* hours at home. Women shouldn't have to choose between being in the office and taking their kids to the doctor.

When Yahoo!, under the leadership of CEO Marissa Mayer, issued a memo against telecommuting to its employees in early 2013, telecommuters and stay-at-home workers around the country raised an uproar. They felt especially offended by lines in the memo such as "Speed and quality are often sacrificed when we work from home."[22] As National Public

Radio reported, a University of Iowa survey found that people who work at home actually put in more time than those who work in the office—approximately five to seven hours more per week. Rebecca Hughes-Parker, a New York-based lawyer and mother of three who works part-time at home, said, "This kind of policy goes backwards in time to when you really had to be chained to a desk and didn't have the flexibility to run to a child's doctor's appointment, answer e-mails on the way if you had to, and then come back. I think it's very scary for people to think those things are going to be taken away from them."[23] By April, Yahoo! softened its stance. Although it didn't change its policy about not working from home, it instituted a new policy that gave both mothers and fathers eight weeks of fully paid leave and up to $500 for expenses such as childcare and laundry.[24]

Giving women and men the option to work at home allows both parents the opportunity to be more actively engaged in the parenting process. On the other hand, it's important to be aware of the needs of your coworkers and communicate with them about your schedule. While some may have no problem accommodating the demands made on them by your duties as a parent, others may feel they are picking up too much of your slack. As a March 2011 survey of 600 employees on work/life balance and flexibility showed, "Many co-workers are left to scramble because a colleague neglected to say that he was leaving early, working from home that day or taking every Friday in August off."[25] Journalist Hannah Seligson wrote in the New York Times, "In theory, flextime seems like an everyone-wins proposition. But one person's work-life balance can be another's work-life overload. Someone, after all, has to make that meeting or hit that deadline. As a result, many Americans who work for companies that embrace flexible hours are confronting a sort of office class warfare. Some employees have come to expect that the demands of their children, in particular, will be accommodated—and not all of their colleagues are happy about it."[26]

For example, what if a coworker says, "Having children is your choice, why should I have to comply with your needs?" Why isn't making the decision to have a family much like an employee saying "I just bought a house, so you'll have to give me a raise so I can pay for it"? Anne-Marie Slaughter, who launched the "having it all" debate in 2012, wrote that a solution to alleviating this tension could be "reason-neutral flexible work." As she explained, "It could be to take care of children or elderly parents, or it could be because an employee simply works better at home part of the time. The great advantage here is that parents, mothers in particular, are not singled out and stigmatized."[27]

Thinking strategically requires effort. It involves projecting what we want our lives to look like in the future and imagining how the choices we make today might help or prevent us from getting to that place. Despite your best efforts, a balance between science, society, and personal goals might be unattainable. In truth, we might achieve only moments of balance instead of a sustained lifetime of balance, but clarifying our objectives and linking them with actions are steps we all can take.

DON'T BE AFRAID OF FEMINISM

I started calling myself a feminist when I was in college, getting involved with various women's causes and groups on campus. This identity became stronger when I was a young activist organizing youth arts and culture programs for the NGO Forum on Women in China in 1995. I encountered women from around the world for whom the core tenets of feminism were a foundation for demanding better access to healthcare, education, jobs, and so on. I realized how lucky I was to live in America, where I felt relatively free to do and say what I wanted compared to women from other countries.

When someone says feminism is no longer necessary, I think, *Tell that to the mother raising five kids who can't get paid as much as a man to do the same job; tell that to the woman who is treated as the aggressor when she is raped; tell that to the girl who isn't allowed to learn how to read, and so on.* It's a Big Lie that we don't need feminism.

You might not want to call yourself a feminist; you might not identify with famous feminists; but can't you get behind what feminism advocates? Feminism encourages a broader democratic framework that counters the fundamentalist backlash, which is a never-ending threat to women around the world every day. As long as a girl can be shot for seeking an education (as happened to Malala Yousafzai in Pakistan in October 2012), as long as a female student can be raped and killed by a group of men on a bus (as happened in India in December 2012), as long as women need to stage a driving protest to ask for their right to drive their own cars (as happened in

Saudi Arabia in June 2011), as long as a woman can ask for contraception coverage and be called a slut (as happened to Sandra Fluke in the United States in March 2012), we need feminism.

Women have been "leaning in," to use Sheryl Sandberg's exhortation, for centuries, but we are too often ignored, held back, or excluded. The world has to be inherently fair for results to come from women leaning in. As Amy Richards explained, "While Anne-Marie Slaughter and Sheryl Sandberg are correct in calling upon women to step up more, they are asking women to enter a broken system. It will take a long time to fix it, and for some women, the suffering they might encounter is not worth it."[28]

If you believe in social justice and the continuing threat to women's freedoms everywhere, feminism is necessary just as civil rights activism and gay rights activism are still necessary. The need for vigilance and more progress never ends and must be kept up every day. As author Caitlin Moran wrote in *How to Be a Woman*, "An old-fashioned feminist 'consciousness-raising' still has enormous value. When the subject turns to abortion, cosmetic intervention, birth, motherhood, sex, love, work, misogyny, fear, or just how you feel in your own skin, women still won't often tell the truth unless they are very, very drunk . . . while chipping in your two cents on what it's *actually* like—rather than what we *pretend* it's like—to be a woman is vital, we still also need a bit of analysis-y, argument-y, 'this needs to change-y' stuff. You know. Feminism."[29]

So don't be afraid to be a feminist. You don't have to join the fight for women's rights, but you can support those rights in whatever way makes sense for you. When I was growing up, there was a tension between feminism—which told women to do what they wanted—and the medical establishment—which told women not to delay motherhood. What we can do moving forward is recast feminism to incorporate more fully the reality of our fertilities.

ADVOCATE FOR A BETTER FUTURE

After communicating with Dr. Pasquale Patrizio for over a year via e-mail, I visited him in person at the Yale Fertility Center in New Haven, Connecticut. When I arrived, his assistant escorted me to his office and explained that he was doing an egg retrieval but would be with me shortly. A few minutes later, he entered wearing blue hospital scrubs and a shower cap. During our conversation, I asked him if there are countries that have gotten it right when it comes to supporting women who need fertility treatments. He said, "Yes, Belgium, Israel, Sweden . . ." because their governments sponsor enough research, insurance is generous, and work policies are more accommodating.[30] I also asked him if he could envision a time when America will be more like those countries with regard to the landscape around fertility treatments. He said, "Definitely." I was surprised by his optimism, but Dr. Patrizio said that with enough pressure from constituencies and enough people voicing their desires for change, reform has to come. He argued that infertility has to be viewed as a disease and that treatments are not elective procedures but medical necessities. He said, "Considering infertility as a non-disease is bogus."[31]

Crystal Wilmhoff of Planned Parenthood Southwest Ohio Region believes that a core issue is "that politics, insurance companies etc. try to control women's fertility."[32] Whether you identify as a feminist or not, you can encourage initiatives to call for better social policies that support people more in their pursuit of parenthood and to increase education and awareness. Jennifer Braunschweiger, deputy editor of *More* magazine, has written about alleviating the burdens on both stay-at-home and working mothers: "All of us should get out there and agitate for whatever political and corporate solutions we believe in; families shouldn't have to figure this out alone. But until then, let's find in ourselves some sympathy for other people's circumstances."[33] And if Dr. Patrizio is right, which I believe he is, there are steps we can all take to advocate for a better future.

The first building block is better education about infertility and the impact of delaying motherhood. Mindy Berkson, the Chicago-based infertility consultant, said, "This messaging needs to be targeted to college age and graduate school women. Advertising and media are venues to disseminate the important educational message."[34]

In addition, we should have nationally mandated insurance coverage for fertility treatments, including egg freezing (we can learn from Israel, which doesn't consider egg freezing elective). Having a child should not be a luxury. The Family Act, giving people a tax credit for fertility treatments, is a must. Some might contend that such tax credits should only be given to couples that have a genetic or medical reason to pursue treatment. But we live in a society that encourages people to delay parenthood for a variety of reasons, including job security and economic stability. RESOLVE has great tools and suggestions for advocacy. You can visit its website at http:// www.resolve.org and sign a pledge committing to help further education and awareness.

Another building block is policy reform. In her book on French parenting, *Bringing up Bébé*, Pamela Druckerman argues that perhaps the United States can learn something from French social policies with regard to parenting. As she explains, for French women, "There's the national paid maternity leave (the United States has none), the subsidized nannies and crèches, the free universal preschool from age three, and myriad tax credits and payments for having kids. All this doesn't ensure that there's equality between men and women. But it does ensure that Frenchwomen can have both a career and kids."[35]

Dr. Arthur Greil agrees that the lack of such social policies hinders prospective mothers in America: "For individual women, the key issue is the balancing act between career and motherhood. But that is a socially constructed issue. Social policies could reduce work/family conflict and make this much less of an issue."[36] Dr. Karina Shreffler explains further, "The United States is the only developed country in the world without at least a minimal amount of paid maternity leave. We also do not have subsidized childcare unless you are close to poverty, and quality infant care costs more than public university tuition. There is research that fertility is linked to the economy, so making it easier for families to have the children that they want to have (if, indeed, they want to have them) would be a key strategy, in my opinion." Many people don't have children because they can't afford them, and this in turn impacts fertility rates, particularly during a recession. Dr. Shreffler said we need "flexibility in work hours, paid maternity leave and sick leave (to care for children in addition to oneself), breastfeeding opportunities, and subsidized quality childcare."[37]

Inequities in pay and job promotion are additional obstacles to women pursuing motherhood. In 1992, Lawrence Perlman, CEO of the Ceridian Corporation, gave a speech titled "A Pregnant CEO: In Whose Lifetime?" in which he said, "If women must choose between having children and being a significant part of their care, or being paid 65 percent of what a male counterpart is earning (who is also 20 times more likely to be promoted into a top job), it is not difficult to see why women might leave their companies to seek better opportunities elsewhere. If companies want stronger career commitment from women, they should hasten to correct pay inequities and create equal opportunities for promotion."[38]

Although family-leave policies have greatly improved over the past few decades, as labor economist Francine Blau said in an interview in the *Atlantic*,

> Especially in very high level jobs, it's how much commitment can you give? Are you working 10 to 15 hours a day? It's not just a question of full time, but above and beyond, 60 hours a week. So it [family-leave policy] could be influential there. It could impact what occupations and industries women go into as well. It might make it more difficult in some that are actually higher paying. So I think that there's no question that if we want to improve outcomes for women, we have to look at these work family issues and see how we can help accommodate balance without major detriment to either sphere.[39]

A partial solution aside from alleviating pay inequity is encouraging men to participate in childcare as well. While parental leave is available to both men and women in some countries, women tend to take it more often. For instance, in some Scandinavian countries, as Francine Blau explains, there's a "use it or lose it" parental leave just for men, meaning that the family gets a certain amount of leave only if the father takes it.[40]

Getting more women into leadership positions can result in more motherhood-friendly reforms. As Laura Dawn, the creative director formerly of MoveOn.org, told me, "We outnumber men and yet we STILL don't have universal paid maternity leave in this country? We need to organize and fight for our rights. Women DO hold up the world—it's time we had a voice in its governance."[41]

While having women at the top does not guarantee that such policies will be enacted, the underrepresentation of women is part of the problem. As Peggy Orenstein writes, citing a Families and Work Institute report, "Having a few token women in top positions doesn't affect the culture of an institution. It's not until women fill half or more of upper-level jobs that companies become more likely to provide near-site day care, elder care resource and referral programs, and that options such as flextime can be pursued without penalty. But here's the rub: Until those humanizing factors are in place, women will have a hard time achieving the numbers necessary to make change."[42]

Around the world, out of 190 heads of state, only nine are women. The landscape of women in leadership positions can be surprising from country to country. For example, in the United States, only 18.3 percent of government seats are held by women in the 113th Congress (up from 17 percent in the 112th), but in Norway, Iceland, Finland, Sweden, Cuba, Nicaragua, South Africa, and Rwanda, at least 40 percent of government seats are held by women.[43] In Saudi Arabia, ranked one of the worst countries in the world for women's rights, King Abdullah has begun opening the doors to some progress by appointing women to the Shura Council, amending the law to ensure that women make up no less than 20 percent of the council, and announcing that women would be able to run and vote in the 2015 elections.[44] Of all the people in parliaments in the world, only 13 percent are women.[45]

In the corporate sector, the statistics are also disheartening. The European Commission estimated that women account for fewer than 15 percent of nonexecutive board positions in companies with more than 250 staff. Some countries have shown improvement. For example, Norway has successfully enforced a 40 percent quota since 2009. British-listed companies rose from 7 percent women in nonexecutive board positions in 1999 to 12.5 percent in 2010. The European Commission wanted to make companies favor female nonexecutive board candidates where they are equally qualified and in 2012 set an objective of having 40 percent women boards by 2020.[46]

A combination of shifting attitudes toward gender, incredible advances in reproductive science, and an opening up of opportunities led many women of my generation to delay motherhood. Together we can advocate for improved education, insurance coverage, and work/life policy reform and build a better future. As a result, the next generations of women will benefit from the realizations of my generation.

ADVICE FOR WOMEN OF DIFFERENT REPRODUCTIVE AGES

The Action Items above can be broken down further to offer specific suggestions for women of different reproductive ages.

(1) If you are up to twenty-one years old:

   (a) Find out the fertility basics. Here are a few resources to start with:

   Association of Reproductive Health Professionals (http://www.arhp.org)

   CDC Division of Reproductive Health (http://www.cdc.gov/reproductivehealth/)

   Guttmacher Institute (http://www.guttmacher.org/)

   Planned Parenthood (http://www.plannedparenthood.org/)

   RESOLVE (http://www.resolve.org)

   There are also many online communities dedicated to fertility, but some of the information is conflicting or incomplete, so remember to balance what you learn online with information from medical professionals.

   (b) Take care of your body. What you do now could affect your future chances of having a child. Be aware that smoking, drinking, and doing drugs could negatively impact your fertility. A healthy diet and exercise are also important.

   (c) Think about your goals. Do you want to be a mother? If so, how do you plan to accomplish it? With a partner? Could you do it on your own? Do you want a career? What kind of career? Do you want to have both a family and a career? How can you achieve balance? What does balance mean for you? How does it relate to your definition of happiness?

(2) If you are between the ages of twenty-one and thirty years old:

   (a) Pay more attention to all of the above. In particular, think more about your goals, as described in 1c.

   (b) Start exploring options for preserving your fertility, such as freezing your eggs. If you are in a committed relationship, you could consider freezing embryos.

(c) If you want to have children with a partner, be open to a partner who will be a good parent. As a friend said to me, the criteria for a mate shouldn't be simply whether the person "makes you breathless or makes you laugh." When considering a serious commitment to a partner that involves having children, think and talk about your respective reproductive goals and parenting approaches.

(d) If you are ready to get pregnant, pay extra attention to your weight and nutrition. Being either obese or too thin can impact your fertility. Look for foods that have vitamins C and E, zinc, and folic acid. Lower your caffeine intake.

(e) Educate yourself. Two great books are *Taking Charge of Your Fertility* and *Fully Fertile*. You could also explore getting a fertility workup with your ob/gyn.

(f) Make sure you have good insurance, preferably a carrier that covers fertility treatments. Be aware that where you live and work is a major factor in your ability to afford having and raising children. For example, only fifteen states in America have mandated coverage for fertility treatments, and certain states have more accommodating parental-leave policies than others. You might want to consider moving or traveling to a different state or country that offers more affordable alternatives for fertility treatments and more family-friendly work environments.

(3) If you are thirty years old and over:

(a) Pay even more attention to all of the above.

(b) If you are above thirty-five years old and having trouble getting pregnant or have had a miscarriage, get yourself to a fertility specialist sooner than even your ob/gyn might advise.

(c) If you are dealing with infertility and thinking of pursuing treatment, educate yourself. A good resource is *Budgeting for Infertility*.

(d) If you have not had a biological child by the age of forty despite pursuing treatment, start considering other options for becoming a mother—for example, egg donation and surrogacy. Think especially about adoption.

(e) If you are over forty-four years old, unless you have already frozen your eggs, think about pursuing the other options for becoming a mother. And be proud to do so!

On May 5, 2013, Cinco de Mayo, I went to see Sonia Sotomayor, the first Hispanic Supreme Court Justice, give a lecture at the PEN World Voices Literary Festival. After the event, I bought her lyrical and poignant memoir, *My Beloved World*, in which she writes, "There are uses to adversity, and they don't reveal themselves until tested. . . . Difficulty can tap unsuspected strengths."[47]

The adversity I experienced and heard about from others motivated me to seek better education and awareness about fertility, better tools to make choices about our futures, and better policies to support us in our pursuit of parenthood. I hope I've left you with some ideas about steps we all can take toward these objectives: (1) share your stories; (2) know your fertility; (3) free yourself from convention; (4) strategize for your goals; (5) don't be afraid of feminism; and (6) advocate for a better future.

EPILOGUE

My personal story is a work in progress, and who knows what the future will bring. I've worked hard on healing myself and honoring the years during which Jay and I were each other's best friend despite and maybe because of what we went through together. Our quest for parenthood and what I learned along the way motivated this book, but the lessons grew bigger and my world larger than I could have envisioned. My attempts to be a mother became part of the puzzle, of the journey, of who I am and what I get to be in this experience. Now, I can't predict how or with whom I will have a child.

But I believe if you're lucky, your life is long and takes you in unexpected directions. We adjust as we move forward. Sometimes you plan ahead, and you will your future into being. Sometimes you plan ahead, and your future doesn't come. But if you stay open to something else, then something else can happen.

Things go up and down; they fall apart and come back together. Each day that passes is one you should be proud to have experienced.

And I'm still here. I remind myself to be grateful for that. It's the greatest gift I ever got.

With my friends who have faced infertility after delaying motherhood, I talk about how hard it can be to see women around our age getting lucky and having kids. We also talk about how much more we can do for ourselves and in our careers because we don't have kids. And we talk about how important it is to honor and care for the people who are already here on this Earth.

The filmmaker Lucy Walker, a close friend who has also struggled with infertility, directed the Academy Award–nominated documentary called *Waste Land* about *catadores* (recyclables pickers) who work in the largest landfill in Brazil. One of the men, Valter, talks about how every can he picks matters, everything anyone does means something, every person is important. He says, "99 is not 100, and that single one will make the difference."

That kind of optimism is often sorely tested, as it was many times while I wrote this book. A six-year-old girl was among the twelve people shot and killed in a movie theater in Aurora, Colorado, in July 2012; twenty kids were among the twenty-eight people shot and killed within minutes in a school in Newtown, Connecticut, in December 2012; an eight-year-old boy was among the three casualties of the bombing at the Boston Marathon in April 2013. And hundreds of kids are killed in areas of conflict around the world every day. I saw a statistic that two hundred million kids wake up every morning and don't go to school; eight hundred million people alive today have grown up illiterate.[1]

After the Newtown shooting, President Obama said: "We've endured too many of these tragedies in the past few years. And each time I learn the news I react not as a President, but as anybody else would—as a parent. And that was especially true today. I know there's not a parent in America who doesn't feel the same overwhelming grief that I do."[2]

But you don't have to be a parent to care about these tragedies.

I hope this book touches people and inspires them to make changes in their world and in their own lives.

Now, in a sense, my journey is beginning again. I feel like I will find fulfillment in ways I could not have anticipated when I started this book. For all the debate about "having it all" in work and life, avoiding "the conflict" of modern motherhood, and "leaning in" to rise to the top of a career, sometimes the journey cannot be reduced to succinct phrases, and the most important goal is to find fulfillment within. Sometimes the best way forward is to begin again.

SUGGESTED RESOURCES

The following list is organized according to subjects discussed in this book: adoption, egg freezing, egg/sperm donation and surrogacy, feminism and the women's movement, fertility, fertility treatment financing, fertility treatments, and motherhood and parenting. I could have gone into much greater detail with some of the sections, but I have provided ideas to get you started on your own research. I will be updating the list at http://www.thebigliebook.com, and I welcome your suggestions.

ADOPTION

(Many thanks to Beth Hall of Pact, An Adoption Alliance for her input on this section.)

The Adoption Guide

http://www.theadoptionguide.com

The Adoption Guide provides lists of adoption agencies, adoption and ART attorneys, and donor and surrogacy professionals, in addition to resources about the adoption process (domestic, foster care, and international), costs, personal stories, and advice from professionals.

American Academy of Adoption Attorneys

http://www.adoptionattorneys.org

The AAAA provides a listing of adoption attorneys by state and has information on why you should hire an adoption attorney and what questions to ask to find the right attorney for your needs.

Child Welfare Information Gateway

http://www.childwelfare.gov

The Child Welfare Information Gateway connects child welfare and related professionals to information, resources, and tools covering topics including child abuse and neglect, foster care, adoption, and more.

Child Welfare League of America

http://www.cwla.org

The CWLA leads and engages its network of public and private agencies and partners to advance policies, best practices, and collaborative strategies that result in better outcomes for vulnerable children, youth, and families.

Creating a Family

http://www.creatingafamily.org

Creating a Family is a nonprofit providing education, resources, and support for those touched by infertility or adoption. The site features a regular blog, radio show, and links to find more information about infertility and adoption as well as service providers in your area.

Dave Thomas Foundation for Adoption

http://www.davethomasfoundation.org

This foundation focuses on finding families for children in foster care and has a wealth of resources on the reality and process of adopting foster children.

Evan B. Donaldson Adoption Institute

http://www.adoptioninstitute.org

The Adoption Institute aims to improve adoption laws, policies, and practices through research, education, and advocacy, and has a variety of events and publications available.

Joint Council on International Adoption

http://www.jointcouncil.org

Through an international coalition of over 260 child welfare organizations, the Joint Council helps orphaned and vulnerable children find permanent and safe families, and provides information for parents on international adoption.

The National Adoption Foundation

http://www.fundyouradoption.org

The NAF focuses on the financial needs of the adoption community and provides financial assistance through grants, loans, and other programs.

North American Council for Adoptable Children

http://www.nacac.org

Founded in 1974 by adoptive parents, NACAC provides advocacy, education, foster care, adoption support, and leadership development in the United States and Canada.

Pact, An Adoption Alliance

http://www.pactadopt.org

Pact is an adoption alliance focusing on adopted children of color and has resources for birth parents and adoptive parents, as well as services for adoptees.

EGG FREEZING

Eggsurance

http://www.eggsurance.com

A reliable online source on egg freezing, Eggsurance provides personal stories, step-by-step guides through the process, interviews with doctors, and recent articles on the topic.

Extend Fertility

http://www.extendfertility.com

Extend Fertility is a company created and run by women dedicated to providing fertility and fertility-preservation information. Its site offers information about egg freezing, affiliated centers across the country, and a regular newsletter.

EGG/SPERM DONATION AND SURROGACY

(Many thanks to Dr. Pasquale Patrizio for his input on this section.)

Donor Egg Bank USA

http://www.donoreggbankusa.com

Donor Egg Bank USA offers frozen eggs from diverse donors around the country. It also provides financing options, including an Assured Refund Plan that gives you six cycles at a fixed price with a money-back guarantee.

The Donor Sibling Registry

http://www.donorsiblingregistry.com

The DSR connects half-siblings conceived as a result of sperm, egg, or embryo donation who are seeking to make mutually desired contact with others with whom they share genetic ties.

Growing Generations

http://www.growinggenerations.com

Growing Generations aims to support and educate surrogates, egg donors, and intended parents. Its site has a great deal of information about the process involved for all parties.

Parents via Egg Donation

http://www.pved.org

This organization provides a community space for parents and parents-to-be to learn and share information about all facets of the egg donation process.

Principles of Oocyte and Embryo Donation edited by Mark V. Sauer

An expanded and updated version of the 1998 textbook, this comprehensive reference book defines the standards of practice that have evolved over the last thirty years and clearly states the outcomes expected from those practices. It also includes opinions from lawyers, ethicists, mental health care professionals, and theologians.

Sperm Bank Directory

http://www.spermbankdirectory.com

This directory provides a list of sperm banks and specialists anywhere in the United States, as well as resources about the process of both donating and banking sperm.

Sperm Donation (Mayo Clinic)

http://www.mayoclinic.com/health/sperm-donation/MY02078

The Mayo Clinic is a great resource for the basic scientific details of what is entailed in the process of sperm donation (and also has information on male infertility issues).

FEMINISM AND THE WOMEN'S MOVEMENT

(Many thanks to Amy Richards for her input on this section.)

Catalyst

http://www.catalyst.org

Catalyst's goal is to expand opportunities for women and business and to create more inclusive workplaces. It is active worldwide and has a wealth of advocacy opportunities, descriptions of existing policies, and an active online community.

Center for American Progress

http://www.americanprogress.org/

A progressive nonpartisan educational institute, CAP is active in developing policy ideas, educating the public, and shaping the national media debate. Its website has a section dedicated to women's rights, where you will find great interviews and analyses.

Elizabeth A. Sackler Center for Feminist Art

http://www.brooklynmuseum.org/eascfa

The Elizabeth A. Sackler Center for Feminist Art is an exhibition and education environment dedicated to feminist art. On permanent view is Judy Chicago's seminal work, *The Dinner Party*, which represents 1,038 women in history. You can check out images and historical information on the website, but if you are in New York City, please make a visit.

Feminist.com

http://www.feminist.com

Feminist.com is an umbrella resource for anything related to feminism. It features links to women-friendly sites and hosts women-owned businesses as well as organizations that can't yet afford or manage their own sites. It is also home to "Ask Amy," where you can get answers from third-wave feminist author Amy Richards.

Feministing

http://www.feministing.com

Feministing is an online community for feminists and their allies. The community aspect of Feministing aims to connect feminists online and off, and to encourage activism.

Feminist Majority Foundation (FMF)

http://www.feminist.org

The FMF is dedicated to women's equality, reproductive health, and nonviolence. The foundation utilizes research and action to empower women economically, socially, and politically.

Free to Be Foundation

http://www.freetobefoundation.org

A subsidiary of the Ms. Foundation for Women, this foundation channels profits from the *Free to Be* book, record, and TV special to projects benefiting children and families.

Full Frontal Feminism: A Young Woman's Guide to Why Feminism Matters by Jessica Valenti

In this book, Valenti aims to reinforce to younger generations why it is critical (and cool) to be a feminist.

Girls Inc.

http://www.girlsinc.org

Girls Inc. is dedicated to inspiring girls between the ages of six and eighteen to become strong, smart, and bold through life-changing programs and experiences that help them navigate gender, economic, and social barriers.

Guerrilla Girls

http://www.guerrillagirls.com

"Reinventing the f-word, feminism," the Guerilla Girls is an anonymous collective of women artists and arts professionals who shake up the male-dominated art world by creating agitprop art for the feminist revolution.

How to Be a Woman by Caitlin Moran

In this memoir/manifesto, Moran cuts to the heart of women's issues today with humor, personal anecdotes, and observations—and reminds us all why feminism is still important.

Makers

http://www.makers.com

This is an extraordinary audio-visual archive featuring interviews of influential women in different fields.

Manifesta: Young Women, Feminism, and the Future by Jennifer Baumgardner and Amy Richards

In this classic of contemporary feminist literature, third-wave feminists Jennifer Baumgardner and Amy Richards take an in-depth look at the successes and stumbling blocks of feminism while inspiring a new generation of female readers. The tenth-anniversary edition has an extensive list of feminism resources.

Ms. Foundation for Women

http://www.forwomen.org

The Ms. Foundation is the first national multi-issue, multiracial public women's fund. It makes grants to projects by and for women in areas such as economic justice; health and safety; AIDS; democracy; and girls, young women, and leadership.

National Organization for Women

http://www.now.org
    NOW advocates for political and social equality for women and is the largest organization of feminist activists in the United States.

National Partnership for Women and Families

http://www.nationalpartnership.org
    The National Partnership aims to eliminate discrimination, create family-friendly workplaces, and ensure that all families have affordable healthcare and economic stability.

Revolution from Within: A Book of Self-Esteem by Gloria Steinem

Steinem wrote this book after the sale of *Ms. Magazine* and her own resignation as its editor. With its author's reflections on the psychological and societal influences on self-esteem, *Revolution from Within* became a pivotal work of the 1990s.

Third Wave Foundation

http://www.thirdwavefoundation.org
    Third Wave is a feminist activist foundation that works nationally to support young women and transgender youth ages fifteen to thirty.

When Everything Changed: The Amazing Journey of American Women from 1960 to the Present by Gail Collins

Mixing oral history and research, Gail Collins's book covers the revolution in women's lives over the last fifty years.

FERTILITY

(Many thanks to Dr. Pasquale Patrizio for his input on this section.)

American Society for Reproductive Medicine (ASRM)

http://www.asrm.org

The ASRM is a nationally and internationally recognized leader in providing information, education, advocacy, and standards in the field of reproductive medicine. It has published *Fertility and Sterility*, a peer-reviewed medical journal in obstetrics and gynecology since 1950, and its website has a wealth of scientific research and data.

The Boston Women's Health Book Collective

http://www.ourbodiesourselves.org

This website is the hub for the nonprofit Boston Women's Health Book Collective, which published *Our Bodies, Ourselves*. The collective promotes accurate, evidence-based information on girls' and women's reproductive health and sexuality, and its website has many community and scientific resources.

Circle + Bloom

http://www.circlebloom.com

Circle + Bloom sells programs and provides resources focusing on the mind-body connection and its relationship to conception, fertility, and general well-being. The website offers a wide array of podcasts and meditation series for women dealing with fertility treatments, egg/embryo donation, and more.

Conquering Infertility by Dr. Alice Domar

Using techniques developed at her clinic, Dr. Domar provides advice and support in this book for infertile women to regain control over their lives and boost their chances of becoming pregnant.

Fertility Plus: Information Written by Patients, for Patients

http://www.fertilityplus.com

A good launching point for conversations with your healthcare provider, Fertility Plus has a community of women trying to get pregnant who share their stories and experiences.

Fertility and Sterility

http://www.fertstert.org

The journal published by ASRM, *Fertility and Sterility* is an excellent resource for the latest scientific research and developments in the field of reproductive medicine.

The Guttmacher Institute

http://www.guttmacher.org

The Guttmacher Institute is the primary authority on statistics related to reproductive health in the United States and worldwide.

How to Get Pregnant by Sherman J. Silber, MD

Revised in 2007, this comprehensive resource for couples trying to conceive includes information on the basic facts of getting pregnant as well as techniques, tests, and procedures involved in treating infertility.

Infertility Family Research Registry

http://www.ifrr-registry.org

The IFRR collects volunteers who want to help improve the understanding of the health of individuals and families dealing with infertility. The registry provides ongoing information about the health of its volunteers (fully controlled by the volunteers themselves) for the purpose of collating solid and reliable data on infertility, and is a hub for additional scientific infertility research study opportunities.

Pew Research Center

http://www.pewresearch.org

A nonpartisan fact tank, the center's website has a wealth of data on the trends and attitudes shaping the United States. In particular, it contains information on birth rates, fertility, and parenthood.

Physicians for Reproductive Choice and Health (PRCH)

http://www.prch.org

PRCH publishes an extensive reference, *PRCH Reproductive Health Resource Guide,* which includes a curriculum on abortion and family planning, as well as a listing of videos, organizations, and facts.

Planned Parenthood

http://www.plannedparenthood.org

The nation's most widespread provider of reproductive health care, Planned Parenthood offers affordable healthcare, sex education, and reproductive health information to women, men, and young people worldwide. Its website offers educational tools for teens, parents, and health professionals.

Redbook's Blogroll: The Best Infertility Blogs

http://www.redbookmag.com/health-wellness/advice/infertility-blogs

Blogs are great places to find active and supportive online communities, and this is an especially great list of some of the most popular infertility blogs.

RESOLVE, the National Infertility Association

http://www.resolve.org

RESOLVE is the nation's largest and most active infertility organization. The website is an excellent source for scientific data on all aspects of infertility, support communities throughout the country, and ways to participate in local and national legislative advocacy efforts.

Taking Charge of Your Fertility by Toni Weschler

This bestseller discusses an alternative to chemical birth control, focusing on the fertility awareness method as a means to manage your own fertility (and either delay or achieve pregnancy).

A Torah Infertility Medium of Exchange (A TIME)

http://www.atime.org
Incorporating viewpoints from rabbis and physicians, A TIME is an international organization that offers advocacy, education, guidance, research, and support to Jewish men, women, and couples struggling with infertility.

The Truth about Trying: Redbook's Infertility Video Series

http://www.redbookmag.com/health-wellness/advice/infertility-video
-series
Featuring a mix of celebrity and user-submitted videos, this series features a wide variety of women's experiences with infertility, fertility treatments, miscarriage, and pregnancy.

FERTILITY TREATMENT FINANCING

Budgeting for Infertility by Evelina Weidman Sterling and Angie Best-Boss

Incorporating hard data, patient anecdotes, and doctor commentary, this book is a practical guide to navigating the costs and process of pursuing fertility treatments. Because it was published in 2009, some of the specifics are not up to date, but it is still a valuable resource.

Fertile Action

http://www.fertileaction.org
Offering education, advocacy, support, and financial aid, Fertile Action is a cancer charity working to ensure that women affected by the disease can become mothers.

Fertile Hope

http://www.fertilehope.org
Fertile Hope is a LIVE**STRONG** initiative dedicated to providing reproductive information and support to cancer patients and survivors whose medical treatments present the risk of infertility.

InterNational Council on Infertility Information Dissemination, Inc. (INCIID)

http://www.inciid.org
INCIID (pronounced "inside") is a nonprofit organization that helps individuals and couples explore their family-building options. The site has links to support about diagnosis, treatment, prevention, adoption, and childfree lifestyles.

National Conference of State Legislature

http://www.ncsl.org/issues-research/health/insurance-coverage-for
-infertility-laws.aspx
This site has detailed descriptions of the exact state laws related to insurance coverage for infertility treatment across the United States.

RESOLVE

http://www.resolve.org/family-building-options/insurance_coverage
RESOLVE is an excellent resource for data on health insurance coverage state by state in the United States, and also has information on employer coverage, the ins and outs of health insurance, and pending federal legislation on the topic.

FERTILITY TREATMENTS

Anonymous Us Project

http://anonymousus.podomatic.com/
The Anonymous Us Project aims to offer a safe space for honest opinions about reproductive technologies and family fragmentation. On the website, you can submit and read stories about those who have experiences based on these technologies.

Center for Genetics and Society

http://www.geneticsandsociety.org
The center is a nonprofit that encourages responsible uses and effective societal governance of new and developing human genetic and reproductive technologies.

Centers for Disease Control and Prevention

http://www.cdc.gov/art
The CDC has comprehensive data on ARTs over the last fifteen years. The website has invaluable research for data on success rates at specific clinics and for age demographics.

European Society of Human Reproduction and Embryology

http://www.eshre.eu
ESHRE facilitates research and the dissemination of research findings in human reproduction and embryology, and uses its work to inform politicians and policy makers throughout Europe.

Lotus Blossom Consulting

http://www.lotusblossomconsulting.com
Founded by Mindy Berkson, LBC is a national infertility consulting

firm (based in Chicago) that provides a comprehensive look at the financial, emotional, physical, and logistical challenges of infertility treatment.

Patients beyond Borders

http://www.patientsbeyondborders.com

Patients beyond Borders is a reliable source of consumer information about international medical and health travel. If you are looking into pursuing IVF abroad, its website has details about the process as well as about particular countries and hospitals.

Society for Assisted Reproductive Technologies

http://www.sart.org

SART is the primary organization of professionals dedicated to ARTs in the United States, and it aims to establish and maintain standards of practice. The website is an excellent resource for IVF success rates and for locating infertility clinics in your area.

MOTHERHOOD AND PARENTING

Babble's Top 100 Mom Blogs of 2012

http://www.babble.com/mom/top-100-mom-blogs

A roundup of the most popular blogs over the entire spectrum of parenthood, this list is a great launching point to find a supportive online community that matches your particular situation, viewpoint, and interests.

BabyCenter

http://www.babycenter.com

An online community with information ranging from getting pregnant all the way through the phases of raising a child, BabyCenter has blogs, parenting news, and a wealth of forums.

Every Mother Counts

http://www.everymothercounts.org

Every Mother Counts is a campaign to end preventable deaths caused by pregnancy and childbirth around the world. They inform, engage, and mobilize new audiences to take action to improve the health and well-being of girls and women worldwide.

National Advocates for Pregnant Women (NAPW)

http://www.advocatesforpregnantwomen.org

Active players in the political scene, NAPW works to secure the human and civil rights, health, and welfare of all women (and focuses on pregnant and parenting women).

Opting In: Having a Child without Losing Yourself by Amy Richards

Feminist author Amy Richards's book addresses parenting and feminism's relationship to motherhood in a blend of research, interviews, historical data, and personal memoir.

Sprout

http://www.sprout-app.com

Developed by *American Baby* magazine and Med ART Studios, Sprout is a great pregnancy app for moms and moms-to-be. It includes stunning images of your baby's development and doctor visit planners.

ACKNOWLEDGMENTS

Aspecial thank you to Jennifer Rubell, who first encouraged me both to write this book and to contact Meg Thompson, who deserves the second special thank you for becoming my agent and champion, along with Susanna Einstein and Molly Reese at Einstein Thompson Literary Agency.

I am honored that my first book is in the excellent hands of Prometheus Books (especially Steven L. Mitchell, Mariel Bard, Julia DeGraf, Mark Hall, Jill Maxick, Lisa Michalski, Catherine Roberts-Abel, and Melissa Shofner) and also under the care of those at Wunderkind PR (especially Elena Stokes and Tanya Farrell).

Reading books was my salvation while I went through the difficult times I recount in this book. I especially thank the authors Sonali Deraniyagala and Cheryl Strayed for their beautiful prose.

A huge thanks to Susan Wilson and Kelsey Ryan for their research assistance and dedication and also for offering their twenty-something perspectives.

Thank you to the many nurses and doctors who have taken great care of me.

Thank you to *all* my friends. Those in particular who shared their personal stories, provided moral support, or gave feedback on my ideas for the book include Kati Agocs, Asif Ahmed, Laurie Anderson, Andrew Andrew, Maureen "Moe" Angelos, Chloe Aridjis, Eva Aridjis, Claude Arpels, Claire Béjanin, Jennie Boddy, Dominique Bousquet, Johanna Burton, Jennifer Braunschweiger, Winsome Brown, Melissa Ceria, Elaine Chen, Gabri Christa, Chiara Clemente, Lisa Cortés, Eisa Davis, Laura Dawn, Adrienne Day, Natalie Dean, Sandi DuBowski, John Fleck, Shari Frilot, Vallejo Gantner, Finian Moore Gerety, Vivien Goldman, Lisa Gottheil, Heather Greene, Tim Griffin, Agnes Gund, Cynthia Hedstrom, Hillary Jordan, Leila Kinney, Susan Kirschbaum, Jenny Laden, Sarah Lash, Karen Lashinsky, Juliet Lashinsky-Revene, Thomas M. Lauderdale, Elizabeth

LeCompte, Chase Madar, Cheri Magid, Rekha Malhotra, Alex and Vida Marashian, Kristin Marting, Suketu Mehta, Alex and Tanya Ager Meillier, Tina Merrill, Liz Mermin, Linda Rattner Metcalfe, Laura Michalchyshyn, Shira Milikowsky, Mike Milley, Unjoo Moon, Satish Moorthy, Felicia Morton, Walter Mosley, Sherwin Parikh, Paige Powell, Roya Rastegar, Caroline Reeves, Tricia Romano, Juan Roselione-Valadez, Orion Ross, Don Rubell, Miguel Sancho, Ahmad Sardar-Afkhami, David Schweizer, Danzy Senna, Lucy Sexton, Shane Sigler, Amy Lou Stein, Catharine Stimpson, Lucy Taylor, Aurelia Thiérrée, Mickalene Thomas, Jennifer Turner, Kate Valk, Carrie Mae Weems, Marianne Weems, Carleigh Welsh, and Soon-Young Yoon. Some also commented on parts or all of my manuscript and helped me write a better book; this group includes Nell Breyer, Isolde Brielmaier, Julia Chaplin, Farai Chideya, Amy Davidson, Jenny Davidson, Joy de Menil, Jennifer Gonnerman, Catherine Gund, Larissa MacFarquhar, Sia Michel, Amy Richards, Mera Rubell, Mary Kaye Schilling, Gabriela Poma Traynor, Lucy Walker, Kim Whitener, and Alex Zafiris.

In addition, I am indebted to the experts and individuals who responded candidly and generously to my inquiries: Mindy Berkson, Victoria Birk Hill, Christy Turlington Burns, Dr. Arthur Greil, Hilary Grove, Beth Hall, Dr. Carole Kowalczyk, Dr. William Kutteh, Dr. Julia McQuillan, Karen Pace, Dr. Pasquale Patrizio, Dr. Sunday Pirkle, Nancy Rosenhaus, Carol Sheingold, Dr. Karina Shreffler, Dr. Irene Souter, and Crystal Wilmhoff. Dr. Patrizio also reviewed some of the chapters.

Most of all, I thank my mother, Therese Selvaratnam; brother, Troy Selvaratnam; and sister-in-law, Mary Skinner, who are always there for me.

In addition to my mother, I dedicate this to the memory of Dr. Khakasa Wapenyi.

Lastly, I thank Jay, for being part of the story that inspired my book.

NOTES AND SOURCES

INTRODUCTION

1. "1 in 3 Campaign," Advocates for Youth, http://www.1in3campaign.org/ (accessed September 24, 2013). "Miscarriage," American Pregnancy Association, http://americanpregnancy.org/pregnancycomplications/miscarriage.html (accessed September 23, 2013). Miriam Zoll and Pamela Tsigdinos, "Selling the Fantasy of Fertility," *New York Times*, September 11, 2013, http://www.nytimes.com/2013/09/12/opinion/selling-the-fantasy-of-fertility.html?emc=eta1&_r=0 (accessed September 14, 2013).

2. Abbie Waters, "IVF Use in America: State IVF Rates and Rankings," http://www.fertilitynation.com/united-states-of-ivf-state-ivf-rates-rankings-map-infographic/ (accessed May 3, 2012).

3. Mindy Berkson, in interview with the author, May 1, 2012.

4. Arthur Greil, PhD, in interview with the author, May 11, 2012.

CHAPTER 1: A WOULD-BE MOTHER'S LAMENT

1. Isolde Brielmaier, in interview with the author, February 21, 2013.

2. Laura Dawn, in interview with the author, February 21, 2013.

3. Michelle Ruiz, "Report: More US Women in Their 40s Never Have Kids," AOL News, June 25, 2010, http://www.aolnews.com/2010/06/25/report-more-us-women-in-their-40s-never-have-kids/ (accessed April 13, 2012).

4. "Women Warned of Infertility Trap," *CNN Health*, April 11, 2002, http://archives.cnn.com/2002/HEALTH/04/11/women.infertility/index.html (accessed March 7, 2012).

5. Charlotte Chandler, "My Dinners with Federico and Michelangelo," *Vanity Fair*, March 2012, http://www.vanityfair.com/hollywood/2012/03/federico-michelangelo-201203 (accessed March 3, 2012).

6. Barbara Ehrenreich, "Why Forced Positive Thinking Is a Total Crock," *AlterNet*, May 20, 2010, http://www.alternet.org/story/146940/barbara_ehrenreich%3A_why_forced_positive_thinking_is_a_total_crock (accessed February 8, 2013).

7. Karen Springen, "The Mysteries of Miscarriage," *Daily Beast*, January 27, 2008, http://www.thedailybeast.com/newsweek/2008/01/27/the-mysteries-of-miscarriage .html (accessed February 15, 2012).

8. Jennifer D'Angelo Friedman, "What Happens to a Woman's Fertility after 40," *SELF*, September 8, 2011, http://www.self.com/blogs/flash/2011/09/what-happens-to -your-fertility.html (accessed February 13, 2012).

9. Peggy Orenstein, "Mourning My Miscarriage," *New York Times*, April 21, 2012, http://www.nytimes.com/2002/04/21/magazine/mourning-my-miscarriage.html (accessed April 22, 2012).

10. Springen, "Mysteries of Miscarriage."

11. Jennifer Wolff Perrine, "This Woman Has a Secret," *SELF*, http://www.self .com/health/2010/08/breaking-the-silence-on-infertility/ (accessed February 13, 2012).

12. "Recurrent Pregnancy Loss," Patient Fact Sheet, American Society for Reproductive Medicine, August 2008, http://www.asrm.org/Recurrent_Pregnancy_Loss/ (accessed February 5, 2012).

13. Alice Lesch Kelly, "Miscarriage: The Hardest Loss," *Conceive*, January 28, 2009, http://www.conceiveonline.com/articles/miscarriage-hardest-loss (accessed April 22, 2012).

14. EMD Serono Inc., "In the Know: Fertility IQ 2011 Survey: Fertility Knowledge Among US Women Aged 25–35: Insights from a New Generation," October 2011.

15. Janet Kornblum, "More Women 40–44 Remaining Childless," *USA Today*, August 19, 2008, http://www.usatoday.com/news/health/2008-08-18-fertility_N.htm (accessed February 18, 2012).

16. Ruiz, "Report: More US Women in Their 40s Never Have Kids."

17. "Census Bureau Reports 'Delayer Boom' as More Educated Women Have Children Later," United States Census Bureau, May 9, 2011, http://www.census.gov/ newsroom/releases/archives/fertility/cb11-83.html (accessed February 8, 2012).

18. Michel Martin, "Birth Rate Declines for Women over 40," NPR, June 29, 2010, http://www.npr.org/templates/story/story.php?storyId=128188446 (accessed February 13, 2012).

19. "2009 Assisted Reproductive Technology Success Rates: National Summary and Fertility Clinic Reports," Centers for Disease Control and Prevention, American Society for Reproductive Medicine, and Society for Assisted Reproductive Technology, 2011.

20. Jean Twenge, "How Long Can You Wait to Have a Baby?" *Atlantic*, June 19, 2013, http://www.theatlantic.com/magazine/archive/2013/07/how-long-can-you-wait-to -have-a-baby/309374/ (accessed August 8, 2013).

21. Ibid.

22. Hilary Grove, in interview with the author, February 21, 2013.

23. "Women Graduates Wait until They Hit 35 before Having Their First Child," *Daily Mail*, October 21, 2012, http://www.dailymail.co.uk/news/article-2220918/Women -graduates-wait-hit-35-having-child.html (accessed October 21, 2012).

24. Julia Chaplin, in interview with the author, April 24, 2012.

25. Judith Shulevitz, "How Older Parenthood Will Upend American Society: The Scary Consequences of the Grayest Generation," *New Republic*, December 6, 2012, http://www.newrepublic.com/article/politics/magazine/110861/how-older-parenthood -will-upend-american-society (accessed December 12, 2012).

26. "Fertility Rate, Total (Births per Woman)," World Bank, http://data.worldbank .org/indicator/SP.DYN.TFRT.IN (accessed March 7, 2012).

27. "The State of World Population 2011," United Nations Population Fund, http://www.unfpa.org/webdav/site/global/shared/documents/publications/2011/ EN-SWOP2011-FINAL.pdf (accessed March 23, 2012).

28. Chris Arsenault, "'Baby Bust' Spells Trouble for Rich Nations," *Al Jazeera*, October 30, 2011, http://www.aljazeera.com/indepth/features/2011/10/201110419532494799 .html (accessed February 8, 2012).

29. Peter Apps, "The Next Challenge: Not Too Many People, but Too Few?" Reuters, October 24, 2011, http://www.reuters.com/article/2011/10/24/population -decline-idUSL5E7LO0VD20111024 (accessed February 13, 2012).

CHAPTER 2: WHAT IS THE BIG LIE?

1. Amy Richards, *Opting In: Having a Child without Losing Yourself* (New York: Farrar, Straus and Giroux, 2008), p. 6.

2. Marlo Thomas, "Mom's Stifled Dreams," *Makers*, http://www.makers.com/ marlo-thomas/moments/moms-stifled-dreams/ (accessed March 17, 2012).

3. Abigail Pogrebin, "How Do You Spell Ms.," *New York*, October 30, 2011, http:// nymag.com/news/features/ms-magazine-2011-11/ (accessed March 4, 2012).

4. Gina Maranto, "Delayed Childbearing," *Atlantic*, June 1, 1995, http://www .theatlantic.com/magazine/archive/1995/06/delayed-childbearing/5964/ (accessed February 8, 2012).

5. April Daniels Hussar, "Survey: Most College Women Want to Be Married by 30," *Self*, August 30, 2012, http://www.self.com/blogs/flash/2012/08/survey-most -college-women-want.html (accessed September 2, 2012).

6. Betty Friedan, *The Feminine Mystique* (New York: W. W. Norton, 2001), p. 78.

7. Liza Mundy, *Everything Conceivable: How Assisted Reproduction Is Changing Our World* (New York: Anchor Books, 2008), p. 323.

8. Nancy Gibbs, "Making Time for a Baby," *Time*, April 15, 2002, http://www .time.com/time/magazine/article/0,9171,1002217,00.html (accessed March 21, 2012).

9. Kate Bolick, "All the Single Ladies," *Atlantic*, September 30, 2011, http://www .theatlantic.com/magazine/archive/2011/11/all-the-single-ladies/8654/ (accessed February 7, 2012).

10. Hussar, "Survey: Most College Women Want to Be Married by 30."

11. Peggy Orenstein, *Flux: Women on Sex, Work, Love, Kids, & Life in a Half-Changed World* (New York: Anchor Books, 2000), p. 16.

12. Amanda Gardner, "U.S. Women Delaying Motherhood, Report Shows," *HealthDay*, August 13, 2012, http://abcnews.go.com/Health/Healthday/story?id=8312506&page=1#.T4xm6ulST80 (accessed April 16, 2012).

13. Pasquale Patrizio, MD, in interview with the author, May 1, 2012.

14. Natalie Angier, *Woman: An Intimate Geography* (New York: Anchor Books, 2000), p. 94.

15. Soon-Young Yoon, in interview with the author, May 11, 2012.

16. Amy Richards, in interview with the author, April 30, 2013.

17. Orenstein, *Flux*, p. 127.

18. Yoon, interview.

19. Debora L. Spar, "Why Women Should Stop Trying to Be Perfect," *Daily Beast*, September 24, 2012, http://www.thedailybeast.com/newsweek/2012/09/23/why-women-should-stop-trying-to-be-perfect.html (accessed October 2, 2012).

20. Marianne Weems, in interview with the author, May 11, 2012.

21. Richards, interview.

22. Ibid.

23. Catherine Gund, in interview with the author, May 1, 2013.

24. Claudia Kalb, "Should You Have Your Baby Now?" *Newsweek*, August 12, 2001, http://www.thedailybeast.com/newsweek/2001/08/12/should-you-have-your-baby-now.html (accessed March 20, 2012).

25. Ibid.

26. Ibid.

27. Cheri Magid, in interview with the author, May 8, 2012.

28. Lindsay Beyerstein, "Anne-Marie Slaughter Has It All," *Duly Noted*, June 21, 2012, http://inthesetimes.com/duly-noted/entry/13429/anne_marie_slaughter_pretty_much_has_it_all/ (accessed June 28, 2012).

29. Jenni Rothenberg Gritz, "Stephen Colbert Solves the 'Having It All' Dilemma in 5 Words," *Atlantic*, July 17, 2012, http://www.theatlantic.com/business/archive/2012/07/stephen-colbert-solves-the-having-it-all-dilemma-in-5-words/259936/ (accessed July 19, 2012).

30. Ayelet Waldman, "Is This Really Goodbye?" *Marie Claire*, October 18, 2012, http://www.marieclaire.com/world-reports/inspirational-women/hillary-clinton-farewell-3 (accessed October 24, 2012).

31. "Townterview Hosted by Bahrain TV," US Department of State, December 3, 2010, http://www.state.gov/secretary/rm/2010/12/152355.htm (accessed October 19, 2012).

32. Sheryl Sandberg, "Why We Have Too Few Women Leaders," TEDWomen, December 2010, http://www.ted.com/talks/sheryl_sandberg_why_we_have_too_few_women_leaders.html (accessed June 28, 2012).

33. Sheryl Sandberg, *Lean In: Women, Work, and the Will to Lead* (New York: Alfred A. Knopf, 2013), p. 162.

34. EMD Serono Inc., "In the Know: Fertility IQ 2011 Survey: Fertility Knowledge among US Women Aged 25–35: Insights from a New Generation," October 2011.

35. Mindy Berkson, in interview with the author, May 1, 2012.

36. "How Birth Control and Abortion Became Politicized," NPR, November 9, 2012, http://www.npr.org/2011/11/09/142097521/how-birth-control-and-abortion-became-politicized (accessed March 18, 2012).

37. EMD Serono Inc., "In the Know: Fertility IQ 2011 Survey."

CHAPTER 3: WHAT THE EXPERTS WISH YOU KNEW

1. Carole Kowalczyk, MD, in interview with the author, April 25, 2012.

2. Amy Richards, *Opting In: Having a Child without Losing Yourself* (New York: Farrar, Straus and Giroux, 2008), p. 54.

3. Evelina Weidman Sterling and Angie Best-Boss, *Budgeting for Infertility* (New York: Fireside, 2009), p. 28.

4. Lillian Schapiro, *Tick Tock* (Lincoln, NE: iUniverse, Inc., 2005), p. 85.

5. William Kutteh, MD, PhD, in interview with the author, April 21, 2012.

6. Joe DeCapua, "Global Infertility Rates Generally Hold Steady," *Voice of America*, December 20, 2012, http://www.voanews.com/content/global-infertility-20dec12/1568597.html (accessed December 22, 2012).

7. Sharon Jayson, "New Face of Infertility: Under 35, Frustrated," *USA Today*, April 23, 2012, http://www.usatoday.com/news/health/story/2012-04-23/infertility-young-women/54482470/1 (accessed May 3, 2012).

8. "Eggsurance Launches Independent Community and Educational Website Devoted to Everything Egg Freezing," May 22, 2012, http://www.marketwire.com/press-release/eggsurance-launches-independent-community-educational-website-devoted-everything-egg-1660037.htm (accessed May 25, 2012).

9. Alex Dobuzinskis, "U.S. Women in 20s Less Likely to Get Pregnant or Have Abortion," Reuters, June 20, 2012, http://www.reuters.com/article/2012/06/20/us-usa-pregnancies-study-idUSBRE85J06820120620 (accessed July 8, 2012).

10. Amanda Gardner, "U.S. Women Delaying Motherhood, Report Shows," Health Day, ABC News, August 13, 2009, http://abcnews.go.com/Health/Healthday/story?id=8312506 (accessed April 3, 2012).

11. Claudia Kalb, "Should You Have Your Baby Now?" *Newsweek*, August 12, 2001, http://www.thedailybeast.com/newsweek/2001/08/12/should-you-have-your-baby-now.html (accessed March 20, 2012).

12. Karen Rowan, "Fertility Decline Surprises Women over 40, Study Finds," Women, *Huffington Post*, December 10, 2012, http://www.huffingtonpost.com/2012/12/10/fertility-decline-women-surprised-over-40-ivf_n_2273122.html (accessed December 15, 2012).

13. Dobuzinskis, "U.S. Women in 20s Less Likely to Get Pregnant or Have Abortion."

14. Lisa Miller, "Parents of a Certain Age," *New York*, September 25, 2011, http://nymag.com/news/features/mothers-over-50-2011-10/ (accessed February 4, 2012).

15. Derek Thompson, "Bye-Bye, Boomers: This Is the Age of the Baby Bust-ers," *Atlantic*, August 22, 2012, http://www.theatlantic.com/business/archive/2012/08/bye-bye-boomers-this-is-the-age-of-the-baby-bust-ers/261424/ (accessed August 30, 2012).

16. Jennifer Wolff Perrine, "This Woman Has a Secret," *SELF*, http://www.self.com/health/2010/08/breaking-the-silence-on-infertility/ (accessed February 13, 2012).

17. Rowan, "Fertility Decline Surprises Women over 40, Study Finds."

18. Mona Lisa Macalino, "What You Don't Know about Infertility," *YourTango*, April 24, 2012, http://www.yourtango.com/2012151161/what-you-dont-know-about-infertility (accessed April 25, 2012).

19. Kate Lunau, "Thirty-Seven and Counting," *Maclean's*, October 27, 2012, http://www2.macleans.ca/2012/10/27/thirty-seven-and-counting/ (accessed December 20, 2012).

20. A survey in the *Guardian* newspaper in the United Kingdom found that half of infertile woman feel their doctor is unsympathetic or ignorant about their condition. Tracy Richardson-Lyne, "Why Do GPs Show So Little Sympathy for Women's Fertility Problems?" *Guardian*, August 29, 2012, http://www.guardian.co.uk/commentisfree/2012/aug/29/gps-no-understanding-womens-fertility (accessed August 30, 2012). A study from New Zealand showed that 74 percent of women coming to a fertility clinic had inadequate fertility awareness. Joshua U. Klein, MD, "Top Doc Reveals 8 Fertility Misconceptions," *CNN Health*, November 7, 2011, http://www.cnn.com/2011/11/07/health/fertility-misconceptions/ (accessed February 8, 2012).

21. Gina Maranto, "Delayed Childbearing," *Atlantic*, June 1, 1995, http://www.theatlantic.com/magazine/archive/1995/06/delayed-childbearing/5964/ (accessed February 8, 2012).

22. "Royal College Warns Women Not to Leave Pregnancy Too Late in Life," 2009, http://www.vitalab.com/infertility-news/royal-college-warns-about-late-pregnancy/ (accessed December 7, 2012).

23. Pasquale Patrizio, MD, in interview with the author, May 1, 2012.

24. Alice G. Walton, "Okay, We Get It: There's No Turning Back the Biological Clock," *Atlantic*, May 1, 2012, http://www.theatlantic.com/health/archive/2012/05/okay-we-get-it-theres-no-turning-back-the-biological-clock/256571/ (accessed May 18, 2012).

25. Sarah Elizabeth Richards, "We Need to Talk about Our Eggs," *New York Times*, October 22, 2012, http://www.nytimes.com/2012/10/23/opinion/we-need-to-talk-about-our-eggs.html (accessed October 28, 2012).

26. Elizabeth Gregory, *Ready: Why Women Are Embracing the New Later Motherhood* (New York: Perseus Books, 2007), p. 174.

27. Richards, *Opting In*, p. 52.

28. Kate Kelland, "Smoking Deaths Triple over Decade: Tobacco Report," Reuters, March 21, 2012, http://www.reuters.com/article/2012/03/21/us-tobacco-global-deaths -idUSBRE82K0C020120321 (accessed April 4, 2012).

29. Mindy Berkson, in interview with the author, May 1, 2012.

30. Carole Kowalczyk, MD, "Understanding Fertility," *Women in Business*, 2012.

31. Julia McQuillan, PhD, in interview with the author, May 11, 2012.

32. Liza Mundy, *Everything Conceivable: How Assisted Reproduction Is Changing Our World* (New York: Anchor Books, 2008), pp. 13, 23.

33. Lindsay Abrams, "It's Not Too Early to Talk about Your Eggs," *Atlantic*, November 9, 2012, http://www.theatlantic.com/health/archive/2012/11/its-not-too-early-to -talk-about-freezing-your-eggs/264992/ (accessed December 8, 2012).

34. Diana Rodriguez, "10 Health Screenings All Women Should Have," *Everyday Health*, April 20, 2012, http://www.everydayhealth.com/womens-health/10-screenings -all-women-should-have.aspx (accessed April 24, 2012).

35. Henri Leridon, "Can Assisted Reproduction Technology Compensate for the Natural Decline in Fertility with Age? A Model Assessment," *Human Reproduction* 18, no. 1 (2004): 1548.

36. Klein, "Top Doc Reveals 8 Fertility Misconceptions."

37. Fiona MacRae, "MEN Are to Blame for Most Cases of Unexplained Infertility— but a New Test Could Help Couples Succeed," *Daily Mail*, November 14, 2012, http://www .dailymail.co.uk/health/article-2232989/MEN-blame-cases-unexplained-infertility--new-test -help-couples-succeed.html (accessed December 10, 2012).

38. Mundy, *Everything Conceivable*, p. 66.

39. Smita Mitra, "Long Journeys to Parenthood," *OutlookIndia.com*, May 7, 2012, http://www.outlookindia.com/article.aspx?280700 (accessed May 23, 2012).

"Infertility on the Rise in Urban Areas, Late Marriage Big Factor," *Hindustan Times*, April 29, 2012, http://www.hindustantimes.com/India-news/NewDelhi/Infertility-on -the-rise-in-urban-areas-late-marriage-big-factor/Article1-848191.aspx (accessed May 23, 2013).

40. Chrissie Russell, "Why It's Time Men Opened up about Infertility," *Irish Independent*, May 28, 2012, http://www.independent.ie/lifestyle/parenting/why-its-time -men-opened-up-about-infertility-3120014.html (accessed June 2, 2012).

41. Tara Parker-Pope, "Can a 'Fertility Diet' Get You Pregnant?" *New York Times*, December 18, 2007, http://www.nytimes.com/2007/12/18/health/nutrition/18well .html (accessed March 2, 2012).

42. Shanna McGoldrick, "Help! I Have a Low Sperm Count," *Sun*, August 23, 2012,

http://www.thesun.co.uk/sol/homepage/woman/health/health/4500607/Your-partner
-cant-conceive-Male-infertility-is-the-most-common-cause.html (accessed December 11, 2012).

43. Benedict Carey, "Father's Age is Linked to Risk of Autism and Schizophrenia," *New York Times*, August 22, 2012, http://www.nytimes.com/2012/08/23/health/fathers -age-is-linked-to-risk-of-autism-and-schizophrenia.html (accessed August 23, 2012).

44. Richard Knox, "Kids of Older Fathers Likelier to Have Genetic Ailments," NPR, August 22, 2012, http://www.npr.org/blogs/health/2012/08/22/159852022/kids-of-older-fathers-likelier-to-have-genetic-ailments (accessed August 30, 2012).

45. Julie Steenhuysen, "Gene Studies Begin to Unravel Autism Puzzle," Reuters, April 4, 2012, http://www.reuters.com/article/2012/04/04/us-autism-usa-genes-idUS BRE83312820120404 (accessed April 20, 2012).

46. Judith Shulevitz, "How Older Parenthood Will Upend American Society," *New Republic*, December 6, 2012, http://www.tnr.com/article/politics/magazine/110861/ how-older-parenthood-will-upend-american-society (accessed December 7, 2012). Carey, "Father's Age is Linked to Risk of Autism and Schizophrenia."

47. Carey, "Father's Age is Linked to Risk of Autism and Schizophrenia."

48. "Supplement Touted as Way to Extend Fertility," CTV News, December 26, 2012, http://www.ctv.ca/CTVNews/Health/20111223/coenzyme-q10-fertility-111226/ (accessed February 12, 2012). "Research with Worms May Shed Light on Women's Fertility," Health, *US News & World Report*, December 6, 2011, http://health.usnews.com/health -news/family-health/womens-health/articles/2011/12/06/research-with-worms-may-shed -light-on-womens-fertility (accessed February 20, 2012). Leigh Ann Woodruff, "Genetic Test to Predict IVF Egg Production in Older Women," *Fertility Authority*, March 19, 2012, http://www.fertilityauthority.com/articles/genetic-test-predict-ivf-egg-production-older -women (accessed April 3, 2012).

49. Noah Charney, "Ingenious Fertility Alternative to IVF," *ARTINFO.com*, January 14, 2013, http://blogs.artinfo.com/secrethistoryofart/2013/01/14/ingenious-fertility -alternative-to-ivf/ (accessed February 23, 2012).

50. Megan Garber, "The IVF Panic: 'All Hell Will Break Loose, Politically and Morally, All Over the World,'" *Atlantic*, June 25, 2012, http://www.theatlantic.com/ technology/archive/2012/06/the-ivf-panic-all-hell-will-break-loose-politically-and -morally-all-over-the-world/258954/ (accessed June 30, 2012).

51. Robert Winston, "The Bravery of Lesley Brown, Mother of the First IVF Baby," *Guardian*, June 21, 2012, http://www.guardian.co.uk/commentisfree/2012/jun/21/lesley -brown-mother-ivf-baby (accessed June 30, 2012).

52. "Fast Facts about Infertility," RESOLVE, June 30, 2011, http://www.resolve .org/about/fast-facts-about-fertility.html (accessed February 3, 2012).

53. Kate Kelland, "British 'Test Tube Baby' Pioneer Robert Edwards Dies," Reuters, April 10, 2013, http://www.reuters.com/article/2013/04/10/us-ivf-edwards-idUSBRE 9390IE20130410 (accessed April 12, 2013).

54. Mundy, *Everything Conceivable*, p. 36.

55. Ibid., p. 37.

56. Saswati Sunderam, PhD, Dmitry M. Kissin, MD, Lisa Flowers, MPA, et al., "Assisted Reproductive Technology Surveillance—United States, 2009," November 2, 2012, http://www.cdc.gov/mmwr/preview/mmwrhtml/ss6107a1.htm (accessed December 4, 2012).

57. Ileana Llorens, "Three Couples Win Free IVF Cycle through Sher Fertility Institute 'I Believe' Contest," *Huffington Post*, June 19, 2012, http://www.huffingtonpost.com/2012/06/19/three-couples-win-free-ivf-contest-sher-fertility_n_1608976.html (accessed July 2, 2012).

58. Miriam Zoll, "Know What You're Doing If You Decide to Wait," *New York Times*, July 10, 2013, http://www.nytimes.com/roomfordebate/2013/07/08/should-women-delay-motherhood/know-what-youre-doing-if-you-decide-to-delay-childbirth (accessed July 12, 2013). According to the CDC's website (http://www.cdc.gov/reproductivehealth/infertility/), its 2011 report on Preliminary ART Success Rates shows the average percentage of fresh, nondonor ART cycles that led to a live birth were 40 percent in women younger than 35 years of age, 32 percent in women aged 35 to 37 years, 22 percent in women aged 38 to 40 years, 12 percent in women aged 41 to 42 years, 5 percent in women aged 43 to 44 years, and 1 percent in women aged 44 years and older.

59. Mundy, *Everything Conceivable*, p. 27.

60. Jenny Hope, "Women over 40 Told: 'Don't Take IVF Success for Granted,'" *Daily Mail*, April 6, 2012, http://www.dailymail.co.uk/health/article-2126057/Women-40-told-Dont-IVF-success-granted.html (accessed April 11, 2012). Walton, "Okay, We Get It: There's No Turning Back the Biological Clock."

61. "Center for Human Reproduction More Than Doubles IVF Pregnancy Rates in Women over 44," PRWeb, June 4, 2012, http://www.prweb.com/releases/prematureovarianaging/failedivf/prweb9567606.htm (accessed June 12, 2012).

62. Robin Marantz Henig and Samantha Henig, "A Daughter Too Young—and Too Old—to Freeze Eggs," *New York Times*, May 15, 2012, http://parenting.blogs.nytimes.com/2012/05/15/a-daughter-too-young-and-too-old-to-freeze-eggs/ (accessed May 27, 2012).

63. Abrams, "It's Not Too Early to Talk about Your Eggs."

64. Joseph Brownstein, "Pregnant Women over 50 'Do Pretty Well,' Study Finds," FoxNews.com, February 3, 2012, http://www.foxnews.com/health/2012/02/03/pregnant-women-over-50-do-pretty-well-study-finds/ (accessed February 12, 2012).

65. Mehmet B. Cetinkaya et al., "Reproductive Outcome of Women 43 Years and beyond Undergoing ART Treatment with Their Own Oocytes in Two Connecticut University Programs," *Journal of Assisted Reproduction and Genetics* 30, no. 5 (June 2013): 673–78, http://link.springer.com/article/10.1007%2Fs10815-013-9981-5 (accessed April 20, 2012).

66. Mundy, *Everything Conceivable*, p. 42.

67. Kate Elizabeth Queram, "Twin Births Rise Brings Concerns," *StarNews Online*, January 19, 2012, http://www.starnewsonline.com/article/20120119/ARTICLES/1201 19641 (accessed February 18, 2012).

68. Jennifer Ludden and Marisa Penaloza, "Taming the Twin Trend from Fertility Treatments," NPR, March 29, 2011, http://www.npr.org/2011/03/30/134960899/taming-ivfs-twin-trend (accessed March 9, 2012).

69. Scott Kirsner, "Michelle Dipp, 36, Reflects Biotech's Next Generation," *Boston Globe*, October 14, 2012, http://bostonglobe.com/business/2012/10/13/michelle-dipp-ovascience-leading-new-generation-biotech-ceo/VqbVwXvcQSRkIVCQapdjhI/story.html (accessed December 2, 2012).

70. Mundy, *Everything Conceivable*, p. 15.

71. Ibid., p. 236.

72. Stacy Lu, "Octuplet Effect: More Choose Single Embryo Transplants for IVF," *TODAY Moms*, June 5, 2012, http://moms.today.msnbc.msn.com/_news/2012/06/05/11396062-octuplet-effect-more-choose-single-embryo-transplants-for-ivf?lite (accessed August 11, 2012).

73. Mundy, *Everything Conceivable*, p. 217.

74. Naomi McAuliffe, "Egg Freezing—For the Woman Who Can Never Win," *Guardian*, November 27, 2012, http://www.guardian.co.uk/commentisfree/2012/nov/27/egg-freezing-women-having-children (accessed December 20, 2012).

75. Jacqueline Mroz, "High Dose of Hormones Faulted in Fertility Care," *New York Times*, July 16, 2012, http://www.nytimes.com/2012/07/17/health/research/high-doses-of-hormones-add-to-ivf-complications.html (accessed August 29, 2012).

76. Michelle Munz, "New Form of in Vitro Fertilization Stirs Debate," *St. Louis Post-Dispatch*, January 26, 2012, http://www.stltoday.com/lifestyles/health-med-fit/fitness/new-form-of-in-vitro-fertilization-stirs-debate/article_1e684439-84f8-50fd-afb9-84aff48b17cb.html (accessed February 7, 2012).

77. Shulevitz, "How Older Parenthood Will Upend American Society." Catherine Pearson, "IVF and Birth Defects Could Be Linked, New Study Finds," *Huffington Post*, October 20, 2012, http://www.huffingtonpost.com/2012/10/20/ivf-birth-defects_n_1989302.html (accessed November 3, 2012).

78. Maia Szalavitz, "The Link between Infertility Treatments and Birth Defects," Health & Family, *Time*, May 7, 2012, http://healthland.time.com/2012/05/07/the-link-between-infertility-treatments-and-birth-defects/ (accessed August 3, 2012).

79. "Birth Defects More Common in IVF Babies: Study," Reuters, April 20, 2012, http://www.reuters.com/article/2012/04/20/us-ivf-idUSBRE83J03M20120420 (accessed April 28, 2012).

80. Stephen Adams, "Discovery to Deliver IVF Joy for Older Women," *Irish*

Independent, October 22, 2012, http://www.independent.ie/lifestyle/parenting/discovery -to-deliver-ivf-joy-for-older-women-3266864.html (accessed October 30, 2012).

81. Ian Sample, "IVF Could Be Revolutionised by New Technique, Says Clinic," *Guardian*, May 16, 2013, http://www.guardian.co.uk/society/2013/may/17/ivf -revolutionised-new-technique-clinic (accessed May 19, 2013).

82. Andrew Parker, "We Designed Our Baby to Be Safe from Cancer," *Sun*, October 7, 2012, http://www.thesun.co.uk/sol/homepage/news/4576137/Nicky-Halford-gives -birth-to-IVF-baby-designed-to-be-safe-from-cancer.html (accessed March 2, 2013).

83. Karen N. Peart, "A New Method for Picking the 'Right' Egg in IVF," *Yale News*, May 31, 2012, http://news.yale.edu/2012/05/31/new-method-picking-right-egg-ivf (accessed June 24, 2012).

84. James Gallagher, "Three-Person IVF 'Is Ethical' to Treat Mitochondrial Disease," BBC News, June 11, 2012, http://www.bbc.co.uk/news/health-18393682 (accessed July 3, 2012). Rebecca Smith, "Children with 'Three Parents' Could Become Reality," *Telegraph*, June 4, 2012, http://www.telegraph.co.uk/health/healthnews/9309023/Children-with -three-parents-could-become-reality.html (accessed July 3, 2012).

85. Robin Banerji, "The Woman Who Lost All Seven Children," BBC News *Magazine*, September 30, 2012, http://www.bbc.co.uk/news/magazine-19648992 (accessed March 3, 2013).

86. Michelle Roberts, "Three-Person IVF Trial 'Success,'" BBC News, October 24, 2012, http://www.bbc.co.uk/news/health-20032216 (accessed October 30, 2012). Malcolm Ritter, "3-Person IVF? Embryos from 2 Women, 1 Man Created in Lab," *Huffington Post*, October 24, 2012, http://www.huffingtonpost.com/2012/10/24/3-person -ivf-embryos-women-man_n_2011546.html (accessed October 30, 2012).

87. Kirsner, "Michelle Dipp, 36, Reflects Biotech's Next Generation."

88. Sunday Pirkle, PhD, in interview with the author, January 8, 2013.

89. Peggy Orenstein, *Flux: Women on Sex, Work, Love, Kids, & Life in a Half-Changed World* (New York: Anchor Books, 2000), p. 146.

90. Kathy Bright, "I'm Still Waiting for the Sting of Adoption to Go Away," Parents, *Huffington Post*, January 25, 2013, http://www.huffingtonpost.com/2013/01/25/adoption -stigma_n_2542717.html (accessed February 2, 2013).

91. Beth Hall, in interview with the author, January 9, 2013.

92. Nancy Rosenhaus, in interview with the author, April 26, 2012.

93. Victoria Birk Hill, in interview with the author, April 25, 2012.

94. "Adoption Can Boost Quality of Life for Infertile Couples, Study Finds," Health, *US News & World Report*, November 19, 2012, http://health.usnews.com/health-news/ news/articles/2012/11/19/adoption-can-boost-quality-of-life-for-infertile-couples-study -finds (accessed December 11, 2012).

95. Mundy, *Everything Conceivable*, pp. 190–91.

96. Craig Young, "Funding Cut Threatens Loveland-Based Program That Encourages

Adoption of Frozen Embryos; Women Tell Adoption Stories," March 10, 2012, http://
www.reporterherald.com/news/loveland-local-news/ci_20149489/funding-cut-threatens
-loveland-based-program-that-encourages (accessed February 6, 2013).

97. Mundy, *Everything Conceivable*, p. 296.

98. Young, "Funding Cut Threatens Loveland-Based Program That Encourages
Adoption of Frozen Embryos." Lindsay Lowe, "Woman Gives Birth Using 19-Year-Old
Embryos: 'He's My Little Miracle,'" *Parade*, August 22, 2013, http://www.parade.com/
66813/linzlowe/woman-gives-birth-using-19-year-old-embryos-hes-my-little-miracle/ (accessed September 2, 2013).

99. "Social Egg Freezing: The Reasons Some Women Freeze Their Eggs," My Fertility
Choices, January 22, 2013, http://myfertilitychoices.com/2013/01/social-egg-freezing-the
-reasons-some-women-freeze-their-eggs/ (accessed February 9, 2013).

100. "Live Births with Egg Freezing Tied to Patient Age and Egg Freezing Method,"
Fertility Authority, http://www.fertilityauthority.com/articles/live-births-egg-freezing-tied
-patient-age-and-egg-freezing-method (accessed January 16, 2013).

101. Susan Donaldson James, "Rabbis Urge Single, Orthodox Women to Freeze
Eggs at 38," ABC News, September 10, 2012, http://abcnews.go.com/Health/rabbis-urge
-single-orthodox-women-freeze-eggs-age/story?id=17185321#.UaeH0CvTXEc (accessed
September 15, 2012).

102. Sarah Elizabeth Richards, *Motherhood, Rescheduled: The New Frontier of Egg Freezing
and the Women Who Tried It* (New York: Simon & Schuster, 2013).

103. Lunau, "Thirty-Seven and Counting."

104. Pasquale Patrizio, MD, in interview with the author, May 1, 2012.

105. "Egg Freezing for Fertility Preservation Priced at $4,900 for the Holidays by
Frozen Egg Bank Inc., a Division of West Coast Fertility Centers in Orange County,
California," PRWeb, November 30, 2012, http://www.prweb.com/releases/prwebEgg
FreezingCalifornia/FertilityPreservation/prweb10184237.htm (accessed January 19, 2013).

106. "New Egg Freezing Technique Offers Hope to Hundreds of Women," ScienceDaily,
June 21, 2006, http://www.sciencedaily.com/releases/2006/06/060621163255.htm (accessed March 5, 2012).

107. Sharon Kirkey, "Freezing of Women's Eggs, Embryos Cause Controversy,"
Health, Canada.com, March 15, 2012, http://o.canada.com/2012/03/15/freezing-of
-womens-eggs-embryos-cause-controversy/ (accessed April 9, 2012).

108. Victoria Vallejo et al., "Social and Psychological Assessment of Women
Undergoing Elective Oocyte Cryopreservation: A 7-Year Analysis," *Open Journal of Obstetrics
and Gynecology* 3 (January 2013), http://www.scirp.org/journal/ojog (accessed March 15,
2013).

109. "Early to Embrace Egg Freezing for Fertility Preservation, a CT Fertility Clinic
Now Sees Its Even Greater Personal and Societal Impact in Donor Egg Banking," PRWeb,

November 1, 2012, http://www.prweb.com/releases/prwebct_fertility_egg_freezing/asrm
_non-experimental/prweb10081736.htm (accessed December 21, 2012).

110. Marie McCullough, "Human Egg-Freezing Gets a Stamp of Approval," *Inquirer*,
Philly.com, October 19, 2012, http://articles.philly.com/2012-10-19/news/34556996_1
_michael-j-glassner-largest-human-cell-egg (accessed October 23, 2012).

111. Michele G. Sullivan, "ASRM: Egg Freezing No Longer 'Experimental,'"
Ob.Gyn. News, October 19, 2012, http://www.obgynnews.com/index.php?id=11146&c
Hash=071010&tx_ttnews[tt_news]=137771 (accessed October 23, 2012).

112. "Freezing Human Eggs for In Vitro Fertilization No Longer Experimental
Procedure," *PBS NewsHour*, October 19, 2012, http://www.pbs.org/newshour/bb/health/
july-dec12/eggs_10-19.html (accessed October 23, 2012).

113. Álison Motluk, "Growth of Egg Freezing Blurs 'Experimental' Label," *Nature*
476 (2011): 382–83, http://www.nature.com/news/2011/110823/full/476382a.html
(accessed October 23, 2012).

114. Ibid.

115. "Eggsurance Launches Independent Community and Educational Website
Devoted to Everything Egg Freezing," Yahoo! Finance, May 22, 2012, http://finance
.yahoo.com/news/eggsurance-launches-independent-community-educational-131500291
.html (accessed June 12, 2012).

116. Doug Brunk, "Fertility Preservation No Longer Experimental," Ob.Gyn. News,
June 14, 2012, http://www.obgynnews.com/news/top-news/single-article/fertility
-preservation-no-longer-experimental-for-cancer-patients/47e02be79468de56e43483da1
38cd478.html (accessed July 16, 2012).

117. McCullough, "Human Egg-Freezing Gets a Stamp of Approval."

118. Rob Stein, "Chance to Pause Biological Clock with Ovarian Transplant Stirs
Debate," NPR, December 24, 2012, http://www.npr.org/blogs/health/2012/12/
24/167705397/chance-to-pause-biological-clock-with-ovarian-transplant-stirs-debate (accessed January 8, 2013).

119. "Chance to Pause Biological Clock with Ovarian Transplant Stirs Debate."

120. Fiona MacRae and Vanessa Allen, "Doctors Carry out First Successful Womb
Transplant," *New Zealand Herald*, May 26, 2012, http://www.nzherald.co.nz/lifestyle/
news/article.cfm?c_id=6&objectid=10808636 (accessed June 9, 2012).

121. Fiona MacRae, "Britain's First Womb Transplant Could Be Carried out in Just
TWO YEARS," *Daily Mail*, July 12, 2012, http://www.dailymail.co.uk/health/article
-2172420/Britain-s-womb-transplant-carried-just-TWO-YEARS.html (accessed July 15, 2012).

122. Ashley Hayes, "First Mother-Daughter Womb Transplants Performed in
Sweden," CNN, September 20, 2012, http://www.cnn.com/2012/09/19/health/uterine
-transplant (accessed September 22, 2012).

123. "Woman Who Underwent 2011 Womb Transplant 6 Weeks Pregnant," CBS/

AP, April 29, 2013, http://www.cbsnews.com/8301-204_162-57581959/woman-who
-underwent-2011-womb-transplant-6-weeks-pregnant/ (accessed April 30, 2013).

124. "IVF Success Rates: Don't Believe Everything You Read, Says Fertility Specialist,"
PRWeb, February 1, 2013, http://www.prweb.com/releases/2013/2/prweb10386327
.htm (accessed February 7, 2013).

125. Motluk, "Growth of Egg Freezing Blurs 'Experimental' Label," pp. 382–83.

126. Toby Harnden, "New Republican Platform Banning All Abortions Could
Also Restrict IVF . . . Which Three of Romney's Sons Have Used to Conceive," *Daily
Mail*, August 21, 2012, http://www.dailymail.co.uk/news/article-2191690/human-life
-amendment--New-Republican-platform-banning-ALL-abortions-restrict-IVF.html (accessed September 4, 2012).

127. Kira Peikoff, "Personhood vs. Stem Cell Research," *Atlanta Journal-Constitution*, May
25, 2012, http://www.ajc.com/news/news/opinion/personhood-vs-stem-cell-research/
nQT65/ (accessed October 13, 2012).

128. Mundy, *Everything Conceivable*, p. 318.

129. David Plotz, "The 'Genius Babies,' and How They Grew," *Slate*, February 8, 2001,
http://www.slate.com/articles/life/seed/2001/02/the_genius_babies_and_how_they
_grew.html (accessed February 15, 2012).

130. Laird Harrison, "California Sperm Donor at Odds with Federal Regulators,"
Reuters, December 20, 2011, http://www.reuters.com/article/2011/12/20/us-sperm
-donor-california-idUSTRE7BJ1F420111220 (accessed February 7, 2012). Benjamin
Wallace, "The Virgin Father," *New York*, February 5, 2012, http://nymag.com/news/
features/trent-arsenault-2012-2/ (accessed February 7, 2012).

131. Jacqueline Mroz, "One Sperm Donor, 150 Offspring," *New York Times*, September
5, 2011, http://www.nytimes.com/2011/09/06/health/06donor.html (accessed February
4, 2012).

132. Rebecca Smith, "British Man 'Fathered 600 Children' at Own Fertility Clinic,"
Telegraph, April 8, 2012, http://www.telegraph.co.uk/news/9193014/British-man
-fathered-600-children-at-own-fertility-clinic.html (accessed April 23, 2012).

133. Mroz, "One Sperm Donor, 150 Offspring."

134. Kerry Grens, "The Black (Egg) Market? IVF Recruiters Are Forgetting about the
Ethics," *MedCity News*, August 9, 2012, http://medcitynews.com/2012/08/the-black-egg
-market-ivf-recruiters-are-forgetting-about-the-ethics/ (accessed August 19, 2012).

CHAPTER 4: DECISIONS, DECISIONS

1. "Merck and RESOLVE Remind Couples That a Conversation with a Specialist
Could Be the Start of Something Small," April 23, 2012, http://www.multivu.com/

mnr/55828-merck-resolve-pregnancy-fertilityguide-national-infertility-awareness-week (accessed May 5, 2012).

2. Jennifer Wolff Perrine, "This Woman Has a Secret," *SELF*, http://www.self .com/health/2010/08/breaking-the-silence-on-infertility/ (accessed March 11, 2012).

3. Janey Adams, "Infertility: It's Not the End of the World," NPR, July 2, 2011, http:// www.npr.org/blogs/babyproject/2011/07/06/137504382/infertility-its-not-the-end-of -the-world/ (accessed April 3, 2012).

4. Natalie Angier, *Woman: An Intimate Geography* (New York: Anchor Books, 2000), p. 13.

5. "Georgia Woman Gives Birth to Her GRANDSON after IVF Treatment Because Her Daughter Couldn't Conceive," *Daily Mail*, October 18, 2012, http://www .dailymail.co.uk/news/article-2217598/Georgia-woman-gives-birth-GRANDSON-IVF -treatment-daughter-conceive.html (accessed December 11, 2012).

6. Lillian Schapiro, *Tick Tock* (Lincoln, NE: iUniverse, Inc., 2005), p. 5.

7. Christine Overall, "Think before You Breed," *New York Times*, June 17, 2012, http://opinionator.blogs.nytimes.com/2012/06/17/think-before-you-breed/ (accessed June 23, 2012).

8. Liza Mundy, *Everything Conceivable: How Assisted Reproduction Is Changing Our World* (New York: Anchor Books, 2008), p. 62.

9. "Couples' Sexual Relationships Can Suffer during IVF, Study Finds," Health, *US News & World Report*, November 2, 2012, http://health.usnews.com/health-news/ news/articles/2012/11/02/couples-sexual-relationships-can-suffer-during-ivf-study-finds (accessed December 18, 2012).

10. "Insurance Coverage in Your State," RESOLVE, http://www.resolve.org/ family-building-options/insurance_coverage/state-coverage.html (accessed April 4, 2012).

11. Fiona McPhillips, "Pals Would Announce Pregnancies and I'd Have to Leave the Room," *Herald*, May 1, 2013, http://www.herald.ie/lifestyle/pals-would-announce -pregnancies-and-id-have-to-leave-the-room-29235717.html (accessed May 6, 2013).

12. Amy Norton, "Failed IVF Attempt Tied to Depression, Anxiety," Reuters, June 27, 2012, http://www.reuters.com/article/2012/06/27/us-ivf-depression-idUSBRE85Q 19120120627 (accessed March 23, 2013).

CHAPTER 5: THE LIMITS OF EVOLUTION

1. Rob Stein, "In Vitro Fertilization Can't Reverse Aging's Effects," *Washington Post*, January 15, 2009, http://articles.washingtonpost.com/2009-01-15/news/36883365_1 _ivf-infertile-women-treatment-cycles (accessed February 8, 2012).

2. Natalie Angier, *Woman: An Intimate Geography* (New York: Anchor Books, 2000), pp. 356–57.

3. Dr. Gerda Lerner, who died on January 2, 2013, at the age of ninety-two, established the first graduate program in women's history in the United States at Sarah Lawrence College in 1972. She was also a founding member of the National Organization for Women. William Grimes, "Gerda Lerner, a Feminist and Historian, Dies at 92," *New York Times*, January 3, 2013, http://www.nytimes.com/2013/01/04/us/gerda-lerner-historian-dies-at-92.html (accessed January 15, 2013).

4. Angier, *Woman: An Intimate Geography*, p. 357.

5. Ibid., p. xiv.

6. Elizabeth Weil, "Puberty Before Age 10: A New 'Normal'?" *New York Times*, March 30, 2012, http://www.nytimes.com/2012/04/01/magazine/puberty-before-age-10-a-new-normal.html (accessed April 2, 2012).

7. Jacque Wilson, "Boys—Like Girls—Hitting Puberty Earlier," CNN, October 23, 2012, http://www.cnn.com/2012/10/20/health/boys-early-puberty/index.html (accessed October 28, 2012).

8. Weil, "Puberty Before Age 10: A New 'Normal'?"

9. Wilson, "Boys—Like Girls—Hitting Puberty Earlier."

10. Caitlin Moran, *How to Be a Woman* (New York: Harper Perennial, 2011), p. 54.

11. Angier, *Woman: An Intimate Geography*, p. 105.

12. Moran, *How to Be a Woman*, p. 18.

13. My mom might not have been wrong about girls being more attractive to boys when they have their periods. Devendra Singh, a psychology professor at the University of Texas in Austin, conducted a study of T-shirts worn by women during their most and least fertile periods. Men responded more strongly to the smell of the "fertile" T-shirts. While studies such as these should be taken with a grain of salt, we do know that we release pheromones, which, though odorless, are hormones that can heighten sexual urges. Perhaps the shift in the way we smell when we are ovulating can contribute to our desirability as well. Melanie Axelrod, "Men Can Smell Fertility, Study Says," ABC News, April 5, 2013, http://abcnews.go.com/Health/story?id=117526&page=1 (accessed April 22, 2013).

14. Leonard Shlain, *Sex, Time and Power: How Women's Sexuality Shaped Human Evolution* (New York: Penguin Books, 2004), p. 55.

15. Ibid., pp. 137–38.

16. Ibid., p. 64.

17. Angier, *Woman: An Intimate Geography*, pp. 179–80.

18. Ibid., p. 109.

19. Shlain, *Sex, Time and Power*, p. 181.

20. Ibid., p. 47.

21. Angier, *Woman: An Intimate Geography*, p. 119.

22. Ibid., p. 222.

23. Ibid., p. 198.

24. Ibid., p. 366.

25. Ibid.

26. Peggy Orenstein, *Flux: Women on Sex, Work, Love, Kids, & Life in a Half-Changed World* (New York: Anchor Books, 2000), p. 25.

27. Ibid., p. 26.

28. Ibid., pp. 283–84.

29. Shlain, *Sex, Time and Power*, p. 49.

30. Angier, *Woman: An Intimate Geography*, pp. 330–31.

31. Shlain, *Sex, Time and Power*, p. 87.

32. Ibid., pp. 356–57.

33. Angier, *Woman: An Intimate Geography*, p. 251.

34. Liza Mundy, *Everything Conceivable: How Assisted Reproduction Is Changing Our World* (New York: Anchor Books, 2008), p. 18.

35. Ibid., pp. 80–81.

36. Martha Beck, *Expecting Adam: A True Story of Birth, Rebirth, and Everyday Magic* (New York: Three Rivers Press, 2011). Priscilla Gilman, *The Anti-Romantic Child: A Memoir of Unexpected Joy* (New York: Harper Perennial, 2011). Kelle Hampton, *Bloom: Finding Beauty in the Unexpected* (New York: William Morrow, 2013).

37. Beck, *Expecting Adam*, p. 6.

38. Jenny Hope, "Children of Mothers over 40 'Are Healthier and More Intelligent and Less Likely to Have Accidents,'" *Daily Mail*, May 21, 2012, http://www.dailymail.co.uk/health/article-2147848/Children-mothers-40-healthier-intelligent.html (accessed May 25, 2012).

39. Michelle Roberts, "Children with Older Fathers and Grandfathers 'Live Longer,'" BBC News, June 11, 2012, http://www.bbc.co.uk/news/health-18392873 (accessed August 9, 2012).

40. Mundy, *Everything Conceivable*, p. 12.

41. Dominique Bousquet, in interview with the author, January 21, 2013.

42. Angier, *Woman: An Intimate Geography*, p. 239.

43. Shlain, *Sex, Time and Power*, p. 87.

44. Angier, *Woman: An Intimate Geography*, p. 237.

45. Shlain, *Sex, Time and Power*, p. 85.

46. Angier, *Woman: An Intimate Geography*, p. 241.

47. Ibid., pp. 235–36.

48. Julia McQuillan, PhD, in interview with the author, May 11, 2012.

49. "Women University Grads Waiting Longer to Have Children," My Fertility Choices, November 5, 2012, http://myfertilitychoices.com/2012/11/women-university-grads-waiting-longer-to-have-children/ (accessed December 10, 2012).

50. Shlain, *Sex, Time and Power*, p. 342.

51. Angier, *Woman: An Intimate Geography*, p. 93.

52. Mundy, *Everything Conceivable*, p. 28.

53. Angier, *Woman: An Intimate Geography*, p. 147.

54. Ibid., pp. 302–305.

55. Ibid.

56. Rebecca J. Hannagan, "Gendered Political Behavior: A Darwinian Feminist Approach," *Sex Roles* 59, no. 7–8 (October 2008): 465–75.

57. Shlain, *Sex, Time and Power*, p. 339.

58. Ibid., p. 349.

59. Roni Caryn Rabin, "Nearly 1 in 5 Women in U.S. Survey Say They Have Been Sexually Assaulted," Health, *New York Times*, December 14, 2011, http://www.nytimes.com/2011/12/15/health/nearly-1-in-5-women-in-us-survey-report-sexual-assault.html (accessed February 9, 2012).

60. Monsoon Bissell, "To the Woman Warrior I Didn't Know," *Daily Beast*, January 5, 2013, http://www.thedailybeast.com/articles/2013/01/05/to-the-woman-warrior-i-did-not-know.html (accessed January 7, 2013).

61. Suchitra Mohanty and Frank Jack Daniel, "Indian Rape Victim's Father Says He Wants Her Named," Reuters, Sunday, January 6, 2013, http://www.reuters.com/article/2013/01/06/us-india-rape-idUSBRE90500B20130106 (accessed January 7, 2013).

62. Michelle Nichols, "Babies as Young as Six Months Victims of Rape in War: U.N. Envoy," Reuters, April 17, 2013, http://www.reuters.com/article/2013/04/17/us-war-rape-un-idUSBRE93G13U20130417 (accessed May 4, 2013).

63. Jonathan Weisman, "Senate Votes Overwhelmingly to Expand Domestic Violence Act," *New York Times*, February 12, 2013, http://www.nytimes.com/2013/02/13/us/politics/senate-votes-to-expand-domestic-violence-act.html (accessed February 15, 2013).

64. Nadia Kounang, "Could 'Personhood' Bills Outlaw IVF?" CNN, August 30, 2012, http://www.cnn.com/2012/08/30/health/ivf-outlawed (accessed December 2, 2012).

65. Ibid.

66. Laura Bassett, "Carolyn Maloney: Rush Limbaugh 'Slut' Comment Is Attempt to Silence Women," *Huffington Post*, March 1, 2012, http://www.huffingtonpost.com/2012/03/01/carolyn-maloney-rush-limbaugh-slut_n_1313243.html (accessed March 8, 2012).

67. Lori Moore, "Rep. Todd Akin: The Statement and the Reaction," *New York Times*, August 20, 2012, http://www.nytimes.com/2012/08/21/us/politics/rep-todd-akin-legitimate-rape-statement-and-reaction.html (accessed August 21, 2012).

68. "Sperm," *Radiolab*, 2008, http://www.radiolab.org/2008/dec/01/ (accessed June 9, 2013).

69. Richard Cowan, "Record Number of Women Sworn into New U.S. Congress," Reuters, January 3, 2013, http://www.reuters.com/article/2013/01/03/us-usa-congress-women-idUSBRE9020KT20130103 (accessed January 8, 2013).

70. Kate Bolick, "All the Single Ladies," *Atlantic*, September 30, 2011, http://www
.theatlantic.com/magazine/archive/2011/11/all-the-single-ladies/8654/ (accessed February 7, 2012).

71. Daniel de Vise, "For Working Mothers in Academia, Tenure Track Is Often a Tough Balancing Act," *Washington Post*, July 11, 2010, http://www.washingtonpost.com/ wp-dyn/content/article/2010/07/10/AR2010071002610.html (accessed February 3, 2012).

72. Mary Ann Mason, "What You Need to Know If You're an Academic," *New York Times*, July 16, 2013, http://www.nytimes.com/roomfordebate/2013/07/08/should -women-delay-motherhood/what-you-need-to-know-if-youre-an-academic-and-want-to -be-a-mom (accessed September 4, 2013).

73. Ibid.

74. Beck, *Expecting Adam*, p. 11.

75. Gilman, *The Anti-Romantic Child*, pp. 30–31.

76. In the top one hundred US universities in 2007, women full professors in math-intensive fields numbered only 4.4 to 12.3 percent, and women were only 16 to 27 percent of assistant professors. Wendy M. Williams and Stephen J. Ceci, "When Scientists Choose Motherhood," *American Scientist* 100, no. 2 (March–April 2012): 138, http://www.american scientist.org/issues/pub/when-scientists-choose-motherhood (accessed May 18, 2012).

77. Lawrence H. Summers, "Remarks at NBER Conference on Diversifying the Science & Engineering Workforce," January 14, 2005, http://www.harvard.edu/president/ speeches/summers_2005/nber.php (accessed March 15, 2013).

78. "Women and Science: A Look at Harvard Pres. Larry Summers," January 25, 2005, http://www.democracynow.org/2005/1/25/women_and_science_a_look_at (accessed May 4, 2012).

79. Denise Grady, "American Woman Who Shattered Space Ceiling," *New York Times*, July 23, 2012, http://www.nytimes.com/2012/07/24/science/space/sally-ride -trailblazing-astronaut-dies-at-61.html (accessed July 29, 2012).

80. In the April 2013 *New York Times* piece about Girls Who Code and other girls' training programs, such as Girl Develop It, Black Girls Code, and Girls Teaching Girls to Code, Reshma Saujani presented disheartening statistics on women in computer science: "Even though women represent more than half the overall work force, they hold less than a quarter of computing and technical jobs, according to the National Center for Women and Information Technology. . . . Women earn just 12 percent of computer science degrees, down from 37 percent in 1984. . . . Roughly 74 percent of girls in middle school express an interest in engineering, science and math. But by the time they get to college, just 0.3 percent choose computer science as a major." Claire Cain Miller, "Opening a Gateway for Girls to Enter the Computer Field," *New York Times*, April 2, 2013, http://dealbook .nytimes.com/2013/04/02/opening-a-gateway-for-girls-to-enter-the-computer-field/ (accessed April 5, 2013).

81. Bolick, "All the Single Ladies."

82. "When There's a Baby between You and the Glass Ceiling," NPR, December 2, 2012, http://www.npr.org/2012/12/23/167923727/when-the-glass-ceiling-is-a-baby-working-through-motherhood (accessed January 15, 2012).

83. Leo Cendrowicz, "Can Mandatory Quotas Bring Gender Equality to Europe's Boardrooms?" *Time*, March 8, 2012, http://www.time.com/time/world/article/0,8599,2108607,00.html (accessed March 10, 2012).

84. Bolick, "All the Single Ladies."

85. Bel Mooney and Sadie Nicholas, "Losing Out at Work, Sidelined by IVF . . . Is the Male of the Species Now Redundant?" *Daily Mail*, October 10, 2012, http://www.dailymail.co.uk/femail/article-2215956/Losing-work-sidelined-IVF--male-species-redundant.html (accessed December 15, 2012).

86. Jordan Weissmann, "Why Are Women Paid Less?" *Atlantic*, October 17, 2012, http://www.theatlantic.com/business/archive/2012/10/why-are-women-paid-less/263776/ (accessed October 28, 2012).

87. "Women Still Confront Yawning Wage Gap—Study," Reuters, April 17, 2012, http://www.reuters.com/article/2012/04/17/wages-gender-gap-idUSL2E8FH9IC20120417 (accessed April 20, 2012).

88. Pauline W. Chen, MD, "Among Doctors, Too, Women Are Paid Less," *New York Times*, June 28, 2012, http://well.blogs.nytimes.com/2012/06/28/among-doctors-too-women-are-paid-less/ (accessed August 11, 2012).

89. Hanna Rosin, "The Gender Wage Gap Lie," *Slate*, August 30, 2013, http://www.slate.com/articles/double_x/doublex/2013/08/gender_pay_gap_the_familiar_line_that_women_make_77_cents_to_every_man_s.html (accessed September 5, 2013).

90. Moran, *How to Be a Woman*, p. 83.

91. Debora L. Spar, "Why Women Should Stop Trying to Be Perfect," *Daily Beast*, September 24, 2012, http://www.thedailybeast.com/newsweek/2012/09/23/why-women-should-stop-trying-to-be-perfect.html (accessed October 2, 2012).

92. Angier, *Woman: An Intimate Geography*, p. 378.

93. Ibid., p. 391.

94. Nick Bostrom, "Nick Bostrom on Our Biggest Problems," *TED Talks*, July 2005, http://www.ted.com/talks/nick_bostrom_on_our_biggest_problems.html (accessed April 8, 2012).

95. James Gallagher, "Is the Six-Million-Dollar Man Possible?" BBC News, March 11, 2012, http://www.bbc.co.uk/news/health-16632764 (accessed March 15, 2012).

96. Simon Tomlinson, "'Women Will Have So Much Choice about When to Have Children': Scientists Can Stop Menopause with Ovary Transplants," *Daily Mail*, March 25, 2012, http://www.dailymail.co.uk/health/article-2120102/Fertility-breakthrough-Scientists-halt-menopause-ovary-transplants.html (accessed March 29, 2012).

97. Kate Lunau, "Thirty-Seven and Counting," *Maclean's*, October 27, 2012, http://www2.macleans.ca/2012/10/27/thirty-seven-and-counting/ (accessed December 20, 2012).

98. Ibid.

99. Angier, *Woman: An Intimate Geography*, p. 392.

100. "The Benefits of State Seat Belt Laws," National Highway Traffic Safety Administration, http://www.policyalmanac.org/economic/archive/seatbelts.shtml (accessed February 24, 2013).

101. "Did You Know . . . ?" *Good Housekeeping*, February 2013, p. 71.

102. Amy Richards, *Opting In: Having a Child without Losing Yourself* (New York: Farrar, Straus and Giroux, 2008), p. 10.

CHAPTER 6: BABY MADNESS AND THE MEDIA

1. Aiyana Baida, "Jennifer Lopez and Casper Smart Expecting via IVF, Surrogate!" *VOXXI*, April 1, 2013, http://www.voxxi.com/jennifer-lopez-expecting-ivf-surrogate/ (accessed April 1, 2013).

2. "Halle Berry Expecting Second Child, First with Olivier Martinez," Reuters, April 5, 2013, http://www.reuters.com/article/2013/04/05/us-halleberry-idUSBRE9340 V220130405 (accessed April 6, 2013).

3. Amy Richards, in interview with the author, April 30, 2013.

4. Alessandra Stanley, "Mother of All Comedy Topics," *New York Times*, March 15, 2013, http://www.nytimes.com/2013/03/17/movies/tina-feys-admission-and-other-comedies-eye-maternity.html (accessed March 18, 2013).

5. Katie Kindelan, "Maria Menounos: 'My Choice' to Freeze My Eggs," ABC News, September 26, 2011, http://abcnews.go.com/blogs/health/2011/09/26/maria-menounos-my-choice-to-freeze-my-eggs/ (accessed February 13, 2012).

6. Rebecca Dana, "The Vitrification Fertility Option," *Newsweek*, January 23, 2012, http://www.thedailybeast.com/newsweek/2012/01/22/the-vitrification-fertility-option.html (accessed February 4, 2012).

7. Thomas Vinciguerra, "He's Not My Grandpa. He's My Dad," *New York Times*, April 12, 2007, http://www.nytimes.com/2007/04/12/fashion/12dads.html (accessed March 19, 2012).

8. "Scientists Warn of Dangers in Delaying Motherhood," *Express Tribune*, April 10, 2012, http://tribune.com.pk/story/362393/scientists-warn-of-dangers-in-delaying-motherhood/ (accessed May 19, 2012).

9. Liza Mundy, *Everything Conceivable: How Assisted Reproduction Is Changing Our World* (New York: Anchor Books, 2008), p. 54.

10. Ibid., p. 55.

11. Ibid., p. 193.

12. Michelle Profis, "Lady Gaga Tells Oprah She Wants a 'Soccer Team' of Kids," PopWatch, *Entertainment Weekly*, March 19, 2012, http://popwatch.ew.com/2012/03/19/lady-gaga-on-oprah/ (accessed March 20, 2012).

13. *Extra* (February 29, 2012).

14. Caitlin Moran, *How to Be a Woman* (New York: Harper Perennial, 2011), pp. 232–33.

15. Katie McDonough, "'I'm Not a Feminist, but . . . ,'" *Salon*, April 6, 2013, http://www.salon.com/2013/04/06/im_not_a_feminist_but/ (accessed April 10, 2013).

16. Maureen O'Connor, "Beyoncé Is a 'Feminist, I Guess,'" *New York*, April 4, 2013, http://nymag.com/thecut/2013/04/beyonc-is-a-feminist-i-guess.html (accessed April 4, 2013).

17. Justine Picardie, "The Real Gwyneth," *Harper's Bazaar*, March 2012, p. 393.

18. Moran, *How to Be a Woman*, p. 77.

19. Sheryl Sandberg, *Lean In: Women, Work, and the Will to Lead* (New York: Alfred A. Knopf, 2013), pp. 157–58.

20. Anya Leon, "Padma Lakshmi: I Don't Parent Alone," *People*, November 3, 2011, http://celebritybabies.people.com/2011/11/03/padma-lakshmi-i-dont-parent-alone/ (accessed February 8, 2012).

21. Charlotte Triggs, "Mariska Hargitay: My Double Adoption Blessing," *People*, October 31, 2011, http://www.people.com/people/archive/article/0,,20538446,00.html (accessed February 3, 2012). Sheila Weller, "My Faith Pulled Me Through," *Good Housekeeping*, April 4, 2012, http://www.goodhousekeeping.com/family/celebrity-interviews/mariska-hargitay-adoption (accessed April 15, 2012).

22. Soraya Roberts, "Hollywood's IVF Stigma's Strong," *Star*, April 29, 2013, http://www.thestar.com/life/parent/2013/04/29/hollywoods_ivf_stigmas_strong.html (accessed April 30, 2013).

23. Jenny Schafer, "Hugh Jackman on Wife's Miscarriages, The Joys of Adoption," *Celebrity Baby Scoop*, December 18, 2012, http://www.celebritybabyscoop.com/2012/12/18/hugh-jackman-on-wifes-miscarriages-the-joys-of-adoption (accessed December 23, 2012).

24. Alasdair Glennie, "I Woke Up and Thought: I Want a Baby. But It Was Too Late, Says Pop Star Lisa Stansfield," *Daily Mail*, October 19, 2012, http://www.dailymail.co.uk/tvshowbiz/article-2220415/I-woke-thought-I-want-baby-But-late-says-pop-star-Lisa-Stansfield.html (accessed February 20, 2012).

25. Syahida Kamarudin, "Hebe Tian Wants to Freeze Her Eggs," *Yahoo! Malaysia*, November 18, 2012, http://my.entertainment.yahoo.com/news/hebe-tian-wants-freeze-her-eggs-233600951.html (accessed December 2, 2012).

26. "Kiran Is a Hands-On Mother: Aamir Khan," *Hindustan Times*, December 3,

2012, http://www.hindustantimes.com/Entertainment/Tabloid/Kiran-is-a-hands-on
-mother-Aamir-Khan/Article1-967736.aspx (accessed December 3, 2012).

27. Leigh Blickley, "Celebrities Who've Used Surrogates to Conceive," *Huffington Post*, February 6, 2013, http://www.huffingtonpost.com/2013/02/06/celebrities-who-have
-used-surrogates_n_2624998.html (accessed February 10, 2013).

28. "Kim Kardashian Would Opt for IVF to Have Baby at 40," *azcentral.com*, June 18, 2012, http://www.azcentral.com/ent/celeb/articles/2012/06/18/20120618kim
-kardashian-would-opt-ivf-baby-40.html (accessed August 15, 2012).

29. Vicki Woods, "Sofia Vergara: Dangerous Curves," *Vogue*, March 2013, http://
www.vogue.com/magazine/article/sofia-vergara-dangerous-curves/ (accessed March 20, 2013).

30. Paloma Corredor, "Sofia Vergara Freezing Her Eggs, IVF a Popular Trend among Women Today," *VOXXI*, April 8, 2013, http://www.voxxi.com/sofia-vergara
-freezing-eggs-ivf-trend/ (accessed April 21, 2013).

31. Lizzie Smith, "'I Chased My Career instead of Chasing Guys': Giuliana Rancic Reveals How Her Infertility 'Blindsided' Her at 35," *Daily Mail*, October 30, 2012, http://
www.dailymail.co.uk/tvshowbiz/article-2225299/I-chase-career-instead-chasing-guys
-Giuliana-Rancic-reveals-infertility-blindsided-her.html (accessed November 2, 2012).

32. Zach Johnson, "Aisha Tyler Opens Up about Infertility Struggle," E! Online, September 13, 2013, http://www.eonline.com/news/458556/aisha-tyler-opens-up-about
-infertility-struggle-on-the-talk-why-she-stopped-ivf-treatments (accessed September 13, 2013). "Aisha Tyler Reveals Struggle with Infertility," *People*, September 12, 2013, http://
celebritybabies.people.com/2013/09/12/aisha-tyler-reveals-infertility-ivf-failure/ (accessed September 13, 2013).

33. Jennifer D'Angelo Friedman, "FOX News Anchor Reveals Infertility Struggle," *SELF*, October 2010, http://www.self.com/health/2010/10/news-anchor-reveals
-infertility-struggle (accessed March 6, 2012).

34. Roger Catlin, "Marlo Thomas: 'It's Amazing the Impact "Free to Be . . ."' Had. Yet Nobody Followed It Up. It's Gone Bad,'" *Salon*, February 26, 2013, http://www
.salon.com/2013/02/26/marlo_thomas_its_amazing_the_impact_free_to_be_had_yet
_nobody_followed_it_up_its_gone_bad/ (accessed February 28, 2013).

35. Ibid.

36. Peggy Orenstein, *Flux: Women on Sex, Work, Love, Kids, & Life in a Half-Changed World* (New York: Anchor Books, 2000), p. 145.

37. Amy Richards, *Opting In: Having a Child without Losing Yourself* (New York: Farrar, Straus and Giroux, 2008), p. 58.

38. Amy Richards, in interview with the author, April 30, 2012.

39. *Glee*, "The Spanish Teacher," February 7, 2012.

40. Megan Angelo, "The *New Girl* Episode That Freaked Out Every Girl in

America," *Glamour*, November 28, 2012, http://www.glamour.com/entertainment/blogs/obsessed/2012/11/the-new-girl-episode-that-frea.html (accessed December 18, 2012).

41. Rajini Vaidyanathan, "The Rise and Rise of New Bollywood," BBC News, June 7, 2012, http://www.bbc.co.uk/news/world-asia-india-18327901 (accessed September 15, 2012).

42. Kinjal Desai, "*Vicky Donor* Lures Ahmedabad Men to Sperm Donation," *DNA*, May 1, 2012, http://www.dnaindia.com/india/report_vicky-donor-lures-ahmedabad-men-to-sperm-donation_1682992 (accessed June 3, 2012).

43. Mansi Tewari, "Vicky Donor Affect: Infertility Specialists in Meerut Get a Boost," *Economic Times*, May 30, 2012, http://articles.economictimes.indiatimes.com/2012-05-30/news/31900430_1_sperm-donation-sperm-banking-meerut (accessed June 3, 2012).

44. Jenny Allen, "Welcome Back, Katie!" *Good Housekeeping*, September 2012, p. 188.

45. Kate Valk, in interview with the author, April 27, 2012.

46. Beth W. Orenstein, "Hot Flashes: Your Favorite Screen Characters Go through 'The Change,'" *Everyday Health*, May 17, 2011, http://www.everydayhealth.com/menopause-pictures/your-favorite-screen-actors-go-through-the-change.aspx (accessed March 20, 2012).

47. Jennifer Wolff Perrine, "This Woman Has a Secret," *SELF*, http://www.self.com/health/2010/08/breaking-the-silence-on-infertility/ (accessed February 13, 2012).

48. Laura Dawn, in interview with the author, February 21, 2013.

49. Emanuella Grinberg, "Sex, Lies and Media: New Wave of Activists Challenge Notions of Beauty," CNN, March 22, 2012, http://www.cnn.com/2012/03/09/living/beauty-media-miss-representation/ (accessed April 3, 2012).

50. Krystina Nellis, "Hollywood Heroines: Here to Stay?" BBC News, August 13, 2012, http://www.bbc.co.uk/news/entertainment-arts-19061388 (accessed March 21, 2013).

51. Tina Fey, *Bossypants* (New York: Reagan Arthur Books, 2011), pp. 143–44.

52. Sarah Elizabeth Richards, "Coming Out of the Fertility Closet," *Time*, August 11, 2013, http://ideas.time.com/2013/08/11/coming-out-of-the-fertility-closet/ (accessed September 4, 2013).

53. Natalie Angier, "The Spirit of Sisterhood Is in the Air and on the Air," *New York Times*, April 23, 2012, http://www.nytimes.com/2012/04/24/science/how-hbos-girls-mirrors-the-spirit-of-sisterhood-in-nature.html (accessed April 25, 2013).

54. Alyssa Rosenberg, "*New Girl*'s Fertility Episode Wants You to Panic about Your Eggs. Don't," *Slate*, November 29, 2012, http://www.slate.com/blogs/xx_factor/2012/11/29/new_girl_latest_episode_may_induce_unnecessary_fertility_panic.html (accessed December 18, 2012).

CHAPTER 7: THE ROLLER COASTER

1. "Adrenal tumor," *Wikipedia*, http://en.wikipedia.org/wiki/Adrenal_tumor (accessed March 25, 2012).

2. Deepak Chopra, "21-Day Meditation Challenge," https://www.chopracentermeditation.com/home (accessed September 17, 2013). (The page for the specific meditation in the "Mind-Body Odyssey" series is no longer active.)

3. Bruce Feiler, "Exit Lines," *New York Times*, December 28, 2012, http://www.nytimes.com/2012/12/30/fashion/finding-the-words-or-not-to-say-goodbye.html (accessed December 29, 2012).

CHAPTER 8: THE GLOBAL LANDSCAPE OF INFERTILITY

1. Mark Lino, "Expenditures on Children by Families, 2011," United States Department of Agriculture, Center for Nutrition Policy and Promotion 1528-2011, June 2012.

2. Jonathan V. Last, "America's Baby Bust," *Wall Street Journal*, February 12, 2013, http://online.wsj.com/article/SB10001424127887323375204578270053387770718.html (accessed February 18, 2013).

3. Rema Rahman, "The World at Seven Billion," BBC News, October 30, 2011, http://www.bbc.co.uk/news/magazine-15494349 (accessed February 7, 2012). Jeff Wise, "About That Overpopulation Problem," *Slate*, January 9, 2013, http://www.slate.com/articles/technology/future_tense/2013/01/world_population_may_actually_start_declining_not_exploding.html (accessed March 12, 2013).

4. Randi Epstein, "IVF for Just $300 Could Be a Reality Soon," *Daily Beast*, August 31, 2013, http://www.thedailybeast.com/articles/2013/08/31/ivf-for-just-300-could-be-a-reality-soon.html (accessed September 13, 2013). "The Baby Bonanza," *Economist*, August 27, 2009, http://www.economist.com/node/14302837 (accessed April 20, 2012). Jack Perkowski, "China's One-Child Policy's Unexpected Issue: Infertility," *Forbes*, May 25, 2012, http://www.forbes.com/sites/jackperkowski/2012/05/25/chinas-one-child-policys-unexpected-issue-infertility/ (accessed October 2, 2012).

5. "The Baby Bonanza."

6. "Highlights and Advance Tables, World Population Prospects: The 2012 Revision," Population Division, UN Department of Economic and Social Affairs, 2013. Joel Kotkin and Harry Siegel, "Where Have All the Babies Gone?" *Daily Beast*, February 19, 2013, http://www.thedailybeast.com/newsweek/2013/02/18/why-the-choice-to-be-childless-is-bad-for-america.html (accessed February 25, 2013).

7. "As Families Change Shape, Societies May, Too," Talk of the Nation, NPR, December 27, 2012, http://www.npr.org/2012/12/27/168149097/as-families-change -shape-societies-may-too (accessed January 4, 2013).

8. Last, "America's Baby Bust." It is worth noting that Japan is known for having a robust aging population. In 2013, both the oldest man and oldest woman in the world were Japanese. Jiroemon Kimura celebrated his 116th birthday in April 2013 (but sadly, he passed away in June 2013), and Misao Okawa was 115 years old. "World's Oldest Person Celebrates His 116th Birthday in Japan," Reuters, April 19, 2013, http://www.reuters.com/ article/2013/04/19/us-japan-oldest-idUSBRE93I0KB20130419 (accessed May 8, 2013). Also, the oldest person to climb Mount Everest, as of May 2013, is a Japanese male octoge- narian, Yuichiro Miura. Gopal Sharma, "Japanese Octogenarian Becomes Oldest to Reach Everest Summit," Reuters, May 23, 2013, http://www.reuters.com/article/2013/05/23/ us-nepal-everest-oldest-idUSBRE94M05420130523 (accessed May 25, 2013).

9. John O'Callaghan, "Tiny Singapore Risks Economic Gloom without Big Baby Boom," Reuters, August 30, 2012, http://www.reuters.com/article/2012/08/30/us -singapore-babies-idUSBRE87T1FS20120830 (accessed September 10, 2012).

10. Edward Wong, "Reports of Forced Abortions Fuel Push to End Chinese Law," New York Times, July 22, 2012, http://www.nytimes.com/2012/07/23/world/asia/ pressure-to-repeal-chinas-one-child-law-is-growing.html (accessed July 29, 2012).

11. Kotkin and Siegel, "Where Have All the Babies Gone?"

12. "Highlights and Advance Tables, World Population Prospects." "As Families Change Shape, Societies May, Too."

13. Wise, "About That Overpopulation Problem."

14. Ibid.

15. Judith Shulevitz, "How Older Parenthood Will Upend American Society: The Scary Consequences of the Grayest Generation," New Republic, December 6, 2012, http://www.newrepublic.com/article/politics/magazine/110861/how-older-parenthood -will-upend-american-society (accessed December 12, 2012). T. J. Mathews, MS, and Brady E. Hamilton, PhD, "Delayed Childbearing: More Women Are Having Their First Child Later in Life," NCHS Data Brief 21 (August 2009).

16. Claudia Kalb, "Should You Have Your Baby Now?" Newsweek, August 12, 2001, http://www.thedailybeast.com/newsweek/2001/08/12/should-you-have-your-baby-now .html (accessed March 20, 2012).

17. Gretchen Livingston and D'Vera Cohn, "The New Demography of American Motherhood," Pew Research Center's Social & Demographic Trends Project (May 6, 2010).

18. Sabrina Tavernise, "Fertility Rate Stabilizes as the Economy Grows," New York Times, September 6, 2013, http://www.nytimes.com/2013/09/06/health/fertility-rate -stabilizes-as-the-economy-grows.html (accessed September 13, 2013). "Birth Data," Centers for Disease Control and Prevention, http://www.cdc.gov/nchs/births.htm

(accessed February 8, 2012). "Baby Bust: Why the U.S. Birth Rate Is Declining," NPR, December 6, 2012, http://www.npr.org/2012/12/06/166655696/baby-bust-why-the-u-s -birth-rate-is-declining (accessed December 12, 2012).

19. "CDC Records Rise in Birth Rate for Women over 40," CNN, April 1, 2011, http://www.cnn.com/2011/HEALTH/04/01/cdc.births.decline/index.html (accessed March 8, 2012).

20. Kate Lunau, "Thirty-Seven and Counting," *Maclean's*, October 27, 2012, http://www2.macleans.ca/2012/10/27/thirty-seven-and-counting/ (accessed December 20, 2012).

21. Amanda Brown, "One Expert Says Couples Are Waiting Too Long to Conceive," Examiner.com, November 6, 2012, http://www.examiner.com/article/one-expert-says -couples-are-waiting-too-long-to-conceive (accessed December 10, 2012).

22. "Ukrainian Women Increasingly Delay Motherhood for Future," forUm, October 25, 2012, http://en.for-ua.com/news/2012/10/25/153839.html (accessed October 28, 2012).

23. Steve Doughty, "The Triple Whammy Baby Boom: Immigration, Recession and Older Mothers Push Birth Rate Numbers up to Their Highest Level in 40 Years," *Daily Mail*, October 17, 2012, http://www.dailymail.co.uk/news/article-2219172/Baby -boom-Catch-generation-older-mothers-delay-having-children-sake-career.html (accessed October 23, 2012).

24. Helen Carroll, "At 60, Britain's Oldest Mum of IVF Twins Finally Admits: I Wish I Had a Man to Help Me," *Daily Mail*, August 14, 2013, http://www.dailymail.co.uk/femail/ article-2393653/At-60-Britains-oldest-mum-IVF-twins-finally-admits-I-wish-I-man-help -me.html (accessed September 14, 2013). Naomi Gryn, "Why I'm Having My First Baby at 51," *Guardian*, November 9, 2012, http://www.theguardian.com/lifeandstyle/2012/ nov/09/having-first-baby-at-51 (accessed September 14, 2013).

25. O'Callaghan, "Tiny Singapore Risks Economic Gloom without Big Baby Boom."

26. Kathryn Greenaway, "Motherhood Delayed: The Pros and Cons of Wait-ing," *Montreal Gazette*, June 22, 2012, http://www.montrealgazette.com/life/Motherhood +delayed/6820983/story.html (accessed July 8, 2012).

27. Laura Dawn, in interview with the author, February 23, 2013.

28. Alex Williams, "Just Wait until Your Mother Gets Home," *New York Times*, August 10,2012,http://www.nytimes.com/2012/08/12/fashion/dads-are-taking-over-as-full-time -parents.html (accessed August 12, 2012).

29. "Thirty-Seven Percent of Working Dads Would Leave Their Jobs if Their Family Could Afford It, CareerBuilder.com's Annual Father's Day Survey Finds," CareerBuilder .com, June 11, 2007, http://msn.careerbuilder.com/share/aboutus/pressreleasesdetail.asp x?id=pr375&sd=6%2F11%2F2007&ed=12%2F31%2F2007 (accessed March 8, 2013).

30. Derek Thompson, "Your Day in a Chart: 10 Cool Facts about How Americans Spend Our Time," *Atlantic*, June 25, 2012, http://www.theatlantic.com/business/archive/2012/06/your-day-in-a-chart-10-cool-facts-about-how-americans-spend-our-time/258967/ (accessed July 7, 2012).

31. Lisa Miller, "The Retro Wife," *New York*, March 17, 2013, http://nymag.com/news/features/retro-wife-2013-3/ (accessed March 18, 2013).

32. "Multitasking a Mom Thing," Reuters, December 2, 2011, http://www.nypost.com/f/print/news/national/multitasking_mom_thing_sOf1zzQLc1ouxF4jxdaHCJ (accessed March 20, 2012).

33. Dina Bakst, "Pregnant, and Pushed Out of a Job," *New York Times*, January 30, 2012, http://www.nytimes.com/2012/01/31/opinion/pregnant-and-pushed-out-of-a-job.html (accessed March 3, 2012).

34. Bonnie Rochman, "The Motherhood Penalty: We're in the Midst of a 'Mom-Cession,'" *Time*, August 17, 2012, http://healthland.time.com/2012/08/17/the-motherhood-penalty-were-in-the-midst-of-a-mom-cession/ (accessed August 25, 2012).

35. Derek Thompson, "The 4 Rich Countries Where Women Out-Earn Men (With 1 Huge Caveat)," *Atlantic*, December 17, 2012, http://www.theatlantic.com/business/archive/2012/12/the-4-rich-countries-where-women-out-earn-men-with-1-huge-caveat/266343/ (accessed December 20, 2012).

36. Gillian Lockwood, MD, "The Egg That Came in from the Cold: ASRM Lifts 'Experimental' Label from Social Egg Freezing," BioNews, November 12, 2012, http://www.bionews.org.uk/page_210873.asp (accessed December 5, 2012).

37. Suzanne Moore, "Extending IVF for Older Women Obscures a Deeper Problem for Society," *Guardian*, February 20, 2013, http://www.guardian.co.uk/commentisfree/2013/feb/20/extending-ivf-older-women-problem (accessed February 28, 2013).

38. "Nearly 1 in 3 Women Delay Motherhood," *Scotsman*, January 10, 2012, http://www.scotsman.com/news/uk/nearly-1-in-3-women-delay-motherhood-1-2556484 (accessed March 15, 2012).

39. "How Millions of Working Women Are Putting off Motherhood Because It Would Cost Too Much," *Daily Mail*, July 23, 2010, http://www.dailymail.co.uk/femail/article-1297073/How-millions-women-putting-motherhood-costs-money.html (accessed February 20, 2012).

40. Sarah O'Meara, "Emotional Infertility: Study Reveals Pain of Single Women Not Having Children," *Huffington Post*, June 9, 2012, http://www.huffingtonpost.co.uk/2012/09/06/single-women-face-emotional-infertility_n_1860925.html (accessed August 17, 2012).

41. Jenny Laden, in interview with the author, May 14, 2013.

42. "China Focus: Increasing Infertility Concerns Chinese Couples," Health, *Xinhua*, December 18, 2012, http://news.xinhuanet.com/english/health/2012-12/18/c_132048349.htm (accessed September 14, 2013).

43. "Over 1,000 Babies Born through Assisted Reproductive Treatment in 10 Years," *Nigerian Tribune*, November 6, 2012, http://tribune.com.ng/index.php/community-news/50354-over-1000-babies-born-through-assisted-reproductive-treatment-in-10-years (accessed December 5, 2012).

44. "Paropakar to Launch IVF Service Today," *Himalayan Times*, April 29, 2012, http://www.thehimalayantimes.com/rssReference.php?headline=Paropakar+to+launch+IVF+service+today&NewsID=330137 (accessed May 8, 2012).

45. "Research and Markets: India IVF Treatment Market Analysis—Infertility in India Is Increasing due to Factors such as Urbanisation, Pollution and Chemical Exposure," *Business Wire*, May 2, 2012, http://www.businesswire.com/news/home/20120502005671/en (accessed May 12, 2012).

46. "5mn Born through IVF since First Test-Tube Baby," AFP, Google News, July 1, 2012, http://www.google.com/hostednews/afp/article/ALeqM5gL6Hjfh8qKm-SpGhL-KVkCVWN1gQ?docId=CNG.aaa6b1a661adda1698923b0be8b5aac9.141 (accessed July 18, 2012). "The World's Number of IVF and ICSI Babies Has Now Reached a Calculated Total of 5 Million," ESHRE, July 2, 2012, http://www.eshre.eu/ESHRE/English/Press-Room/Press-Releases/Press-releases-2012/5-million-babies/page.aspx/1606 (accessed July 13, 2012).

47. Liza Mundy, *Everything Conceivable: How Assisted Reproduction Is Changing Our World* (New York: Anchor Books, 2008), p. 11.

48. Julieanne Strachan, "Frozen Egg Birth Rate Remains Low," *Sydney Morning Herald*, July 1, 2012, http://www.smh.com.au/national/frozen-egg-birth-rate-remains-low-20120630-219d1.html (accessed July 17, 2012).

49. "ART Fact Sheet," ESHRE, http://www.eshre.eu/ESHRE/English/Guidelines-Legal/ART-fact-sheet/page.aspx/1061 (accessed March 2, 2012).

50. Victoria Lambert, "Why DO So Many Women Pretend the Menopause Doesn't Exist?" *Daily Mail*, July 11, 2012, http://www.dailymail.co.uk/femail/article-2172274/Why-DO-women-pretend-menopause-doesnt-exist.html (accessed August 5, 2012).

51. Viva Sarah Press, "IVF Baby Boom in Israel," ISRAEL21c, May 13, 2012, http://israel21c.org/news/ivf-baby-boom-in-israel/ (accessed May 16, 2012).

52. Michele Catanzaro, "Human-Rights Court Orders World's Last IVF Ban to Be Lifted," *Nature*, December 28, 2012, http://blogs.nature.com/news/2012/12/human-rights-court-orders-worlds-last-ivf-ban-to-be-lifted.html (accessed January 5, 2012).

53. The number of ART cycles/million population per year in countries with higher than average utilization rates include Denmark, 2,726; Belgium, 2,562; the Czech Republic, 1,851; Slovenia, 1,840; Sweden, 1,800; Finland, 1,701; and Norway, 1,780. Countries with below-average ART cycles/million population include Austria, 747; Germany, 830; Italy, 863; and the United Kingdom, 879. "The World's Number of IVF and ICSI Babies Has Now Reached a Calculated Total of 5 Million."

54. "5,000 Women Give Birth in Beijing by IVF," *People's Daily* Online, March 11, 2013, http://english.peopledaily.com.cn/90882/8162799.html (accessed March 18, 2013).

55. Scott Kirsner, "Michelle Dipp, 36, Reflects Biotech's Next Generation," *Boston Globe*, October 14, 2012, http://bostonglobe.com/business/2012/10/13/michelle-dipp -ovascience-leading-new-generation-biotech-ceo/VqbVwXvcQSRkIVCQapdjhI/story .html (accessed December 2, 2012).

56. The number of ART procedures in 2011 per 1 million women were the following in the highest-ranked states: Massachusetts, 7,260; New York, 6,848; the District of Columbia, 6,146; New Jersey, 5,345; Connecticut, 4,893; Maryland, 4,142; Illinois, 3,851; and Delaware, 3,558. Saswati Sunderam, PhD, et al., "Assisted Reproductive Technology Surveillance—United States, 2009," November 2, 2012, Centers for Disease Control and Prevention, http://www.cdc.gov/mmwr/preview/mmwrhtml/ss6107a1.htm (accessed December 4, 2012).

57. Before driving much of the funding for IVF research, women also drove the funding for development of the Pill. In the 1950s, Katharine Dexter McCormick, one of MIT's first female students, almost singlehandedly funded the human testing required by the FDA. Mundy, *Everything Conceivable*, p. 30.

58. Miriam Zoll and Pamela Tsigdinos, "Selling the Fantasy of Fertility," *New York Times*, September 11, 2013, http://www.nytimes.com/2013/09/12/opinion/selling-the -fantasy-of-fertility.html?emc=eta1&_r=0 (accessed September 14, 2013). "Can You Trick the Biological Clock?" *WAtoday*, April 18, 2012, http://www.watoday.com.au/world/ science/can-you-trick-the-biological-clock-20120418-1x6if.html (accessed May 23, 2012).

59. "Fertility," Merck, http://merck.online-report.eu/2011/ar/merckserono/ therapeuticareas/fertility.html (accessed March 8, 2012).

60. Iva Skoch, "Should IVF Be Affordable for All?" *Newsweek*, July 21, 2010, http:// www.thedailybeast.com/newsweek/2010/07/20/should-ivf-be-affordable-for-all.html (accessed February 10, 2012).

61. Douglas Quenqua, "Clinic Raffles Could Make You a Winner, and Maybe a Mother," *New York Times*, October 20, 2012, http://www.nytimes.com/2012/10/21/ health/ethical-questions-raised-by-in-vitro-raffle.html (accessed December 2, 2012).

62. Skoch, "Should IVF Be Affordable for All?"

63. Jack Perkowski, "China's One-Child Policy's Unexpected Issue: Infertility," *Forbes*, May 25, 2012, http://www.forbes.com/sites/jackperkowski/2012/05/25/chinas -one-child-policys-unexpected-issue-infertility/ (accessed May 28, 2012).

64. "Health Matters International Introduces Innovative Program to Help Women with the High Costs of Fertility Drugs and Associated IVF Treatments," PRWeb, April 21, 2012, http://www.prweb.com/releases/In-Vitro/Fertilization/prweb9360931.htm (accessed May 1, 2012).

65. Stephanie Cary, "Nonprofits Join Forces to Help Cancer Survivors with Fertility Preservation," *Daily Breeze*, June 6, 2012, http://www.dailybreeze.com/lifeandculture/

ci_20797424/nonprofits-join-forces-help-cancer-survivors-fertility-preservation (accessed June 17, 2012).

66. Susan Johnston, "Can You Afford Fertility Treatments?" *US News & World Report*, August 20, 2012, http://money.usnews.com/money/personal-finance/articles/2012/08/20/can-you-afford-fertility-treatments_print.html (accessed October 3, 2012).

67. Peggy Orenstein, *Waiting for Daisy: A Tale of Two Continents, Three Religions, Five Infertility Doctors, An Oscar®, an Atomic Bomb, a Romantic Night, and One Woman's Quest to Become a Mother* (New York: Bloomsbury, 2007), p. 195.

68. Skoch, "Should IVF Be Affordable for All?"

69. Alan Zarembo, "An Ethics Debate over Embryos on the Cheap," *Los Angeles Times*, November 19, 2012, http://articles.latimes.com/2012/nov/19/local/la-me-embryo-20121120 (accessed December 7, 2012).

70. Mundy, *Everything Conceivable*, p. 238.

71. Helia Ebrahimi, "Care Fertility Group in £60m Auction," *Telegraph*, June 6, 2012, http://www.telegraph.co.uk/finance/newsbysector/pharmaceuticalsandchemicals/9312443/Care-Fertility-Group-in-60m-auction.html (accessed July 20, 2012).

72. Sophie Borland, "Half of Women Delay Starting a Family Because They Don't Want to Give up Their Freedom," *Daily Mail*, September 4, 2012, http://www.dailymail.co.uk/news/article-2198428/Half-women-delay-starting-family-dont-want-freedom.html (accessed September 29, 2012).

73. Laura Donnelly, "Couple Sue for IVF in Landmark 'Age Discrimination' Case," *Telegraph*, December 1, 2012, http://www.telegraph.co.uk/health/healthnews/9716432/Couple-sue-for-IVF-in-landmark-age-discrimination-case.html (accessed December 9, 2012). Sophie Borland, "Woman, 37, Sues Health Minister after She Was Told She Is 'Too Old' for IVF," *Daily Mail*, December 2, 2012, http://www.dailymail.co.uk/news/article-2241871/Woman-37-sues-health-minister-Jeremy-Hunt-told-old-IVF.html (accessed December 9, 2012).

74. Malkah Fleisher, "Israeli IVF Success Doubles in Decade," *Jewish Press*, May 14, 2012, http://www.jewishpress.com/news/israeli-ivf-success-doubles-in-decade/2012/05/14/ (accessed May 22, 2012).

75. Dina Krafy, "Where Families Are Prized, Help Is Free," *New York Times*, July 17, 2011, http://www.nytimes.com/2011/07/18/world/middleeast/18israel.html (accessed August 5, 2012).

76. Dan Even, "Israeli Health Ministry Considers Cutting Fertility Treatment Subsidies for Older Women," *Haaretz*, June 4, 2012, http://www.haaretz.com/news/national/israeli-health-ministry-considers-cutting-fertility-treatment-subsidies-for-older-women-1.434194 (accessed July 17, 2012).

77. Michelle Goldberg, "Should Frozen Sperm Be Used to Create Posthumous Grandchildren?" *Jewish Journal*, March 22, 2011, http://www.jewishjournal.com/science

_and_technology/article/should_frozen_sperm_be_used_to_create_posthumous
_grandchildren_20110322 (accessed May 19, 2012).

78. Ibid.

79. PMA Rasheed, "Monetary Aid Eases IVF Woes," *Gulf Today*, November 23, 2012, http://www.gulftoday.ae/portal/cd204c96-f960-47bf-8aba-f147c2646a84.aspx (accessed December 11, 2012).

80. "Over 1,000 Babies Born through Assisted Reproductive Treatment in 10 Years."

81. "Opposition Party Backs IVF Ban in Poland," Polskie Radio, June 27, 2012, http://www.thenews.pl/1/9/Artykul/104060,Opposition-party-backs-IVF-ban-in-Poland (accessed July 12, 2012).

82. Fiona Dillon, "Desperate Couples Rush for Cut-Price Czech IVF," *Herald.ie*, May 28, 2012, http://www.herald.ie/news/desperate-couples-rush-for-cutprice-czech-ivf-3121211.html (accessed June 3, 2012).

83. F. Shenfield et al., "Cross Border Reproductive Care in Six European Countries," *Human Reproduction* 25, no. 6 (2010): 1361–68.

84. Smita Mitra, "Long Journeys to Parenthood," *OutlookIndia.com*, May 7, 2012, http://www.outlookindia.com/article.aspx?280700 (accessed May 23, 2012).

85. Scott Carney, "Inside India's Rent-a-Womb Business," *Mother Jones*, March/April 2010, http://www.motherjones.com/politics/2010/02/surrogacy-tourism-india-nayna-patel (accessed May 11, 2012).

86. Nilanjana Bhowmick, "Why People Are Angry about India's New Surrogacy Rules," *Time*, February 15, 2013, http://world.time.com/2013/02/15/why-people-are-angry-about-indias-new-surrogacy-laws/ (accessed March 8, 2012).

87. Shekhar Bhatia, "'Baby Factory' Proliferation Worries Indian Government," *Vancouver Sun*, June 9, 2012, http://www2.canada.com/vancouversun/news/archives/story.html?id=7fe06ee4-4b41-4ca9-acec-8cdfbe7df943 (accessed July 14, 2012). "Britons Paying up to £25k to Buy Children from Indian 'Baby Factories' as Authorities Plan Clampdown on Unregulated Fertility Industry," *Daily Mail*, May 27, 2012, http://www.dailymail.co.uk/news/article-2150748/Britons-paying-25k-buy-children-booming-Indian-baby-factories-authorities-plan-clampdown-unregulated-fertility-industry.html (accessed July 14, 2012).

88. Chaitra Arjunpuri, "India's Growing 'Rent-a-Womb' Industry," Al Jazeera, February 3, 2013, http://www.aljazeera.com/indepth/features/2013/01/2013128122419799224.html (accessed February 9, 2013).

89. "Understanding the Hague Convention," Intercountry Adoption, http://adoption.state.gov/hague_convention/overview.php (accessed March 8, 2012).

90. John Leland, "For Adoptive Parents, Questions without Answers," *New York Times*, September 16, 2011, http://www.nytimes.com/2011/09/18/nyregion/chinas-adoption-scandal-sends-chills-through-families-in-united-states.html (accessed March 19, 2012).

91. Alessandra Prentice, "Two U.S. Mothers Speak of Russian Adoption Joy," Reuters, February 11, 2013, http://www.reuters.com/article/2013/02/11/us-russia-usa -adoption-idUSBRE91A0YL20130211 (accessed February 24, 2012). Ben Brumfield and Elise Labott, "Russia Lashes out at U.S. Human Rights Blacklist," CNN, April 13, 2013, http://www.cnn.com/2013/04/13/world/europe/russia-magnitsky-ban (accessed April 29, 2013).

92. David M. Herszenhorn and Erik Eckholm, "Putin Signs Bill That Bars U.S. Adoptions, Upending Families," *New York Times*, December 27, 2012, http://www.nytimes .com/2012/12/28/world/europe/putin-to-sign-ban-on-us-adoptions-of-russian-children .html (accessed January 3, 2013).

93. Elissa Gootman, "So Eager for Grandchildren, They're Paying the Egg-Freezing Clinic," *New York Times*, May 13, 2012, http://www.nytimes.com/2012/05/14/us/eager -for-grandchildren-and-putting-daughters-eggs-in-freezer.html (accessed May 15, 2012).

94. "Egg Freezing for Fertility Preservation Priced at $4,900 for the Holidays by Frozen Egg Bank Inc., a Division of West Coast Fertility Centers in Orange County, California," PRWeb, November 30, 2012, http://www.prweb.com/releases/prwebEgg FreezingCalifornia/FertilityPreservation/prweb10184237.htm (accessed December 6, 2012).

95. Cary, "Nonprofits Join Forces to Help Cancer Survivors with Fertility Preservation."

96. Ibid.

97. "Push for Insurance to Cover Egg Freezing," WCAX, October 26, 2012, http://www.wcax.com/story/19926286/push-for-insurance-to-cover-fertilotiy-treatment (accessed December 7, 2012).

98. Sharon Kirkey, "Freezing Eggs, Embryos Poses Legal Concerns," *Vancouver Sun*, March 17, 2012, http://www2.canada.com/vancouversun/news/archives/story .html?id=82fa00c2-bfff-48f3-82d2-27b54b429ae8 (accessed March 25, 2012).

99. Anna Magee, "Fertility Miracle or Cruel Myth?" *Daily Mail*, November 7, 2012, http://www.dailymail.co.uk/femail/article-2229454/Fertility-miracle-cruel-myth -Freezing-eggs-dream-come-true-high-fliers-wanting-delay-motherhood-A-decade -produced-just-12-babies-So-women-spending-fortune-it.html (accessed December 12, 2012). Sophie Borland, "Freezing Eggs When Women Turn 30 'Is an Insurance Policy for Later Babies,'" *Daily Mail*, October 24, 2012, http://www.dailymail.co.uk/news/article -2222766/Freezing-eggs-women-turn-30-insurance-policy-later-babies.html (accessed October 29, 2012). Kara Dolman, "Ice Ice Baby . . . Why More London Women Are Freezing Their Eggs for the Future," *London Evening Standard*, October 30, 2012, http:// www.standard.co.uk/lifestyle/london-life/ice-ice-baby-why-more-london-women-are -freezing-their-eggs-for-the-future-8252800.html (accessed November 2, 2012).

100. Susan Donaldson James, "Rabbis Urge Single, Orthodox Women to Freeze Eggs at 38," ABC News, September 10, 2012, http://abcnews.go.com/Health/rabbis-urge

-single-orthodox-women-freeze-eggs-age/story?id=17185321#.UaeH0CvTXEc (accessed September 15, 2012).

101. Elizabeth Cohen, "Egg Freezing Changing Fertility Treatments," CNN, November 8, 2012, http://www.cnn.com/2012/10/22/health/frozen-egg-banks/index .html (accessed December 12, 2012).

102. Jay Newton-Small, "Frozen Assets: Why American Sperm Is a Hot Commodity," *Time*, April 5, 2012, http://healthland.time.com/2012/04/05/frozen-assets-why-u-s -sperm-is-a-hot-commodity/ (accessed April 9, 2012).

103. For more about bloodlines and genetics, see Masha Gessen's excellent book *Blood Matters*. Masha Gessen, *Blood Matters: From Inherited Illness to Designer Babies, How the World and I Found Ourselves in the Future of the Gene* (Orlando, FL: Harcourt Books, 2008).

104. Jacqueline Mroz, "One Sperm Donor, 150 Offspring," *New York Times*, September 5, 2011, http://www.nytimes.com/2011/09/06/health/06donor.html (accessed February 4, 2012).

105. Ibid.

106. "Donor Compensation, Reimbursement and Benefits in Kind," *Human Fertilisation & Embryology Authority*, http://www.hfea.gov.uk/6177.html (accessed March 17, 2013).

107. Victoria Macdonald, "I Couldn't Be a Mother . . . Until I Went to Spain," *Telegraph*, July 11, 2010, http://www.telegraph.co.uk/health/7883281/I-couldnt-be-a -mother...-until-I-went-to-Spain.html (accessed July 26, 2012).

108. Jasmeet Sidhu, "How to Buy a Daughter," *Slate*, September 14, 2012, http:// www.pulse.me/s/dhvor#/www.slate.com/articles/health_and_science/medical_examiner/ 2012/09/sex_selection_in_babies_through_pgd_americans_are_paying_to_have _daughters_rather_than_sons_.html (accessed September 23, 2012).

109. Tanya Westthorp, "Couples Go to Asia to Select Baby Gender," Lifestyle, PerthNow, April 2, 2013, http://www.perthnow.com.au/lifestyle/parenting/couples-go -to-asia-to-select-baby-gender/story-fnhqgv0m-1226610697956 (accessed April 14, 2013).

110. Chris Arsenault, "Millions of Aborted Girls Imbalance India," Al Jazeera, October 30, 2011, http://www.aljazeera.com/indepth/features/2011/10/201110415385524923 .html (accessed February 17, 2012). Nita Halla, "'Wife-Sharing' Haunts Indian Villages as Girls Decline," Reuters, October 27, 2011, http://www.reuters.com/article/2011/10/27/ us-india-women-exploitation-idUSTRE79Q1WX20111027 (accessed February 17, 2012).

111. Arsenault, "Millions of Aborted Girls Imbalance India."

112. Hilary White, "Eugenics Threat Growing in IVF Industry: British Fertility Expert," LifeSiteNews.com, April 8, 2013, http://www.lifesitenews.com/news/eugenics -threat-growing-in-ivf-industry-british-fertility-expert/ (accessed April 20, 2013).

113. Andrew Solomon, *Far from the Tree: Parents, Children, and the Search for Identity* (New York: Scribner, 2012), pp. 683–84.

114. Chloe Hadjimatheou, "The Greek Parents Too Poor to Care for Their Children," BBC News, January 9, 2012, http://www.bbc.co.uk/news/magazine-16472310 (accessed February 14, 2012).

115. Barbie Latza Nadeau, "Italy Has Europe's Highest Percentage of Children in Poverty, Says UNICEF," *Daily Beast*, March 4, 2012, http://www.thedailybeast.com/articles/2012/03/04/italy-has-europe-s-highest-percentage-of-children-in-poverty-says-unicef.html (accessed March 19, 2012).

116. Barbie Latza Nadeau, "Europe's Growing Crisis of Abandoned Babies," *Daily Beast*, July 11, 2012, http://www.thedailybeast.com/articles/2012/07/11/europe-s-growing-crisis-of-abandoned-babies.html (accessed July 25, 2012).

117. James Gallagher, "Funding of IVF in the UK 'Is Feeble,'" BBC News, July 2, 2012, http://www.bbc.co.uk/news/health-18675858 (accessed July 21, 2012).

118. Stephen Adams, "Thousands Denied IVF because of British Restrictions," *Telegraph*, July 2, 2012, http://www.telegraph.co.uk/health/healthnews/9369851/Thousands-denied-IVF-because-of-British-restrictions.html (accessed July 21, 2012).

119. "Insurance Coverage in Your State," RESOLVE, http://www.resolve.org/family-building-options/insurance_coverage/state-coverage.html (accessed February 13, 2012). "State Laws Related to Insurance Coverage for Infertility Treatment," National Conference of State Legislature, http://www.ncsl.org/issues-research/health/insurance-coverage-for-infertility-laws.aspx (accessed February 13, 2012).

120. Robert Pear, "Gender Gap Persists in Cost of Health Insurance," *New York Times*, March 19, 2012, http://www.nytimes.com/2012/03/19/health/policy/women-still-pay-more-for-health-insurance-data-shows.html (accessed April 2, 2012).

121. Dov Fox and I. Glenn Cohen, "It Is Time for the U.S. to Cover IVF (for Gays and Lesbians Too)," *Huffington Post*, March 18, 2013, http://www.huffingtonpost.com/dov-fox/it-is-time-for-the-us-to-_b_2900323.html (accessed April 3, 2013). K. R. Omurtag and T. L. Toth, "The Cost Effectiveness and Health Incomes of in Vitro Fertilization (IVF) as a Mandated Benefit," *Fertility and Sterility* 88, no. 1 (September 2007): S122.

122. Evelina Weidman Sterling and Angie Best-Boss, *Budgeting for Infertility* (New York: Fireside, 2009), p. 166.

123. Jennifer Wolff Perrine, "This Woman Has a Secret," *SELF*, http://www.self.com/health/2010/08/breaking-the-silence-on-infertility/ (accessed February 13, 2012).

124. Mundy, *Everything Conceivable*, p. xiv.

125. "Fast Facts about Infertility," RESOLVE, June 30, 2011, http://www.resolve.org/about/fast-facts-about-fertility.html (accessed February 3, 2012).

126. Pasquale Patrizio, MD, in interview with the author, May 1, 2012.

127. Sterling, *Budgeting for Infertility*, p. xii.

128. Ibid., p. 177.

129. "A United Front: Dr. Dan Gehlbach Offers Support for Family Act of 2011 and Families Facing Infertility," PRWeb, August 7, 2012, http://www.prweb.com/releases/mrcfamilyact/08/prweb9766588.htm (accessed August 18, 2012).

130. "Family Act of 2011 Takes a Positive Step Forward," *Fertility Authority*, http://

www.fertilityauthority.com/articles/family-act-2011-takes-positive-step-forward (accessed February 20, 2012).

131. Jessica Silver-Greenberg, "In Vitro a Fertile Niche for Lenders," *Wall Street Journal*, February 24, 2012, http://online.wsj.com/article/SB10001424052970203960804577241270123249832.html (accessed February 28, 2012).

132. Linda Carroll, "Growing IVF Loan Business Helps Families Finance Their Fertility," *Today*, July 12, 2012, http://todayhealth.today.com/_news/2012/07/12/12701879-growing-ivf-loan-business-helps-families-finance-their-fertility (accessed August 16, 2012).

133. Cassie Murdoch, "Is Your Fertility Doctor Taking Kickbacks?" *Slate*, July 13, 2012, http://www.slate.com/blogs/xx_factor/2012/07/13/ivf_loans_predatory_lending_hits_the_fertility_market.html (accessed July 15, 2012).

134. Ibid.

135. Rasheed, "Monetary Aid Eases IVF Woes." Manal Ismail, "IVF Loans: The Cost of Borrowing for Babies," *National*, December 9, 2012, http://www.thenational.ae/news/uae-news/health/ivf-loans-the-cost-of-borrowing-for-babies (accessed January 14, 2012).

136. Louise Peacock, "What's Wrong with Offering IVF Treatment as a Prize?" *Telegraph*, October 25, 2012, http://www.telegraph.co.uk/women/womens-life/9631684/Whats-wrong-with-offering-IVF-treatment-as-a-prize.html (accessed December 3, 2012).

137. Tracey Minella, "Win a Free Basic Micro-IVF Cycle in Long Island IVF's 'Extreme Family-Building Makeover' Contest!" Long Island IVF, April 23, 2012, http://blog.longislandivf.com/2012/win-a-free-basic-micro-ivf-cycle-in-long-island-ivfs-extreme-family-building-makeover-contest/ (accessed April 29, 2012).

138. Quenqua, "Clinic Raffles Could Make You a Winner, and Maybe a Mother."

139. Bonnie Rochman, "Baby Contest: Couples Compete for Free IVF—Is This Exploitation of Generosity?" *Time*, June 20, 2012, http://ideas.time.com/2012/06/20/baby-contest-couples-compete-for-free-ivf-is-this-exploitation-or-generosity/ (accessed July 8, 2012).

140. KJ Dell'Antonia, "Crowdfunding Fertility Treatments," *New York Times*, May 20, 2012, http://parenting.blogs.nytimes.com/2012/05/20/hold-crowdfunding-fertility/ (accessed June 7, 2012). Johnston, "Can You Afford Fertility Treatments?"

141. Ruth Walker, "IVF Treatment: Shopping Abroad," *Scotsman*, November 11, 2012, http://www.scotsman.com/scotland-on-sunday/scotland/ivf-treatment-shopping-abroad-1-2628043 (accessed January 15, 2013). Sydney Lupkin, "IVF: When Insurance Companies Won't Pay," ABC News, October 29, 2012, http://abcnews.go.com/Health/couples-extremes-pay-ivf/story?id=17575724#.UNHnfLZUYa8 (accessed December 14, 2012).

142. Christina Ng, "Texas Couple Auctioning Football Card to Pay for IVF," ABC News, October 17, 2012, http://abcnews.go.com/US/texas-couple-auctioning-football-card-pay-ivf/story?id=17500767#.UJK1iIVUYa8 (accessed October 24, 2012).

143. "Houston Couple Hoping Sale of Rare Sanders/Payton Trading Card Funds

Last Chance at in Vitro Fertilization," Associated Press, October 22, 2012, http://www
.thespec.com/sports-story/2248128-houston-couple-hoping-sale-of-rare-sanders-payton
-trading-card-funds-l/ (accessed October 24, 2012).

144. "Families Struggling with Infertility Given Hope by Cade Foundation's Race
for the Family®," PRNewswire, June 14, 2012, http://www.prnewswire.com/news
-releases/families-struggling-with-infertility-given-hope-by-cade-foundations-race-for-the
-family-159032855.html (accessed July 6, 2012).

145. Mundy, *Everything Conceivable*, p. xv.

146. Epstein, "IVF for Just $300 Could Be a Reality Soon."

CHAPTER 9: FRIENDS WITH KIDS
AND FRIENDS WITHOUT

1. Maureen Angelos, in interview with the author, February 21, 2013.

2. Gabriela Poma Traynor, in interview with the author, March 23, 2013.

3. Andrew Solomon, *Far from the Tree: Parents, Children, and the Search for Identity* (New
York: Scribner, 2012), p. 21.

4. Ibid., p. 470.

5. Jennifer Senior, "All Joy and No Fun: Why Parents Hate Parenting," *New York*,
July 4, 2010, http://nymag.com/news/features/67024/ (accessed March 14, 2013).

6. Mary Kaye Schilling, in interview with the author, May 2, 2012.

7. Elaine Chen, in interview with the author, May 22, 2012.

8. Jenny Davidson, in interview with the author, May 1, 2012.

9. Caitlin Moran, *How to Be a Woman* (New York: Harper Perennial, 2011), p. 234.

10. Michelle Ruiz, "Report: More US Women in Their 40s Never Have Kids," AOL
News, June 25, 2010, http://www.aolnews.com/2010/06/25/report-more-us-women-in
-their-40s-never-have-kids/ (accessed April 13, 2012).

11. Katie Gard, "Why Staying Childless Is NOT the Path of Least Resistance,"
Huffington Post, March 21, 2013, http://www.huffingtonpost.com/katie-gard-/childless-not
-the-path-of-least-resistance_b_2918034.html (accessed March 25, 2013).

12. Jonathan V. Last, "America's Baby Bust," *Wall Street Journal*, February 12, 2013,
http://online.wsj.com/article/SB10001424127887323375204578270053387770718
.html (accessed February 18, 2013).

13. Gretchen Livingston and D'Vera Cohn, "Childless Up among All Women; Down
among Women with Advanced Degrees," Pew Research Center Social & Demographic
Trends, June 25, 2010, http://www.pewsocialtrends.org/2010/06/25/childlessness-up
-among-all-women-down-among-women-with-advanced-degrees/ (accessed April 8, 2012).

14. Michel Martin, "Birth Rate Declines for Women over 40," NPR, June 29, 2010, http://

www.npr.org/templates/story/story.php?storyId=128188446 (accessed February 13, 2012).

15. Kate Valk, in interview with the author, April 27, 2012.

16. Schilling, interview.

17. "Supreme Court Justice Sonia Sotomayor Regrets Not Having Borne or Adopted Children in Memoir, 'My Beloved World,'" *NY Daily News*, Associated Press, December 10, 2012, http://www.nydailynews.com/news/national/sotomayor-regrets-borne-adopted -children-memoir-article-1.1217303 (accessed January 4, 2012).

18. "Sotomayor's Life in Pictures," CNN, May 26, 2009, http://www.cnn.com/2009/POLITICS/05/26/gallery.sotomayor.life/index.html (accessed February 17, 2013).

19. Schilling, interview.

20. Natalie Dean, in interview with the author, May 1, 2012.

21. Jennie Boddy, in interview with the author, March 23, 2013.

22. Angelos, interview.

23. Samantha Brick, "My Baby Envy Has Destroyed Decades-Old Friendships," *Daily Mail*, November 17, 2012, http://www.dailymail.co.uk/home/you/article-2232800/Samantha-Brick-My-baby-envy-destroyed-decades-old-friendships.html (accessed December 12, 2012).

24. Laura Dawn, in interview with the author, February 23, 2013.

25. Schilling, interview.

26. Amy Richards, in interview with the author, April 30, 2012.

27. Dawn, interview.

28. Dean, interview.

29. Hope Reese, "'Anger Boiled Up, and Betty Friedan Was There': 'Feminine Mystique' at 50," *Atlantic*, January 28, 2013, http://www.theatlantic.com/sexes/archive/2013/01/anger-boiled-up-and-betty-friedan-was-there-feminine-mystique-at-50/272575 (accessed February 2, 2013).

30. Mary Elizabeth Williams, "Motherhood Is Not a Job," *Salon*, April 27, 2012, http://www.salon.com/2012/04/27/motherhood_is_not_a_job (accessed May 3, 2012).

31. Emily Matchar, "How Parenting Became a DIY Project," *Atlantic*, February 4, 2013, http://www.theatlantic.com/sexes/archive/2013/02/how-parenting-became-a-diy -project/272792/ (accessed February 9, 2013).

32. Sheryl Sandberg, *Lean In: Women, Work, and the Will to Lead* (New York: Alfred A. Knopf, 2013), p. 15.

33. Caitlin Moran, *How to Be a Woman* (New York: Harper Perennial, 2011), pp. 223–24.

34. Dawn, interview.

35. Tina Merrill, in interview with the author, May 1, 2012.

36. Hilary Grove, in interview with the author, February 21, 2013.

37. Dean, interview.

38. Erin Callan, "Is There Life After Work?" *New York Times*, March 9, 2013, http://www.nytimes.com/2013/03/10/opinion/sunday/is-there-life-after-work.html (accessed March 15, 2013).

39. Karen Rowan, "Best Age to Raise Kids? Older Parents Say 30s," FoxNews.com, March 9, 2012, http://www.foxnews.com/health/2012/03/09/best-age-to-raise-kids-older-parents-say-30s/ (accessed March 10, 2012).

40. Nancy Cook, "For Richer (Not for Poorer): The Inequality Crisis of Marriage," *Atlantic*, March 14, 2012, http://www.theatlantic.com/business/archive/2012/03/marriages-inequality-crisis/254523/ (accessed March 23, 2012).

41. Gladys Martinez, PhD, Kimberly Daniels, PhD, and Anjani Chandra, PhD, "Fertility of Men and Women Aged 15–44 Years in the United States: National Survey of Family Growth, 2006–2010," *National Health Statistics Report* 51 (April 12, 2012).

42. Jason DeParle and Sabrina Tavernise, "For Women under 30, Most Births Occur Outside Marriage," *New York Times*, February 17, 2012, http://www.nytimes.com/2012/02/18/us/for-women-under-30-most-births-occur-outside-marriage.html (accessed February 20, 2012).

43. Lisa Belkin, "With More Single Fathers, a Changing Family Picture," *New York Times*, June 2, 2011, http://parenting.blogs.nytimes.com/2011/06/02/with-more-single-fathers-a-changing-family-picture/ (accessed May 30, 2013).

44. Mireya Navarro, "The Bachelor Life Includes a Family," *New York Times*, September 5, 2008, http://www.nytimes.com/2008/09/07/fashion/07single.html (accessed March 16, 2013).

45. Aparna Mathur, Hao Fu, and Peter Hansen, "The Mysterious and Alarming Rise of Single Parenthood in America," *Atlantic*, September 3, 2013, www.theatlantic.com/business/archive/2013/09/the-mysterious-and-alarming-rise-of-single-parenthood-in-america/279203/ (accessed September 16, 2013).

46. Stacia L. Brown, "How Unwed Mothers Feel about Being Unwed Mothers," *Atlantic*, March 23, 2013, http://www.theatlantic.com/sexes/archive/2013/03/how-unwed-mothers-feel-about-being-unwed-mothers/274301/ (accessed March 29, 2013).

47. DeParle, "For Women under 30, Most Births Occur Outside Marriage."

48. Phoebe Maltz Bovy, "There's No Perfect Age to Find a Husband," *Atlantic*, February 1, 2013, http://www.theatlantic.com/sexes/archive/2013/02/theres-no-perfect-age-to-find-a-husband/272789/ (accessed February 5, 2013).

49. Lori Gottlieb, *Marry Him: The Case for Settling for Mr. Good Enough* (New York: New American Library, 2010), pp. 42–43.

50. Ibid., p. 60.

51. Lisa Miller, "The Retro Wife," *New York*, March 17, 2013, http://nymag.com/news/features/retro-wife-2013-3/ (accessed March 18, 2013).

52. Sandberg, *Lean In*, p. 167.

53. Sonia Sotomayor, *My Beloved World* (New York: Alfred A. Knopf, 2013), p. 30.

54. Jennifer Braunschweiger, "Why the Mommy Wars Rage On," *More*, April 2013, http://www.more.com/reinvention-money/careers/why-mommy-wars-rage-0 (accessed April 28, 2013).

55. Ibid.

56. Lilian V. Faulhaber, "How the I.R.S. Hurts Mothers," *New York Times*, April 3, 2013, http://www.nytimes.com/2013/04/04/opinion/lean-in-what-about-child-care.html (accessed April 8, 2013).

57. Judith Warner, "The Opt-Out Generation Wants Back In," *New York Times Magazine*, August 7, 2013, http://www.nytimes.com/2013/08/11/magazine/the-opt-out -generation-wants-back-in.html (accessed August 8, 2013).

58. Ibid.

59. Ibid.

60. Ibid.

61. Jordan Weissmann, "The Overhyped Rise of Stay-at-Home Dads," *Atlantic*, September 3, 2013, http://www.theatlantic.com/business/archive/2013/09/the -overhyped-rise-of-stay-at-home-dads/279279/ (accessed September 16, 2013).

62. Elizabeth Wurtzel, "1% Wives Are Helping Kill Feminism and Make the War on Women Possible," *Atlantic*, June 15, 2012, http://www.theatlantic.com/politics/ archive/2012/06/1-wives-are-helping-kill-feminism-and-make-the-war-on-women -possible/258431/ (accessed June 22, 2012).

63. Gabri Christa, in interview with the author, April 24, 2012.

64. Moran, *How to Be a Woman*, p. 233.

65. Poma Traynor, interview.

66. Merrill, interview.

67. Caroline Reeves, in interview with the author, April 23, 2013.

68. Peggy Orenstein, *Flux: Women on Sex, Work, Love, Kids, & Life in a Half-Changed World* (New York: Anchor Books, 2000), p. 95.

69. Amy Richards, *Opting In: Having a Child without Losing Yourself* (New York: Farrar, Straus and Giroux, 2008), p. 202.

70. Ibid., p. 205.

71. Grove, interview.

72. Davidson, interview.

73. Schilling, interview.

74. Chen, interview.

75. Angelos, interview.

76. Liz Mermin, in interview with the author, May 1, 2012.

77. Dean, interview.

78. Jackie Kuchinich and Martha T. Moore, "Hilary Rosen Says Ann Romney

Never Worked a 'Day in Her Life,'" *USA Today*, April 12, 2012, http://usatoday30.usa today.com/news/politics/story/2012-04-12/ann-romney-hilary-rosen-work/54235706/1 (accessed April 16, 2012).

79. Kristen A. Lee, "Mitt Romney's Advice to College Graduates: Marry Young, Have a 'Quiver Full of Kids,'" *Daily News*, April 30, 2013, http://www.nydailynews.com/romney-advice-college-grads-marry-young-kids-article-1.1331517 (accessed May 2, 2013).

80. Mary Elizabeth Williams, "End the Mom War," *Salon*, April 13, 2012, http://www.salon.com/2012/04/13/end_the_mom_war/ (accessed April 17, 2012).

81. Richards, *Opting In*, p. 155.

82. Frank Bruni, "A Childless Bystander's Baffled Hymn," *New York Times*, March 30, 2013, http://www.nytimes.com/2013/03/31/opinion/sunday/bruni-a-childless-bystanders-baffled-hymn.html (accessed April 5, 2013).

83. Amy Chua, *Battle Hymn of the Tiger Mother* (New York: Penguin Press, 2011), p. 101.

84. Ibid., p. 69.

85. Ibid., p. 228.

86. Amy Chua, "Why Chinese Mothers Are Superior," *Wall Street Journal*, January 8, 2011, http://online.wsj.com/article/SB10001424052748704111504576059713528698754.html (accessed February 7, 2012).

87. Pamela Druckerman, *Bringing Up Bébé: One American Mother Discovers the Wisdom of French Parenting* (New York: Penguin Press, 2012), p. 3.

88. Erika Brown Ekiel, "Bringing Up Bebe? No Thanks. I'd Rather Raise a Billionaire," *Forbes*, March 7, 2012, http://www.forbes.com/sites/forbeswomanfiles/2012/03/07/bringing-up-bebe-no-thanks-id-rather-raise-a-billionaire/ (accessed March 19, 2012).

89. KJ Dell'Antonia, "The Eternal, Internal Mommy Wars," *New York Times*, April 23, 2012, http://parenting.blogs.nytimes.com/2012/04/23/the-eternal-internal-mommy-wars/ (accessed April 28, 2012).

90. Amy Allen, "'Mommy Wars' Redux: A False Conflict," *New York Times*, May 27, 2012, http://opinionator.blogs.nytimes.com/2012/05/27/the-mommy-wars-redux-a-false-conflict/ (accessed June 4, 2012).

91. Braunschweiger, "Why the Mommy Wars Rage On."

92. Moran, *How to Be a Woman*, pp. 237–38.

CHAPTER 10: THE POWER OF OPTIMISM

1. Cheryl Strayed, *Wild* (New York: Vintage Books, 2013), p. 6.

2. Siddhartha Mukherjee, *The Emperor of All Maladies: A Biography of Cancer* (New York: Scribner, 2011), p. 469.

3. Ibid., p. 470.

4. A. D. Domar, P. C. Zuttermeister, and R. Friedman, "The Psychological Impact of Infertility: A Comparison with Patients with Other Medical Conditions," *Journal of Psychosomatic Obstetrics and Gynaecology* 14 (1993): 45–52, http://www.ncbi.nlm.nih.gov/entrez/query.fcgi?cmd=Retrieve&db=PubMed&dopt=Citation&list_uids=8142988 (accessed March 16, 2013).

5. S. R. Leiblum, A. Aviv, and R. Hamer, "Life after Infertility Treatment: A Long-Term Investigation of Marital and Sexual Function," *Human Reproduction* 13, no. 12 (1998): 3569–74, http://humrep.oxfordjournals.org/content/13/12/3569.full.pdf (accessed March 16, 2013).

6. Esben Agerbo, Preben Bo Mortensen, and Trine Munk-Olsen, "Childlessness, Parental Mortality and Psychiatric Illness: A Natural Experiment Based on In Vitro Fertility Treatment and Adoption," *Journal of Epidemiology and Community Health* 67, no. 4 (2012): 374, http://jech.bmj.com/content/early/2012/11/08/jech-2012-201387.short (accessed April 25, 2013).

7. Lucy Freem, MD, "Childlessness Resulting from Failed IVF Is Associated with Decreased Lifespan," BioNews, December 10, 2012, http://www.bionews.org.uk/page_224477.asp (accessed February 21, 2013).

8. "The Psychological Impact of Infertility and Its Treatment," *Harvard Mental Health Letter*, May 2009, http://www.health.harvard.edu/newsletters/Harvard_Mental_Health_Letter/2009/May/The-psychological-impact-of-infertility-and-its-treatment (accessed May 3, 2013).

9. Cora de Klerk, "The Psychological Impact of IVF Treatment," 2008, http://repub.eur.nl/res/pub/20792/The%20Psychological%20Impact%20of%20IVF%20Treatment%20-%20Cora%20de%20Klerk.pdf (accessed April 30, 2013). B. J. Berg, J. F. Wilson, and P. J. Weingartner, "Psychological Sequelae of Infertility Treatment: The Role of Gender and Sex-Role Identification," *Social Science & Medicine* 33, no. 9 (1991): 1071–80. "Participants in RESOLVE's monthly discussion meetings, which always included both women and men, often talked about how the experience of infertility is 'different for women.' Men, it was frequently said with humor, are 'about a trimester behind' their wives in coming to the decision to seek a diagnosis for infertility, to seek treatment for infertility, to move from low-tech to high-tech treatment, and to begin considering adoption or a child-free life. Women are also more likely to research the treatment options 'obsessively,' according to the experiences reported at RESOLVE meetings, and to be more eager to get back on the 'treadmill of infertility' after any treatment that does not result in a pregnancy. In fact, trying several cycles of IVF back to back was not uncommon. Women, it would seem, are differently invested than men in becoming parents," from Karey Harwood, *The Infertility Treadmill* (Chapel Hill: University of North Carolina Press, 2007), p. 72.

10. Sarah Elizabeth Richards, "Alimony for Your Eggs," *New York Times*, September 6, 2013, http://www.nytimes.com/2013/09/07/opinion/alimony-for-your-eggs.html (ac-

cessed September 16, 2013).

11. Michael Ondaatje, "The Time around Scars," *The Cinnamon Peeler* (New York: Vintage, 1997).

12. Tracy Clark-Flory, "Cheryl Strayed: 'Tackle Love,'" *Salon*, July 7, 2012, http://www.salon.com/2012/07/08/cheryl_strayed_tackle_love/ (accessed March 16, 2013).

13. Pema Chödrön, *When Things Fall Apart* (Boston: Shambhala, 1997), p. 46.

14. Sonali Deraniyagala, *Wave* (New York: Alfred A. Knopf, 2013), p. 37.

CHAPTER 11: ACTION ITEMS FOR THE FUTURE

1. Natalie Dean, in interview with the author, May 1, 2012.

2. Caroline Reeves, in interview with the author, April 23, 2013.

3. Arthur Greil, PhD, in interview with the author, May 11, 2012.

4. Crystal Wilmhoff, in interview with the author, May 29, 2012.

5. "Online Support Communities," RESOLVE, http://www.resolve.org/resources/online-support-communities.html (accessed April 7, 2013).

6. "About the Anonymous Us Project," *Anonymous Us*, http://anonymousus.podomatic.com/ (accessed September 9, 2013).

7. Wilmhoff, interview.

8. Claudia Kalb, "Have Another 'Fertilitini,'" *Newsweek*, January 26, 2009, http://www.thedailybeast.com/newsweek/2009/01/26/have-another-fertilitini.html (accessed March 6, 2013).

9. Tina Merrill, in interview with the author, May 1, 2012.

10. Gail Sheehy, *Passages: Predictable Crises of Adult Life* (New York: Random House, 2006), p. 119.

11. Ibid., p. 122.

12. Victoria Birk Hill, in interview with the author, April 25, 2012.

13. William Kutteh, MD, PhD, in interview with the author, April 21, 2012.

14. *PBS NewsHour*, October 19, 2012.

15. Karina Shreffler, PhD, in interview with the author, May 21, 2012.

16. Jenny Davidson, PhD, in interview with the author, May 1, 2012.

17. Catherine Gund, in interview with the author, May 3, 2013.

18. Peggy Orenstein, *Flux: Women on Sex, Work, Love, Kids, & Life in a Half-Changed World* (New York: Anchor Books, 2000), p. 202.

19. Soon-Young Yoon, in interview with the author, May 11, 2012.

20. Amy Richards, *Opting In: Having a Child without Losing Yourself* (New York: Farrar, Straus and Giroux, 2008), p. 24.

21. Matt Richtel, "Housecleaning, Then Dinner? Silicon Valley Perks Come Home,"

New York Times, October 19, 2012, http://www.nytimes.com/2012/10/20/us/in-silicon-valley-perks-now-begin-at-home.html (accessed April 8, 2013).

22. Jennifer Ludden, "Stay-at-Home Workers Defend Choice after Yahoo Ban," NPR, March 1, 2013, http://www.npr.org/2013/03/01/173186526/stay-at-home-workers-defend-choice-after-yahoo-ban (accessed March 14, 2013).

23. Ibid.

24. Eyder Peralta, "Yahoo's Marissa Mayer Expands Parental Leave," NPR, April 30, 2013, http://www.npr.org/blogs/thetwo-way/2013/04/30/180150731/yahoos-marissa-mayer-expands-parental-leave (accessed May 2, 2013).

25. Hannah Seligson, "When the Work-Life Scales Are Unequal," *New York Times*, September 1, 2012, http://www.nytimes.com/2012/09/02/business/straightening-out-the-work-life-balance.html (accessed December 4, 2012).

26. Ibid.

27. Anne-Marie Slaughter, "There Are Lots of Ways to Help Make Men and Women Truly Equal," *Atlantic*, March 18, 2013, http://www.theatlantic.com/sexes/archive/2013/03/there-are-lots-of-ways-to-help-make-men-and-women-truly-equal/274084/ (accessed March 22, 2013).

28. Amy Richards, in interview with the author, April 30, 2013.

29. Caitlin Moran, *How to Be a Woman* (New York: Harper Perennial, 2011), p. 11.

30. Pasquale Patrizio, MD, in interview with the author, May 1, 2012.

31. Patrizio, interview.

32. Wilmhoff, interview.

33. Jennifer Braunschweiger, "Why the Mommy Wars Rage On," *More*, April 2013, http://www.more.com/reinvention-money/careers/why-mommy-wars-rage-0 (accessed April 28, 2013).

34. Mindy Berkson, in interview with the author, May 1, 2012.

35. Pamela Druckerman, *Bringing Up Bébé: One American Mother Discovers the Wisdom of French Parenting* (New York: Penguin Press, 2012), p. 192.

36. Greil, interview.

37. Shreffler, interview.

38. Megan Garber, "A Pregnant CEO: In Whose Lifetime?" *Atlantic*, July 17, 2012, http://www.theatlantic.com/technology/archive/2012/07/a-pregnant-ceo-in-whose-lifetime/259919/ (accessed July 25, 2012).

39. Jordan Weissmann, "Why Are Women Paid Less?" *Atlantic*, October 17, 2012, http://www.theatlantic.com/business/archive/2012/10/why-are-women-paid-less/263776 (accessed October 21, 2012).

40. Ibid.

41. Laura Dawn, in interview with the author, February 23, 2013.

42. Orenstein, *Flux*, p. 289.

43. Anjali Mullany, "Women and Leadership," *Fast Company*, July 6, 2012, http://www.fastcompany.com/1842212/thread-women-and-leadership (accessed July 10, 2012). "Women in Elective Office 2013," Center for American Women and Politics fact sheet, Eagleton Institute of Politics, Rutgers, the State University of New Jersey, http://www.cawp.rutgers.edu/fast_facts/levels_of_office/documents/elective.pdf (accessed September 9, 2013).

44. Isobel Coleman, "Saudi Arabia's Timid Flirtation with Women's Rights," *Atlantic*, January 16, 2013, http://www.theatlantic.com/international/archive/2013/01/saudi-arabias-timid-flirtation-with-womens-rights/267245/ (accessed February 8, 2013).

45. Michelle Nichols, "Fewer Women in Parliaments after Arab Spring: Study," Reuters, March 2, 2012, http://www.reuters.com/article/2012/03/02/us-women-parliament-un-idUSTRE82112O20120302 (accessed March 24, 2012).

46. Claire Davenport, "EU Wants Direct Action to Get Women into Boardrooms," Reuters, November 13, 2012, http://www.reuters.com/article/2012/11/13/us-eu-gender-idUSBRE8AC0PE20121113 (accessed December 5, 2012).

47. Sonia Sotomayor, *My Beloved World* (New York: Alfred A. Knopf, 2013), p. 11.

EPILOGUE

1. Calvin Yang, "Using Books to Build a Ladder out of Poverty," *New York Times*, April 29, 2013, http://www.nytimes.com/2013/04/29/world/asia/using-books-to-build-a-ladder-out-of-poverty.html (accessed May 8, 2013).

2. Megan Slack, "President Obama Speaks on the Shooting in Connecticut," *White House Blog*, December 14, 2012, http://www.whitehouse.gov/blog/2012/12/14/president-obama-speaks-shooting-connecticut (accessed December 17, 2012).

BIBLIOGRAPHY

"About the Anonymous Us Project." *Anonymous Us*. http://anonymousus.podomatic.com/ (accessed September 9, 2013).

Abrams, Lindsay. "It's Not Too Early to Talk about Your Eggs." *Atlantic*, November 9, 2012. http://www.theatlantic.com/health/archive/2012/11/its-not-too-early-to-talk -about-freezing-your-eggs/264992/ (accessed December 8, 2012).

Adams, Janey. "Infertility: It's Not the End of the World." NPR, July 2, 2011. http://www .npr.org/blogs/babyproject/2011/07/06/137504382/infertility-its-not-the-end-of -the-world/ (accessed April 3, 2012).

Adams, Stephen. "Discovery to Deliver IVF Joy for Older Women." *Irish Independent*, October 22, 2012. http://www.independent.ie/lifestyle/parenting/discovery-to -deliver-ivf-joy-for-older-women-3266864.html (accessed October 30, 2012).

———. "Thousands Denied IVF because of British Restrictions." *Telegraph*, July 2, 2012. http://www.telegraph.co.uk/health/healthnews/9369851/Thousands-denied-IVF -because-of-British-restrictions.html (accessed July 21, 2012).

"Adoption Can Boost Quality of Life for Infertile Couples, Study Finds." Health, *US News & World Report*, November 19, 2012. http://health.usnews.com/health-news/news/ articles/2012/11/19/adoption-can-boost-quality-of-life-for-infertile-couples-study -finds (accessed December 11, 2012).

"Adrenal tumor." *Wikipedia*. http://en.wikipedia.org/wiki/Adrenal_tumor (accessed March 25, 2012).

Agerbo, Esben, Preben Bo Mortensen, and Trine Munk-Olsen. "Childlessness, Parental Mortality and Psychiatric Illness: A Natural Experiment Based on in Vitro Fertility Treatment and Adoption." *Journal of Epidemiology and Community Health* 67, no. 4 (2012): 374. http://jech.bmj.com/content/early/2012/11/08/jech-2012-201387.short (accessed April 25, 2013).

"Aisha Tyler Reveals Struggle with Infertility." *People*, September 12, 2013. http://celebrity babies.people.com/2013/09/12/aisha-tyler-reveals-infertility-ivf-failure/ (accessed September 13, 2013).

Allen, Amy. "'Mommy Wars' Redux: A False Conflict." *New York Times*, May 27, 2012. http://opinionator.blogs.nytimes.com/2012/05/27/the-mommy-wars-redux-a-false -conflict/ (accessed June 4, 2012).

Allen, Jenny. "Welcome Back, Katie!" *Good Housekeeping*, September 2012.

Angelo, Megan. "The *New Girl* Episode That Freaked Out Every Girl in America."

Glamour, November 28, 2012. http://www.glamour.com/entertainment/blogs/obsessed/2012/11/the-new-girl-episode-that-frea.html (accessed December 18, 2012).

Angelos, Maureen. In interview with the author. February 21, 2013.

Angier, Natalie. "The Spirit of Sisterhood Is in the Air and on the Air." *New York Times*, April 23, 2012. http://www.nytimes.com/2012/04/24/science/how-hbos-girls-mirrors-the-spirit-of-sisterhood-in-nature.html (accessed April 25, 2013).

————. *Woman: An Intimate Geography*. New York: Anchor Books, 2000.

Apps, Peter. "The Next Challenge: Not Too Many People, but Too Few?" Reuters, October 24, 2011. http://www.reuters.com/article/2011/10/24/population-decline-idUSL5E7LO0VD20111024 (accessed February 13, 2012).

Arjunpuri, Chaitra. "India's Growing 'Rent-a-Womb' Industry." Al Jazeera, February 3, 2013. http://www.aljazeera.com/indepth/features/2013/01/2013128122419799224.html (accessed February 9, 2013).

Arsenault, Chris. "'Baby Bust' Spells Trouble for Rich Nations." Al Jazeera, October 30, 2011. http://www.aljazeera.com/indepth/features/2011/10/201110419532494799.html (accessed February 8, 2012).

————. "Millions of Aborted Girls Imbalance India." Al Jazeera, October 30, 2011. http://www.aljazeera.com/indepth/features/2011/10/201110415385524923.html (accessed February 17, 2012).

"ART Fact Sheet." ESHRE. http://www.eshre.eu/ESHRE/English/Guidelines-Legal/ART-fact-sheet/page.aspx/1061 (accessed March 2, 2012).

"As Families Change Shape, Societies May, Too." Talk of the Nation, NPR, December 27, 2012. http://www.npr.org/2012/12/27/168149097/as-families-change-shape-societies-may-too (accessed January 4, 2013).

Axelrod, Melanie. "Men Can Smell Fertility, Study Says." ABC News, April 5, 2013. http://abcnews.go.com/Health/story?id=117526&page=1 (accessed April 22, 2013).

"The Baby Bonanza." *Economist*, August 27, 2009. http://www.economist.com/node/14302837 (accessed April 20, 2012).

"Baby Bust: Why the U.S. Birth Rate Is Declining." NPR, December 6, 2012. http://www.npr.org/2012/12/06/166655696/baby-bust-why-the-u-s-birth-rate-is-declining (accessed December 12, 2012).

Baida, Aiyana. "Jennifer Lopez and Casper Smart Expecting via IVF, Surrogate!" *VOXXI*, April 1, 2013. http://www.voxxi.com/jennifer-lopez-expecting-ivf-surrogate/ (accessed April 1, 2013).

Bakst, Dina. "Pregnant, and Pushed Out of a Job." *New York Times*, January 30, 2012. http://www.nytimes.com/2012/01/31/opinion/pregnant-and-pushed-out-of-a-job.html (accessed March 3, 2012).

Banerji, Robin. "The Woman Who Lost All Seven Children." *BBC News Magazine*, September 30, 2012. http://www.bbc.co.uk/news/magazine-19648992 (accessed March 3, 2013).

Bassett, Laura. "Carolyn Maloney: Rush Limbaugh 'Slut' Comment Is Attempt to Silence Women." *Huffington Post*, March 1, 2012. http://www.huffingtonpost.com/2012/03/01/carolyn-maloney-rush-limbaugh-slut_n_1313243.html (accessed March 8, 2012).

Beck, Martha. *Expecting Adam: A True Story of Birth, Rebirth, and Everyday Magic.* New York: Three Rivers Press, 2011.

Belkin, Lisa. "With More Single Fathers, a Changing Family Picture." *New York Times*, June 2, 2011. http://parenting.blogs.nytimes.com/2011/06/02/with-more-single-fathers-a-changing-family-picture/ (accessed May 30, 2013).

"The Benefits of State Seat Belt Laws." National Highway Traffic Safety Administration. http://www.policyalmanac.org/economic/archive/seatbelts.shtml (accessed February 24, 2013).

Berg, B. J., J. F. Wilson, and P. J. Weingartner. "Psychological Sequelae of Infertility Treatment: The Role of Gender and Sex-Role Identification." *Social Science & Medicine* 33, no. 9 (1991): 1071–80.

Berkson, Mindy. In interview with the author, May 1, 2012.

Beyerstein, Lindsay. "Anne-Marie Slaughter Has It All." *Duly Noted*, June 21, 2012. http://inthesetimes.com/duly-noted/entry/13429/anne_marie_slaughter_pretty_much_has_it_all/ (accessed June 28, 2012).

Bhatia, Shekar. "'Baby Factory' Proliferation Worries Indian Government." *Vancouver Sun*, June 9, 2012. http://www2.canada.com/vancouversun/news/archives/story.html?id=7fe06ee4-4b41-4ca9-acec-8cdfbe7df943 (accessed July 14, 2012).

Bhowmick, Nilanjana. "Why People Are Angry about India's New Surrogacy Rules." *Time*, February 15, 2013. http://world.time.com/2013/02/15/why-people-are-angry-about-indias-new-surrogacy-laws/ (accessed March 8, 2012).

Birk Hill, Victoria. In interview with the author. April 25, 2012.

"Birth Defects More Common in IVF Babies: Study." Reuters, April 20, 2012. http://www.reuters.com/article/2012/04/20/us-ivf-idUSBRE83J03M20120420 (accessed April 28, 2012).

Bissell, Monsoon. "To the Woman Warrior I Didn't Know." *Daily Beast*, January 5, 2013. http://www.thedailybeast.com/articles/2013/01/05/to-the-woman-warrior-i-did-not-know.html (accessed January 7, 2013).

Blickley, Leigh. "Celebrities Who've Used Surrogates to Conceive." *Huffington Post*, February 6, 2013. http://www.huffingtonpost.com/2013/02/06/celebrities-who-have-used-surrogates_n_2624998.html (accessed February 10, 2013).

Boddy, Jennie. In interview with the author, March 23, 2013.

Bolick, Kate. "All the Single Ladies." *Atlantic*, September 30, 2011. http://www.theatlantic

.com/magazine/archive/2011/11/all-the-single-ladies/8654/ (accessed February 7, 2012).

Borland, Kate. "Half of Women Delay Starting a Family Because They Don't Want to Give Up Their Freedom." *Daily Mail*, September 4, 2012. http://www.dailymail.co.uk/news/article-2198428/Half-women-delay-starting-family-dont-want-freedom.html (accessed September 29, 2012).

Borland, Sophie. "Freezing Eggs When Women Turn 30 'Is an Insurance Policy for Later Babies.'" *Daily Mail*, October 24, 2012. http://www.dailymail.co.uk/news/article-2222766/Freezing-eggs-women-turn-30-insurance-policy-later-babies.html (accessed October 29, 2012).

———. "Woman, 37, Sues Health Minister after She Was Told She Is 'Too Old' for IVF." *Daily Mail*, December 2, 2012. http://www.dailymail.co.uk/news/article-2241871/Woman-37-sues-health-minister-Jeremy-Hunt-told-old-IVF.html (accessed December 9, 2012).

Bostrom, Nick. "Nick Bostrom on Our Biggest Problems." *TED Talks*, July 2005. http://www.ted.com/talks/nick_bostrom_on_our_biggest_problems.html (accessed April 8, 2012).

Bousquet, Dominique. In interview with the author, January 21, 2013.

Braunschweiger, Jennifer. "Why the Mommy Wars Rage On." *More*, April 2013. http://www.more.com/reinvention-money/careers/why-mommy-wars-rage-0 (accessed April 28, 2013).

Brick, Samantha. "My Baby Envy Has Destroyed Decades-Old Friendships." *Daily Mail*, November 17, 2012. http://www.dailymail.co.uk/home/you/article-2232800/Samantha-Brick-My-baby-envy-destroyed-decades-old-friendships.html (accessed December 12, 2012).

Brielmaier, Isolde. In interview with the author, February 21, 2013.

Bright, Kathy. "I'm Still Waiting for the Sting of Adoption to Go Away." Parents, *Huffington Post*, January 25, 2013. http://www.huffingtonpost.com/2013/01/25/adoption-stigma_n_2542717.html (accessed February 2, 2013).

"Britons Paying up to £25k to Buy Children from Indian 'Baby Factories' as Authorities Plan Clampdown on Unregulated Fertility Industry." *Daily Mail*, May 27, 2012. http://www.dailymail.co.uk/news/article-2150748/Britons-paying-25k-buy-children-booming-Indian-baby-factories-authorities-plan-clampdown-unregulated-fertility-industry.html (accessed July 14, 2012).

Brown, Amanda. "One Expert Says Couples Are Waiting Too Long to Conceive." Examiner.com, November 6, 2012. http://www.examiner.com/article/one-expert-says-couples-are-waiting-too-long-to-conceive (accessed December 10, 2012).

Brown, Stacia L. "How Unwed Mothers Feel about Being Unwed Mothers." *Atlantic*, March 23, 2013. http://www.theatlantic.com/sexes/archive/2013/03/how-unwed-mothers-feel-about-being-unwed-mothers/274301/ (accessed March 29, 2013).

Brown Ekiel, Erika. "Bringing Up Bebe? No Thanks. I'd Rather Raise a Billionaire/" *Forbes*, March 7, 2012. http://www.forbes.com/sites/forbeswomanfiles/2012/03/07/bringing-up-bebe-no-thanks-id-rather-raise-a-billionaire/ (accessed March 19, 2012).

Brownstein, Joseph. "Pregnant Women over 50 'Do Pretty Well,' Study Finds." FoxNews .com, February 3, 2012. http://www.foxnews.com/health/2012/02/03/pregnant -women-over-50-do-pretty-well-study-finds/ (accessed February 12, 2012).

Brumfield, Ben, and Elise Labott. "Russia Lashes out at U.S. Human Rights Blacklist." CNN, April 13, 2013. http://www.cnn.com/2013/04/13/world/europe/russia -magnitsky-ban (accessed April 29, 2013).

Bruni, Frank. "A Childless Bystander's Baffled Hymn." *New York Times*, March 30, 2013. http://www.nytimes.com/2013/03/31/opinion/sunday/bruni-a-childless -bystanders-baffled-hymn.html (accessed April 5, 2013).

Brunk, Doug. "Fertility Preservation No Longer Experimental." Ob.Gyn. News, June 14, 2012. http://www.obgynnews.com/news/top-news/single-article/fertility-preservation -no-longer-experimental-for-cancer-patients/47e02be79468de56e43483da138cd478 .html (accessed July 16, 2012).

Callan, Eric. "Is There Life after Work?" *New York Times*, March 9, 2013. http://www .nytimes.com/2013/03/10/opinion/sunday/is-there-life-after-work.html (accessed March 15, 2013).

"Can You Trick the Biological Clock?" *WAtoday*, April 18, 2012. http://www.watoday.com .au/world/science/can-you-trick-the-biological-clock-20120418-1x6if.html (accessed May 23, 2012).

Cain Miller, Claire. "Opening a Gateway for Girls to Enter the Computer Field." *New York Times*, April 2, 2013. http://dealbook.nytimes.com/2013/04/02/opening-a-gateway -for-girls-to-enter-the-computer-field/ (accessed April 5, 2013).

Carey, Benedict. "Father's Age Is Linked to Risk of Autism and Schizophrenia." *New York Times*, August 22, 2012. http://www.nytimes.com/2012/08/23/health/fathers-age -is-linked-to-risk-of-autism-and-schizophrenia.html (accessed August 28, 2012).

Carney, Scott. "Inside India's Rent-a-Womb Business." *Mother Jones*, March/April 2010. http://www.motherjones.com/politics/2010/02/surrogacy-tourism-india-nayna -patel (accessed May 11, 2012).

Carroll, Helen. "At 60, Britain's Oldest Mum of IVF Twins Finally Admits: I Wish I Had a Man to Help Me." *Daily Mail*, August 14, 2013. http://www.dailymail.co.uk/femail/ article-2393653/At-60-Britains-oldest-mum-IVF-twins-finally-admits-I-wish-I-man -help-me.html (accessed September 14, 2013).

Carroll, Linda. "Growing IVF Loan Business Helps Families Finance Their Fertility." *Today*, July 12, 2012. http://todayhealth.today.com/_news/2012/07/12/12701879 -growing-ivf-loan-business-helps-families-finance-their-fertility (accessed August 16, 2012).

Cary, Stephanie. "Nonprofits Join Forces to Help Cancer Survivors with Fertility Preservation." *Daily Breeze*, June 6, 2012. http://www.dailybreeze.com/lifeandculture/ci_20797424/nonprofits-join-forces-help-cancer-survivors-fertility-preservation (accessed June 17, 2012).

Catanzaro, Michele. "Human-Rights Court Orders World's Last IVF Ban to Be Lifted." *Nature*, December 28, 2012. http://blogs.nature.com/news/2012/12/human-rights-court-orders-worlds-last-ivf-ban-to-be-lifted.html (accessed January 5, 2012).

Catlin, Roger. "Marlo Thomas: 'It's amazing the Impact "Free to Be . . ." Had. Yet Nobody Followed It Up. It's Gone Bad.'" *Salon*, February 26, 2013. http://www.salon.com/2013/02/26/marlo_thomas_its_amazing_the_impact_free_to_be_had_yet_nobody_followed_it_up_its_gone_bad/ (accessed February 28, 2013).

"CDC Records Rise in Birth Rate for Women over 40." CNN, April 1, 2011. http://www.cnn.com/2011/HEALTH/04/01/cdc.births.decline/index.html (accessed March 8, 2012).

Cendrowicz, Leo. "Can Mandatory Quotas Bring Gender Equality to Europe's Boardrooms?" *Time*, March 8, 2012. http://www.time.com/time/world/article/0,8599,2108607,00.html (accessed March 10, 2012).

"Census Bureau Reports 'Delayer Boom' as More Educated Women Have Children Later." United States Census Bureau, May 9, 2011. http://www.census.gov/newsroom/releases/archives/fertility/cb11-83.html (accessed February 8, 2012).

"Center for Human Reproduction More Than Doubles IVF Pregnancy Rates in Women Over 44." PRWeb, June 4, 2012. http://www.prweb.com/releases/prematureovarianaging/failedivf/prweb9567606.htm (accessed June 12, 2012).

Cetinkaya, Mehmet B., Linda J. Siano, Claudio Benadiva, Denny Sakkas, and Pasquale Patrizio. "Reproductive Outcome of Women 43 Years and Beyond Undergoing ART Treatment with Their Own Oocytes in Two Connecticut University Programs." *Journal of Assisted Reproduction and Genetics* 30, no. 5 (June 2013): 673–78. http://link.springer.com/article/10.1007%2Fs10815-013-9981-5 (accessed April 20, 2012).

"Chance to Pause Biological Clock with Ovarian Transplant Stirs Debate." NPR, December 24, 2012. http://www.npr.org/templates/transcript/transcript.php?storyId=167705397 (accessed January 8, 2013).

Chandler, Charlotte. "My Dinners with Federico and Michelangelo." *Vanity Fair*, March 2012. http://www.vanityfair.com/hollywood/2012/03/federico-michelangelo-201203 (accessed March 3, 2012).

Chaplin, Julia. In interview with the author, April 24, 2012.

Charney, Noah. "Ingenious Fertility Alternative to IVF." *ARTINFO.com*, January 14, 2013. http://blogs.artinfo.com/secrethistoryofart/2013/01/14/ingenious-fertility-alternative-to-ivf/ (accessed February 23, 2012).

Chen, Elaine. In interview with the author, May 22, 2012.

Chen, Pauline W., MD, "Among Doctors, Too, Women Are Paid Less." *New York Times*, June

28, 2012. http://well.blogs.nytimes.com/2012/06/28/among-doctors-too-women-are-paid-less/ (accessed August 11, 2012).

"China Focus: Increasing Infertility Concerns Chinese Couples." Health. *Xinhua*, December 18, 2012. http://news.xinhuanet.com/english/health/2012-12/18/c_132048349.htm (accessed September 14, 2013).

Chödrön, Pema. *When Things Fall Apart*. Boston: Shambhala, 1997.

Chopra, Deepak. "21-Day Meditation Challenge." https://www.chopracentermeditation.com/ (accessed September 17, 2013). (The page for the specific meditation in the "Mind-Body Odyssey" series is no longer active.)

Christa, Gabri. In interview with the author, April 24, 2012.

Chua, Amy. *Battle Hymn of the Tiger Mother*. New York: Penguin Press, 2011.

———. "Why Chinese Mothers Are Superior." *Wall Street Journal*, January 8, 2011. http://online.wsj.com/article/SB10001424052748704111504576059713528698754.html (accessed February 7, 2012).

Clark-Flory, Tracy. "Cheryl Strayed: 'Tackle Love.'" *Salon*, July 7, 2012. http://www.salon.com/2012/07/08/cheryl_strayed_tackle_love/ (accessed March 16, 2013).

Cohen, Elizabeth. "Egg Freezing Changing Fertility Treatments." CNN, November 8, 2012. http://www.cnn.com/2012/10/22/health/frozen-egg-banks/index.html (accessed December 12, 2012).

Coleman, Isobel. "Saudi Arabia's Timid Flirtation with Women's Rights." *Atlantic*, January 16, 2013. http://www.theatlantic.com/international/archive/2013/01/saudi-arabias-timid-flirtation-with-womens-rights/267245/ (accessed February 8, 2013).

Cook, Nancy. "For Richer (Not for Poorer): The Inequality Crisis of Marriage." *Atlantic*, March 14, 2012. http://www.theatlantic.com/business/archive/2012/03/marriages-inequality-crisis/254523/ (accessed March 23, 2012).

Corredor, Paloma. "Sofia Vergara Freezing Her Eggs, IVF a Popular Trend among Women Today." *VOXXI*, April 8, 2013. http://www.voxxi.com/sofia-vergara-freezing-eggs-ivf-trend/ (accessed April 21, 2013).

"Couples' Sexual Relationships Can Suffer during IVF, Study Finds." Health, *US News & World Report*, November 2, 2012. http://health.usnews.com/health-news/news/articles/2012/11/02/couples-sexual-relationships-can-suffer-during-ivf-study-finds (accessed December 18, 2012).

Cowan, Richard. "Record Number of Women Sworn into New U.S. Congress." Reuters, January 3, 2013. http://www.reuters.com/article/2013/01/03/us-usa-congress-women-idUSBRE9020KT20130103 (accessed January 8, 2013).

Dana, Rebecca. "The Vitrification Fertility Option." *Newsweek*, January 23, 2012. http://www.thedailybeast.com/newsweek/2012/01/22/the-vitrification-fertility-option.html (accessed February 4, 2012).

D'Angelo Friedman, Jennifer. "FOX News Anchor Reveals Infertility Struggle." *SELF*,

October 2010. http://www.self.com/health/2010/10/news-anchor-reveals-infertility
-struggle (accessed March 6, 2012).

———. "What Happens to a Woman's Fertility after 40." *SELF*, September 8, 2011.
http://www.self.com/blogs/flash/2011/09/what-happens-to-your-fertility.html (accessed February 13, 2012).

Daniels Hussar, April. "Survey: Most College Women Want to Be Married by 30." *SELF*,
August 30, 2012. http://www.self.com/blogs/flash/2012/08/survey-most-college
-women-want.html (accessed September 2. 2012).

Davenport, Claire. "EU Wants Direct Action to Get Women into Boardrooms." Reuters,
November 13, 2012. http://www.reuters.com/article/2012/11/13/us-eu-gender-id
USBRE8AC0PE20121113 (accessed December 5, 2012).

David, Sami S., MD, and Jill Blakeway, LAc. *Making Babies: A Proven 3-Month Program for
Maximum Fertility*. New York: Little, Brown, 2009.

Davidson, Jenny, PhD. In interview with the author, May 1, 2012.

Dawn, Laura. In interview with the author, February 21, 2013.

Dean, Natalie. In interview with the author, May 1, 2012.

DeCapua, Joe. "Global Infertility Rates Generally Hold Steady." *Voice of America*, December
20, 2012. http://www.voanews.com/content/global-infertility-20dec12/1568597.html
(accessed December 22, 2012).

de Klerk, Cora. "The Psychological Impact of IVF Treatment." 2008. http://repub.eur.nl/
res/pub/20792/The%20Psychological%20Impact%20of%20IVF%20Treatment
%20-%20Cora%20de%20Klerk.pdf (accessed April 30, 2013).

Dell'Antonia, KJ. "Crowdfunding Fertility Treatments." *New York Times*, May 20, 2012.
http://parenting.blogs.nytimes.com/2012/05/20/hold-crowdfunding-fertility/ (accessed June 7, 2012).

———. "The Eternal, Internal Mommy Wars." *New York Times*, April 23, 2012. http://
parenting.blogs.nytimes.com/2012/04/23/the-eternal-internal-mommy-wars/ (accessed April 28, 2012).

DeParle, Jason, and Sabrina Tavernise. "For Women under 30, Most Births Occur
Outside Marriage." *New York Times*, February 17, 2012. http://www.nytimes.com/
2012/02/18/us/for-women-under-30-most-births-occur-outside-marriage.html (accessed February 20, 2012).

Deraniyagala, Sonali. *Wave*. New York: Alfred A. Knopf, 2013.

Desai, Kinjal. "*Vicky Donor* Lures Ahmedabad Men to Sperm Donation." *DNA*, May 1, 2012.
http://www.dnaindia.com/india/report_vicky-donor-lures-ahmedabad-men-to
-sperm-donation_1682992 (accessed June 3, 2012).

de Vise, Daniel. "For Working Mothers in Academia, Tenure Track Is Often a Tough Balancing Act." *Washington Post*, July 11, 2010. http://www.washingtonpost.com/wp-dyn/
content/article/2010/07/10/AR2010071002610.html (accessed February 3, 2012).

Dillon, Fiona. "Desperate Couples Rush for Cut-Price Czech IVF." *Herald.ie*, May 28, 2012. http://www.herald.ie/news/desperate-couples-rush-for-cutprice-czech-ivf-3121211 .html (accessed June 3, 2012).

Dobuzinskis, Alex. "U.S. Women in 20s Less Likely to Get Pregnant or Have Abortion." Reuters, June 20, 2012. http://www.reuters.com/article/2012/06/20/us-usa -pregnancies-study-idUSBRE85J06820120620 (accessed July 8, 2012).

Dolman, Kara. "Ice Ice Baby . . . Why More London Women Are Freezing Their Eggs for the Future." *London Evening Standard*, October 30, 2012. http://www.standard.co.uk/ lifestyle/london-life/ice-ice-baby-why-more-london-women-are-freezing-their-eggs -for-the-future-8252800.html (accessed November 2, 2012).

Domar, A. D., P. C. Zuttermeister, and R. Friedman. "The Psychological Impact of Infertility: A Comparison with Patients with Other Medical Conditions." *Journal of Psychosomatic Obstetrics and Gynaecology* 14 (1993): 45–52. http://www.ncbi.nlm.nih.gov/ entrez/query.fcgi?cmd=Retrieve&db=PubMed&dopt=Citation&list_uids=8142988 (accessed March 16, 2013).

Donaldson James, Susan. "Rabbis Urge Single, Orthodox Women to Freeze Eggs at 38." ABC News, September 10, 2012. http://abcnews.go.com/Health/rabbis-urge-single -orthodox-women-freeze-eggs-age/story?id=17185321#.UaeH0CvTXEc (accessed September 15, 2012).

Donnelly, Laura. "Couple Sue for IVF in Landmark 'Age Discrimination' Case." *Telegraph*, December 1, 2012. http://www.telegraph.co.uk/health/healthnews/9716432/ Couple-sue-for-IVF-in-landmark-age-discrimination-case.html (accessed December 9, 2012).

"Donor Compensation, Reimbursement and Benefits in Kind." *Human Fertilisation & Embryology Authority*. http://www.hfea.gov.uk/6177.html (accessed March 17, 2013).

Doughty, Steve. "The Triple Whammy Baby Boom: Immigration, Recession and Older Mothers Push Birth Rate Numbers up to Their Highest Level in 40 Years." *Daily Mail*, October 17, 2012. http://www.dailymail.co.uk/news/article-2219172/Baby-boom -Catch-generation-older-mothers-delay-having-children-sake-career.html (accessed October 23, 2012).

Druckerman, Pamela. *Bringing Up Bébé: One American Mother Discovers the Wisdom of French Parenting*. New York: Penguin Press, 2012.

"Early to Embrace Egg Freezing for Fertility Preservation, a CT Fertility Clinic Now Sees Its Even Greater Personal and Societal Impact in Donor Egg Banking." PRWeb, November 1, 2012. http://www.prweb.com/releases/prwebct_fertility_egg_freezing/ asrm_non-experimental/prweb10081736.htm (accessed December 21, 2012).

Ebrahimi, Helia. "Care Fertility Group in £60M Auction." *Telegraph*, June 6, 2012. http://www.telegraph.co.uk/finance/newsbysector/pharmaceuticalsandchemicals/ 9312443/Care-Fertility-Group-in-60m-auction.html (accessed July 20, 2012).

"Egg Freezing for Fertility Preservation Priced at $4,900 for the Holidays by Frozen Egg Bank Inc., a Division of West Coast Fertility Centers in Orange County, California." PRWeb, November 30, 2012. http://www.prweb.com/releases/prwebEggFreezing California/FertilityPreservation/prweb10184237.htm (accessed January 19, 2013).

"Eggsurance Launches Independent Community and Educational Website Devoted to Everything Egg Freezing." Yahoo! Finance, May 22, 2012. http://www.marketwire .com/press-release/eggsurance-launches-independent-community-educational -website-devoted-everything-egg-1660037.htm (accessed May 25, 2012).

Ehrenreich, Barbara. "Why Forced Positive Thinking Is a Total Crock." *AlterNet*, May 20, 2010. http://www.alternet.org/story/146940/barbara_ehrenreich%3A_why_forced _positive_thinking_is_a_total_crock (accessed February 8, 2013).

EMD Serono, Inc. "In the Know: Fertility IQ 2011 Survey: Fertility Knowledge among US Women Aged 25–35: Insights from a New Generation." October 2011.

Epstein, Randi. "IVF for Just $300 Could Be a Reality Soon." *Daily Beast*, August 31, 2013. http://www.thedailybeast.com/articles/2013/08/31/ivf-for-just-300-could-be-a-reality -soon.html (accessed September 13, 2013).

Even, Dan. "Israeli Health Ministry Considers Cutting Fertility Treatment Subsidies for Older Women." *Haaretz*, June 4, 2012. http://www.haaretz.com/news/national/ israeli-health-ministry-considers-cutting-fertility-treatment-subsidies-for-older-women -1.434194 (accessed July 17, 2012).

Extra. February 29, 2012.

"Families Struggling with Infertility Given Hope by Cade Foundation's Race for the Family." PRNewswire, June 14, 2012. http://www.prnewswire.com/news-releases/families -struggling-with-infertility-given-hope-by-cade-foundations-race-for-the-family -159032855.html (accessed July 6, 2012).

"Family Act of 2011 Takes a Positive Step Forward." *Fertility Authority*. http://www .fertilityauthority.com/articles/family-act-2011-takes-positive-step-forward (accessed February 20, 2012).

"Fast Facts about Infertility." RESOLVE, June 30, 2011. http://www.resolve.org/about/ fast-facts-about-fertility.html (accessed February 3, 2012).

Faulhaber, Lilian V. "How the I.R.S. Hurts Mothers." *New York Times*, April 3, 2013. http://www.nytimes.com/2013/04/04/opinion/lean-in-what-about-child-care.html (accessed April 8, 2013).

Feiler, Bruce. "Exit Lines." *New York Times*, December 28, 2012. http://www.nytimes .com/2012/12/30/fashion/finding-the-words-or-not-to-say-goodbye.html (accessed December 29, 2012).

"Fertility." Merck. http://merck.online-report.eu/2011/ar/merckserono/therapeutic areas/ fertility.html (accessed March 8, 2012).

"Fertility Rate, Total (Births per Woman)." World Bank. http://data.worldbank.org/ indicator/SP.DYN.TFRT.IN (accessed March 7, 2012).

Fey, Tina. *Bossypants*. New York: Reagan Arthur Books, 2011.

"5,000 Women Give Birth in Beijing by IVF." *People's Daily* Online, March 11, 2013. http://english.peopledaily.com.cn/90882/8162799.html (accessed March 18, 2013).

Fleisher, Malkah. "Israeli IVF Success Doubles in Decade." *Jewish Press*, May 14, 2012. http://www.jewishpress.com/news/israeli-ivf-success-doubles-in-decade/2012/05/14/ (accessed May 22, 2012).

"5mn Born through IVF since First Test-Tube Baby." AFP, Google News, July 1, 2012. http://www.google.com/hostednews/afp/article/ALeqM5gL6Hjfh8qKm-SpGhL-KVkCVWN1gQ?docId=CNG.aaa6b1a661adda1698923b0be8b5aac9.141 (accessed July 18, 2012).

Fox, Dov, and I. Glenn Cohen. "It Is Time for the U.S. to Cover IVF (for Gays and Lesbians Too)." *Huffington Post*, March 18, 2013. http://www.huffingtonpost.com/dov-fox/it-is-time-for-the-us-to-_b_2900323.html (accessed April 3, 2013).

Freem, Lucy, MD. "Childlessness Resulting from Failed IVF Is Associated with Decreased Lifespan." BioNews, December 10, 2012. http://www.bionews.org.uk/page_224477.asp (accessed February 21, 2013).

"Freezing Human Eggs for In Vitro Fertilization No Longer Experimental Procedure." *PBS NewsHour*, October 19, 2012. http://www.pbs.org/newshour/bb/health/july-dec12/eggs_10-19.html (accessed October 23, 2012).

Friedan, Betty. *The Feminine Mystique*. New York: W. W. Norton, 2001.

Garber, Megan. "The IVF Panic: 'All Hell Will Break Loose, Politically and Morally, All Over the World.'" *Atlantic*, June 25, 2012. http://www.theatlantic.com/technology/archive/2012/06/the-ivf-panic-all-hell-will-break-loose-politically-and-morally-all-over-the-world/258954/ (accessed June 30, 2012).

———. "A Pregnant CEO: In Whose Lifetime?" *Atlantic*, July 17, 2012. http://www.theatlantic.com/technology/archive/2012/07/a-pregnant-ceo-in-whose-lifetime/259919/ (accessed July 25, 2012).

Gard, Katie. "Why Staying Childless Is NOT the Path of Least Resistance." *Huffington Post*, March 21, 2013. http://www.huffingtonpost.com/katie-gard-/childless-not-the-path-of-least-resistance_b_2918034.html (accessed March 25, 2013).

Gardner, Amanda. "U.S. Women Delaying Motherhood, Report Shows." HealthDay, ABC News, August 13, 2009. http://abcnews.go.com/Health/Healthday/story?id=8312506&page=1#.T4xm6ulST80 (accessed April 16, 2012).

Gallagher, James. "Funding of IVF in the UK 'Is Feeble.'" BBC News, July 2, 2012. http://www.bbc.co.uk/news/health-18675858 (accessed July 21, 2012).

———. "Is the Six-Million-Dollar Man Possible?" BBC News, March 11, 2012. http://www.bbc.co.uk/news/health-16632764 (accessed March 15, 2012).

———. "Three-Person IVF 'Is Ethical' to Treat Mitochondrial Disease." BBC News, June 11, 2012. http://www.bbc.co.uk/news/health-18393682 (accessed July 3, 2012).

"Georgia Woman Gives Birth to Her GRANDSON after IVF Treatment Because Her Daughter Couldn't Conceive." *Daily Mail*, October 18, 2012. http://www.dailymail .co.uk/news/article-2217598/Georgia-woman-gives-birth-GRANDSON-IVF -treatment-daughter-conceive.html (accessed December 11, 2012).

Gessen, Masha. *Blood Matters: From Inherited Illness to Designer Babies, How the World and I Found Ourselves in the Future of the Gene.* Orlando, FL: Harcourt Books, 2008.

Gibbs, Nancy. "Making Time for a Baby." *Time*, April 15, 2002. http://www.time.com/ time/magazine/article/0,9171,1002217,00.html (accessed March 21, 2012).

Gilman, Priscilla. *The Anti-Romantic Child: A Memoir of Unexpected Joy.* New York: Harper Perennial, 2011.

Glee. "The Spanish Teacher." February 7, 2012.

Glennie, Alasdair. "I Woke Up and Thought: I Want a Baby. But It Was Too Late, Says Pop Star Lisa Stansfield." *Daily Mail*, October 19, 2012. http://www.dailymail.co.uk/ tvshowbiz/article-2220415/I-woke-thought-I-want-baby-But-late-says-pop-star-Lisa -Stansfield.html (accessed February 20, 2012).

Goldberg, Michelle. "Should Frozen Sperm Be Used to Create Posthumous Grandchildren?" *Jewish Journal*, March 22, 2011 http://www.jewishjournal.com/science_and _technology/article/should_frozen_sperm_be_used_to_create_posthumous _grandchildren_20110322 (accessed May 19, 2012).

Gootman, Elissa. "So Eager for Grandchildren, They're Paying the Egg-Freezing Clinic." *New York Times*, May 13, 2012. http://www.nytimes.com/2012/05/14/us/eager-for -grandchildren-and-putting-daughters-eggs-in-freezer.html (accessed May 15, 2012).

Gottlieb, Lori. *Marry Him: The Case for Settling for Mr. Good Enough.* New York: New American Library, 2010.

Grady, Denise. "American Woman Who Shattered Space Ceiling." *New York Times*, July 23, 2012. http://www.nytimes.com/2012/07/24/science/space/sally-ride-trailblazing -astronaut-dies-at-61.html (accessed July 29, 2012).

Greenaway, Kathryn. "Motherhood Delayed: The Pros and Cons of Waiting." *Montreal Gazette*, June 22, 2012. http://www.montrealgazette.com/life/Motherhood +delayed/6820983/story.html (accessed July 8, 2012).

Gregory, Elizabeth. *Ready: Why Women Are Embracing the New Later Motherhood* (New York: Perseus Books, 2007).

Greil, Arthur, PhD. In interview with the author, May 11, 2012.

Grens, Kerry. "The Black (Egg) Market? IVF Recruiters Are Forgetting about the Ethics." *MedCity News*, August 9, 2012. http://medcitynews.com/2012/08/the-black-egg -market-ivf-recruiters-are-forgetting-about-the-ethics/ (accessed August 19, 2012).

Grimes, William. "Gerda Lerner, a Feminist and Historian, Dies at 92." *New York Times*, January 3, 2013. http://www.nytimes.com/2013/01/04/us/gerda-lerner-historian -dies-at-92.html (accessed January 15, 2013).

Grinberg, Emanuella. "Sex, Lies and Media: New Wave of Activists Challenge Notions of Beauty." CNN, March 22, 2012. http://www.cnn.com/2012/03/09/living/beauty-media-miss-representation/ (accessed April 3, 2012).

Grove, Hilary. In interview with the author, February 21, 2013.

Gryn, Naomi. "Why I'm Having My First Baby at 51." *Guardian*, November 9, 2012. http://www.theguardian.com/lifeandstyle/2012/nov/09/having-first-baby-at-51 (accessed September 14, 2013).

Gund, Catherine. In interview with the author, May 1, 2013.

Hadjimatheou, Chloe. "The Greek Parents Too Poor to Care for Their Children." BBC News, January 9, 2012. http://www.bbc.co.uk/news/magazine-16472310 (accessed February 14, 2012).

Hall, Beth. In interview with the author, January 9, 2013.

Halla, Nita. "'Wife-Sharing' Haunts Indian Villages as Girls Decline." Reuters, October 27, 2011. http://www.reuters.com/article/2011/10/27/us-india-women-exploitation-idUSTRE79Q1WX20111027 (accessed February 17, 2012).

"Halle Berry Expecting Second Child, First with Olivier Martinez." Reuters, April 5, 2013. http://www.reuters.com/article/2013/04/05/us-halleberry-idUSBRE9340V2201 30405 (accessed April 6, 2013).

Hampton, Kelle. *Bloom: Finding Beauty in the Unexpected.* New York: William Morrow, 2013.

Hannagan, Rebecca J. "Gendered Political Behavior: A Darwinian Feminist Approach." *Sex Roles* 59, no. 7–8 (October 2008): 465–75.

Harnden, Toby. "New Republican Platform Banning ALL Abortions Could Also Restrict IVF . . . Which Three of Romney's Sons Have Used to Conceive." *Daily Mail*, August 21, 2012. http://www.dailymail.co.uk/news/article-2191690/human-life-amendment--New-Republican-platform-banning-ALL-abortions-restrict-IVF.html (accessed September 4, 2012).

Harrison, Laird. "California Sperm Donor at Odds with Federal Regulators." Reuters, December 20, 2011. http://www.reuters.com/article/2011/12/20/us-sperm-donor-california-idUSTRE7BJ1F420111220 (accessed February 7, 2012).

Harwood, Karey, *The Infertility Treadmill.* Chapel Hill: University of North Carolina Press, 2007.

Hayes, Ashley. "First Mother-Daughter Womb Transplants Performed in Sweden," CNN, September 20, 2012. http://www.cnn.com/2012/09/19/health/uterine-transplant (accessed September 22, 2012).

"Health Matters International Introduces Innovative Program to Help Women with the High Costs of Fertility Drugs and Associated IVF Treatments." PRWeb, April 21, 2012. http://www.prweb.com/releases/In-Vitro/Fertilization/prweb9360931.htm (accessed May 1, 2012).

Herszenhorn, David M., and Erik Eckholm. "Putin Signs Bill That Bars U.S. Adoptions, Upending Families." *New York Times*, December 27, 2012. http://www.nytimes .com/2012/12/28/world/europe/putin-to-sign-ban-on-us-adoptions-of-russian -children.html (accessed January 3, 2013).

"Highlights and Advance Tables, World Population Prospects: The 2012 Revision." Population Division, UN Department of Economic and Social Affairs, 2013.

Hope, Jenny. "Children of Mothers over 40 'Are Healthier and More Intelligent and Less Likely to Have Accidents.'" *Daily Mail*, May 21, 2012. http://www.dailymail.co.uk/ health/article-2147848/Children-mothers-40-healthier-intelligent.html (accessed May 25, 2012).

———. "Women over 40 Told: 'Don't Take IVF Success for Granted.'" *Daily Mail*, April 6, 2012. http://www.dailymail.co.uk/health/article-2126057/Women-40-told-Dont -IVF-success-granted.html (accessed April 11, 2012).

"Houston Couple Hoping Sale of Rare Sanders/Payton Trading Card Funds Last Chance at in vitro Fertilization." Associated Press, October 22, 2012. http://www.thespec .com/sports-story/2248128-houston-couple-hoping-sale-of-rare-sanders-payton -trading-card-funds-l/ (accessed October 24, 2012).

"How Birth Control and Abortion Became Politicized." NPR, November 9, 2012. http:// www.npr.org/2011/11/09/142097521/how-birth-control-and-abortion-became -politicized (accessed March 18, 2012).

"How Millions of Working Women Are Putting Off Motherhood Because It Would Cost Too Much." *Daily Mail*, July 23, 2010. http://www.dailymail.co.uk/femail/article -1297073/How-millions-women-putting-motherhood-costs-money.html (accessed February 20, 2012).

"Infertility on the Rise in Urban Areas, Late Marriage Big Factor." *Hindustan Times*, April 29, 2012. http://www.hindustantimes.com/India-news/NewDelhi/Infertility-on-the -rise-in-urban-areas-late-marriage-big-factor/Article1-848191.aspx (accessed May 23, 2013).

"Insurance Coverage in Your State." RESOLVE. http://www.resolve.org/family- building -options/insurance_coverage/state-coverage.html (accessed April 4, 2012).

Ismail, Manal. "IVF Loans: The Cost of Borrowing for Babies." *National*, December 9, 2012. http://www.thenational.ae/news/uae-news/health/ivf-loans-the-cost-of -borrowing-for-babies (accessed January 14, 2012).

"IVF Success Rates: Don't Believe Everything You Read, Says Fertility Specialist." PRWeb, February 1, 2013. http://www.prweb.com/releases/2013/2/prweb10386327.htm (accessed February 7, 2013).

Jayson, Sharon. "New Face of Infertility: Under 35, Frustrated." *USA Today*, April 23, 2012. http://www.usatoday.com/news/health/story/2012-04-23/infertility-young -women/54482470/1 (accessed May 3, 2012).

Johnson, Zach. "Aisha Tyler Opens Up about Infertility Struggle," E! Online, September 13,

2013. http://www.eonline.com/news/458556/aisha-tyler-opens-up-about-infertility
-struggle-on-the-talk-why-she-stopped-ivf-treatments (accessed September 13, 2013).

Johnston, Susan. "Can You Afford Fertility Treatments?" *US News & World Report*, August
20, 2012. http://money.usnews.com/money/personal-finance/articles/2012/08/
20/can-you-afford-fertility-treatments_print.html (accessed October 3, 2012).

Kalb, Claudia. "Have Another 'Fertilitini.'" *Newsweek*, January 26, 2009. http://www
.thedailybeast.com/newsweek/2009/01/26/have-another-fertilitini.html (accessed
March 6, 2013).

———. "Should You Have Your Baby Now?" *Newsweek*, August 12, 2001. http://www
.thedailybeast.com/newsweek/2001/08/12/should-you-have-your-baby-now.html
(accessed March 20, 2012).

Kamarudin, Syahida. "Hebe Tian Wants to Freeze Her Eggs." *Yahoo! Malaysia*, November
18, 2012. http://my.entertainment.yahoo.com/news/hebe-tian-wants-freeze-her-eggs
-233600951.html (accessed December 2, 2012).

Kelland, Kate. "Smoking Deaths Triple over Decade: Tobacco Report." Reuters, March
21, 2012. http://www.reuters.com/article/2012/03/21/us-tobacco-global-deaths-id
USBRE82K0C020120321 (accessed April 4, 2012).

"Kim Kardashian Would Opt for IVF to Have Baby at 40." *azcentral.com*, June 18, 2012. http:
//www.azcentral.com/ent/celeb/articles/2012/06/18/20120618kim
-kardashian-would-opt-ivf-baby-40.html (accessed August 15, 2012).

Kindelan, Katie. "Maria Menounos: 'My Choice' to Freeze My Eggs." ABC News,
September 26, 2011. http://abcnews.go.com/blogs/health/2011/09/26/maria
-menounos-my-choice-to-freeze-my-eggs/ (accessed February 13, 2012).

"Kiran Is a Hands-On Mother: Aamir Khan." *Hindustan Times*, December 3, 2012. http://
www.hindustantimes.com/Entertainment/Tabloid/Kiran-is-a-hands-on-mother
-Aamir-Khan/Article1-967736.aspx (accessed December 3, 2012).

Kirkey, Sharon. "Freezing Eggs, Embryos Poses Legal Concerns." *Vancouver Sun*, March 17,
2012. http://www2.canada.com/vancouversun/news/archives/story.html?id=82fa
00c2-bfff-48f3-82d2-27b54b429ae8 (accessed March 25, 2012).

———. "Freezing of Women's Eggs, Embryos Cause Controversy." Health, Canada
.com, March 15, 2012. http://o.canada.com/2012/03/15/freezing-of-womens-eggs
-embryos-cause-controversy/ (accessed April 9, 2012).

Kirsner, Scott. "Michelle Dipp, 36, Reflects Biotech's Next Generation." *Boston Globe*,
October 14, 2012. http://bostonglobe.com/business/2012/10/13/michelle-dipp
-ovascience-leading-new-generation-biotech-ceo/VqbVwXvcQSRkIVCQapdjhI/
story.html (accessed December 2, 2012).

Klein, Joshua U., MD. "Top Doc Reveals 8 Fertility Misconceptions." *CNN Health*, November
7, 2011. http://www.cnn.com/2011/11/07/health/fertility-misconceptions/ (accessed
February 8, 2012).

Knapp, Caroline. *Drinking: A Love Story*. New York: Dial Press, 1997.

Knox, Richard. "Kids of Older Fathers Likelier to Have Genetic Ailments." NPR, August 22, 2012. http://www.npr.org/blogs/health/2012/08/22/159852022/kids-of-older-fathers-likelier-to-have-genetic-ailments (accessed August 30, 2012).

Kornblum, Janet. "More Women 40–44 Remaining Childless." *USA Today*, August 19, 2008. http://www.usatoday.com/news/health/2008-08-18-fertility_N.htm (accessed February 18, 2012).

Kotkin, Joel, and Harry Siegel. "Where Have All the Babies Gone?" *Daily Beast*, February 19, 2013. http://www.thedailybeast.com/newsweek/2013/02/18/why-the-choice-to-be-childless-is-bad-for-america.html (accessed February 25, 2013).

Kounang, Nadia. "Could 'Personhood' Bills Outlaw IVF?" CNN, August 30, 2012. http://www.cnn.com/2012/08/30/health/ivf-outlawed (accessed December 2, 2012).

Kowalczyk, Carole, MD. In interview with the author, April 25, 2012.

Krafy, Dina. "Where Families Are Prized, Help Is Free." *New York Times*, July 17, 2011. http://www.nytimes.com/2011/07/18/world/middleeast/18israel.html (accessed August 5, 2012).

Kuchinich, Jackie, and Martha T. Moore. "Hilary Rosen Says Ann Romney Never Worked a 'Day in Her Life.'" *USA Today*, April 12, 2012. http://usatoday30.usatoday.com/news/politics/story/2012-04-12/ann-romney-hilary-rosen-work/54235706/1 (accessed April 16, 2012).

Kutteh, William, MD, PhD. In interview with the author, April 21, 2012.

Laden, Jenny. In interview with the author, May 14, 2013.

Lambert, Victoria. "Why DO So Many Women Pretend the Menopause Doesn't Exist?" *Daily Mail*, July 11, 2012. http://www.dailymail.co.uk/femail/article-2172274/Why-DO-women-pretend-menopause-doesnt-exist.html (accessed August 5, 2012).

Last, Jonathan V. "America's Baby Bust." *Wall Street Journal*, February 12, 2013. http://online.wsj.com/article/SB10001424127887323375204578270053387770718.html (accessed February 18, 2013).

Latza Nadeau, Barbie. "Europe's Growing Crisis of Abandoned Babies." *Daily Beast*, July 11, 2012. http://www.thedailybeast.com/articles/2012/07/11/europe-s-growing-crisis-of-abandoned-babies.html (accessed July 25, 2012).

———. "Italy Has Europe's Highest Percentage of Children in Poverty, Says UNICEF." *Daily Beast*, March 4, 2012. http://www.thedailybeast.com/articles/2012/03/04/italy-has-europe-s-highest-percentage-of-children-in-poverty-says-unicef.html (accessed March 19, 2012).

Lee, Kirsten A. "Mitt Romney's Advice to College Graduates: Marry Young, Have a 'Quiver Full of Kids.'" *Daily News*, April 30, 2013. http://www.nydailynews.com/romney-advice-college-grads-marry-young-kids-article-1.1331517 (accessed May 2, 2013).

Leiblum, S. R., A. Aviv, and R. Hamer. "Life after Infertility Treatment: A Long-Term Investigation of Marital and Sexual Function." *Human Reproduction* 13, no. 12 (1998): 3569–74. http://humrep.oxfordjournals.org/content/13/12/3569.full.pdf (accessed March 16, 2013).

Leland, John. "For Adoptive Parents, Questions without Answers." *New York Times*, September 16, 2011. http://www.nytimes.com/2011/09/18/nyregion/chinas-adoption-scandal-sends-chills-through-families-in-united-states.html (accessed March 19, 2012).

Leon, Anya. "Padma Lakshmi: I Don't Parent Alone." *People*, November 3, 2011. http://celebritybabies.people.com/2011/11/03/padma-lakshmi-i-dont-parent-alone/ (accessed February 8, 2012).

Leridon, Henri. "Can Assisted Reproduction Technology Compensate for the Natural Decline in Fertility with Age? A Model Assessment," *Human Reproduction* 18, no. 1 (2004): 1548.

Lesch Kelly, Alice. "Miscarriage: The Hardest Loss." *Conceive*, January 28, 2009. http://www.conceiveonline.com/articles/miscarriage-hardest-loss (accessed April 22, 2012).

Lino, Mark. "Expenditures on Children by Families, 2011." United States Department of Agriculture, Center for Nutrition Policy and Promotion 1528–2011, June 2012.

"Live Births with Egg Freezing Tied to Patient Age and Egg Freezing Method." *Fertility Authority*. http://www.fertilityauthority.com/articles/live-births-egg-freezing-tied-patient-age-and-egg-freezing-method (accessed January 16, 2013).

Livingston, Gretchen, and D'Vera Cohn. "Childless Up among All Women; Down among Women with Advanced Degrees." Pew Research Center Social & Demographic Trends, June 25, 2010. http://www.pewsocialtrends.org/2010/06/25/childlessness-up-among-all-women-down-among-women-with-advanced-degrees/ (accessed April 8, 2012).

———. "The New Demography of American Motherhood." Pew Research Center's Social & Demographic Trends Project, May 6, 2010.

Llorens, Ileana. "Three Couples Win Free IVF Cycle through Sher Fertility Institute 'I Believe' Contest." *Huffington Post*, June 19, 2012. http://www.huffingtonpost.com/2012/06/19/three-couples-win-free-ivf-contest-sher-fertility_n_1608976.html (accessed July 2, 2012).

Lockwood, Gillian, MD. "The Egg That Came in from the Cold: ASRM Lifts 'Experimental' Label from Social Egg Freezing." BioNews, November 12, 2012. http://www.bionews.org.uk/page_210873.asp (accessed December 5, 2012).

Lowe, Lindsay. "Woman Gives Birth Using 19-Year-Old Embryos: 'He's My Little Miracle.'" *Parade*, August 22, 2013. http://www.parade.com/66813/linzlowe/woman-gives-birth-using-19-year-old-embryos-hes-my-little-miracle/ (accessed September 2, 2013).

Lu, Stacy. "Octuplet Effect: More Choose Single Embryo Transplants for IVF." *TODAY Moms*, June 5, 2012. http://moms.today.msnbc.msn.com/_news/2012/06/05/11396062

-octuplet-effect-more-choose-single-embryo-transplants-for-ivf?lite (accessed August 11, 2012).

Ludden, Jennifer. "Stay-at-Home Workers Defend Choice after Yahoo Ban." NPR, March 1, 2013. http://www.npr.org/2013/03/01/173186526/stay-at-home-workers-defend-choice-after-yahoo-ban (accessed March 14, 2013).

Ludden, Jennifer, and Marisa Penaloza. "Taming the Twin Trend from Fertility Treatments." NPR, March 29, 2011. http://www.npr.org/2011/03/30/134960899/taming-ivfs-twin-trend (accessed March 9, 2012).

Lunau, Kate. "Thirty-Seven and Counting." *Maclean's*, October 27, 2012. http://www2.macleans.ca/2012/10/27/thirty-seven-and-counting/ (accessed December 20, 2012).

Lupkin, Sydney. "IVF: When Insurance Companies Won't Pay." ABC News, October 29, 2012. http://abcnews.go.com/Health/couples-extremes-pay-ivf/story?id=17575724#.UNHnfLZUYa8 (accessed December 14, 2012).

Macalino, Mona Lisa. "What You Don't Know about Infertility." *YourTango*, April 24, 2012. http://www.yourtango.com/2012151161/what-you-dont-know-about-infertility (accessed April 25, 2012).

Macdonald, Victoria. "I Couldn't Be a Mother . . . Until I Went to Spain." *Telegraph*, July 11, 2010. http://www.telegraph.co.uk/health/7883281/I-couldnt-be-a-mother...-until-I-went-to-Spain.html (accessed July 26, 2012).

MacRae, Fiona. "Britain's First Womb Transplant Could Be Carried Out in Just TWO YEARS." *Daily Mail*, July 12, 2012. http://www.dailymail.co.uk/health/article-2172420/Britain-s-womb-transplant-carried-just-TWO-YEARS.html (accessed July 15, 2012).

———. "MEN Are to Blame for Most Cases of Unexplained Infertility—But a New Test Could Help Couples Succeed." *Daily Mail*, November 14, 2012. http://www.dailymail.co.uk/health/article-2232989/MEN-blame-cases-unexplained-infertility--new-test-help-couples-succeed.html (accessed December 10, 2012).

MacRae, Fiona, and Vanessa Allen. "Doctors Carry Out First Successful Womb Transplant." *New Zealand Herald*, May 26, 2012. http://www.nzherald.co.nz/lifestyle/news/article.cfm?c_id=6&objectid=10808636 (accessed June 9, 2012).

Magee, Anna. "Fertility Miracle or Cruel Myth?" *Daily Mail*, November 7, 2012. http://www.dailymail.co.uk/femail/article-2229454/Fertility-miracle-cruel-myth-Freezing-eggs-dream-come-true-high-fliers-wanting-delay-motherhood-A-decade-produced-just-12-babies-So-women-spending-fortune-it.html (accessed December 12, 2012).

Magid, Cheri. In interview with the author, May 8, 2012.

Maltz Bovy, Phoebe. "There's No Perfect Age to Find a Husband." *Atlantic*, February 1, 2013. http://www.theatlantic.com/sexes/archive/2013/02/theres-no-perfect-age-to-find-a-husband/272789/ (accessed February 5, 2013).

Maranto, Gina. "Delayed Childbearing." *Atlantic*, June 1, 1995. http://www.theatlantic

.com/magazine/archive/1995/06/delayed-childbearing/5964/ (accessed February 8, 2012).

Marantz Henig, Robin, and Samantha Henig, "A Daughter Too Young—and Too Old—to Freeze Eggs." *New York Times*, May 15, 2012. http://parenting.blogs.nytimes.com/2012/05/15/a-daughter-too-young-and-too-old-to-freeze-eggs/ (accessed May 27, 2012).

Martin, Michel. "Birth Rate Declines for Women Over 40." NPR, June 29, 2010. http://www.npr.org/templates/story/story.php?storyId=128188446 (accessed February 13, 2012).

Martinez, Gladys, PhD, Kimberly Daniels, PhD, and Anjani Chandra, PhD. "Fertility of Men and Women Aged 15–44 Years in the United States: National Survey of Family Growth, 2006–2010." *National Health Statistics Report* 51 (April 12, 2012).

Mason, Mary Ann. "What You Need to Know If You're an Academic." *New York Times*, July 16, 2013. http://www.nytimes.com/roomfordebate/2013/07/08/should-women-delay-motherhood/what-you-need-to-know-if-youre-an-academic-and-want-to-be-a-mom (accessed September 4, 2013).

Matchar, Emily. "How Parenting Became a DIY Project." *Atlantic*, February 4, 2013. http://www.theatlantic.com/sexes/archive/2013/02/how-parenting-became-a-diy-project/272792/ (accessed February 9, 2013).

Mathews, T. J., MS, and Brady E. Hamilton, PhD. "Delayed Childbearing: More Women Are Having Their First Child Later in Life." *NCHS Data Brief* 21 (August 2009).

Mathur, Aparna, Hao Fu, and Peter Hansen. "The Mysterious and Alarming Rise of Single Parenthood in America." *Atlantic*, September 3, 2013. www.theatlantic.com/business/archive/2013/09/the-mysterious-and-alarming-rise-of-single-parenthood-in-america/279203/ (accessed September 16, 2013).

McAuliffe, Naomi. "Egg Freezing—For the Woman Who Can Never Win." *Guardian*, November 27, 2012. http://www.guardian.co.uk/commentisfree/2012/nov/27/egg-freezing-women-having-children (accessed December 20, 2012).

McCullough, Marie. "Human Egg-Freezing Gets a Stamp of Approval." *Inquirer*, Philly.com, October 19, 2012. http://articles.philly.com/2012-10-19/news/34556996_1_michael-j-glassner-largest-human-cell-egg (accessed October 23, 2012).

McDonough, Katie. "'I'm Not a Feminist, but . . . ,'" *Salon*, April 6, 2013. http://www.salon.com/2013/04/06/im_not_a_feminist_but/ (accessed April 10, 2013).

———. "Women May 'Evolve' out of Menopause, Says Scientist." *Salon*, May 29, 2013. http://www.salon.com/2013/05/29/women_may_evolve_out_of_menopause_says_scientist (accessed May 31, 2013).

McGoldrick, Shanna. "Help! I Have a Low Sperm Count." *Sun*, August 23, 2012. http://www.thesun.co.uk/sol/homepage/woman/health/health/4500607/Your-partner-cant-conceive-Male-infertility-is-the-most-common-cause.html (accessed December 11, 2012).

McPhillips, Fiona. "Pals Would Announce Pregnancies and I'd Have to Leave the Room." May 1, 2013. http://www.herald.ie/lifestyle/pals-would-announce-pregnancies-and -id-have-to-leave-the-room-29235717.html (accessed May 6 2013).

McQuillan, Julia, PhD. In interview with the author, May 11, 2012.

"Merck and RESOLVE Remind Couples That a Conversation with a Specialist Could Be the Start of Something Small," April 23, 2012. http://www.multivu.com/mnr/55828 -merck-resolve-pregnancy-fertilityguide-national-infertility-awareness-week (accessed May 5, 2012).

Mermin, Liz. In interview with the author, May 1, 2012.

Merrill, Tina. In interview with the author, May 1, 2012.

Miller, Lisa. "Parents of a Certain Age," *New York*, September 25, 2011. http://nymag .com/news/features/mothers-over-50-2011-10/ (accessed February 4, 2012).

———. "The Retro Wife." *New York*, March 17, 2013. http://nymag.com/news/features/ retro-wife-2013-3/ (accessed March 18, 2013).

Minella, Tracey. "Win a Free Basic Micro-IVF Cycle in Long Island IVF's 'Extreme Family-Building Makeover' Contest!" Long Island IVF, April 23, 2012. http://blog .longislandivf.com/2012/win-a-free-basic-micro-ivf-cycle-in-long-island-ivfs-extreme -family-building-makeover-contest/ (accessed April 29, 2012).

"Miscarriage." American Pregnancy Association. http://americanpregnancy.org/ pregnancycomplications/miscarriage.html (accessed September 23, 2013).

Mitra, Smita. "Long Journeys to Parenthood." *OutlookIndia.com*, May 7, 2012. http://www .outlookindia.com/article.aspx?280700 (accessed May 23, 2012).

Mohanty, Suchitra, and Frank Jack Daniel. "Indian Rape Victim's Father Says He Wants Her Named." Reuters, Sunday, January 6, 2013. http://www.reuters.com/article/2013/01/06/ us-india-rape-idUSBRE90500B20130106 (accessed January 7, 2013).

Mooney, Bel, and Sadie Nicholas. "Losing Out at Work, Sidelined by IVF . . . Is the Male of the Species Now Redundant?" *Daily Mail*, October 10, 2012. http://www.dailymail .co.uk/femail/article-2215956/Losing-work-sidelined-IVF--male-species-redundant .html (accessed December 15, 2012).

Moore, Lori. "Rep. Todd Akin: The Statement and the Reaction." *New York Times*, August 20, 2012. http://www.nytimes.com/2012/08/21/us/politics/rep-todd-akin -legitimate-rape-statement-and-reaction.html (accessed August 21, 2012).

Moore, Suzanne. "Extending IVF for Older Women Obscures a Deeper Problem for Society." *Guardian*, February 20, 2013. http://www.guardian.co.uk/commentisfree/ 2013/feb/20/extending-ivf-older-women-problem (accessed February 28, 2013).

Moran, Caitlin. *How to Be a Woman*. New York: Harper Perennial, 2011.

Motluk, Alison. "Growth of Egg Freezing Blurs 'Experimental' Label." *Nature* 476 (2011): 382–83. http://www.nature.com/news/2011/110823/full/476382a.html (accessed October 23, 2012).

Mroz, Jacqueline. "High Dose of Hormones Faulted in Fertility Care." *New York Times*, July 16, 2012. http://www.nytimes.com/2012/07/17/health/research/high-doses -of-hormones-add-to-ivf-complications.html (accessed August 29, 2012).

———. "One Sperm Donor, 150 Offspring." *New York Times*, September 5, 2011. http://www.nytimes.com/2011/09/06/health/06donor.html (accessed February 4, 2012).

Mukherjee, Siddhartha. *The Emperor of All Maladies: A Biography of Cancer*. New York: Scribner, 2011.

Mullany, Anjali. "Women and Leadership." *Fast Company*, July 6, 2012. http://www.fast company.com/1842212/thread-women-and-leadership (accessed July 10, 2012).

"Multitasking a Mom Thing." Reuters, December 2, 2011. http://www.nypost.com/f/ print/news/national/multitasking_mom_thing_sOf1zzQLc1ouxF4jxdaHCJ (accessed March 20, 2012).

Mundy, Liza. *Everything Conceivable: How Assisted Reproduction Is Changing Our World*. New York: Anchor Books, 2008.

Munz, Michelle. "New Form of in Vitro Fertilization Stirs Debate." *St. Louis Post-Dispatch*, January 26, 2012. http://www.stltoday.com/lifestyles/health-med-fit/fitness/new -form-of-in-vitro-fertilization-stirs-debate/article_1e684439-84f8-50fd-afb9-84aff48b 17cb.html (accessed February 7, 2012).

Murdoch, Cassie. "Is Your Fertility Doctor Taking Kickbacks?" *Slate*, July 13, 2012. http:// www.slate.com/blogs/xx_factor/2012/07/13/ivf_loans_predatory_lending_hits _the_fertility_market.html (accessed July 15, 2012).

Navarro, Mireya. "The Bachelor Life Includes a Family." *New York Times*, September 5, 2008. http://www.nytimes.com/2008/09/07/fashion/07single.html (accessed March 16, 2013).

"Nearly 1 in 3 Women Delay Motherhood." *Scotsman*, January 10, 2012. http://www .scotsman.com/news/uk/nearly-1-in-3-women-delay-motherhood-1-2556484 (accessed March 15, 2012).

Nellis, Krystina. "Hollywood Heroines: Here to Stay?" BBC News, August 13, 2012. http:// www.bbc.co.uk/news/entertainment-arts-19061388 (accessed March 21, 2013).

"New Egg Freezing Technique Offers Hope to Hundreds of Women." ScienceDaily, June 21, 2006. http://www.sciencedaily.com/releases/2006/06/060621163255.htm (accessed March 5, 2012).

Ng, Christina. "Texas Couple Auctioning Football Card to Pay for IVF." ABC News, October 17, 2012. http://abcnews.go.com/US/texas-couple-auctioning-football -card-pay-ivf/story?id=17500767#.UJK1iIVUYa8 (accessed October 24, 2012).

Nichols, Michelle. "Babies as Young as Six Months Victims of Rape in War: U.N. Envoy." Reuters, April 17, 2013. http://www.reuters.com/article/2013/04/17/us-war-rape -un-idUSBRE93G13U20130417 (accessed May 4, 2013).

———. "Fewer Women in Parliaments after Arab Spring: Study." Reuters, March 2, 2012.

http://www.reuters.com/article/2012/03/02/us-women-parliament-un-idUSTRE 821112O20120302 (accessed March 24, 2012).

Norton, Amy. "Failed IVF Attempt Tied to Depression, Anxiety." Reuters, June 27, 2012. http://www.reuters.com/article/2012/06/27/us-ivf-depression-idUSBRE85Q1912 0120627 (accessed March 23, 2013).

O'Callaghan, John. "Tiny Singapore Risks Economic Gloom without Big Baby Boom." Reuters, August 30, 2012. http://www.reuters.com/article/2012/08/30/us -singapore-babies-idUSBRE87T1FS20120830 (accessed September 10, 2012).

O'Connor, Maureen. "Beyoncé Is a 'Feminist, I Guess.'" *New York*, April 4, 2013. http:// nymag.com/thecut/2013/04/beyonc-is-a-feminist-i-guess.html (accessed April 4, 2013).

O'Meara, Sarah. "Emotional Infertility: Study Reveals Pain of Single Women Not Having Children." *Huffington Post*, June 9, 2012. http://www.huffingtonpost.co .uk/2012/09/06/single-women-face-emotional-infertility_n_1860925.html (accessed August 17, 2012).

Omurtag, K. R., and T. L. Toth, "The Cost Effectiveness and Health Incomes of in Vitro Fertilization (IVF) as a Mandated Benefit." *Fertility and Sterility* 88, no. 1 (September 2007): S122.

Ondaatje, Michael. *The Cinnamon Peeler*. New York: Vintage, 1997.

"1 in 3 Campaign." Advocates for Youth. http://www.1in3campaign.org/ (accessed September 24, 2013).

"Online Support Communities." RESOLVE. http://www.resolve.org/resources/online -support-communities.html (accessed April 7, 2013).

"Opposition Party Backs IVF Ban in Poland." Polskie Radio, June 27, 2012. http://www .thenews.pl/1/9/Artykul/104060,Opposition-party-backs-IVF-ban-in-Poland (ac- cessed July 12, 2012).

Orenstein, Beth W. "Hot Flashes: Your Favorite Screen Characters Go through 'The Change.'" *Everyday Health*, May 17, 2011. http://www.everydayhealth.com/ menopause-pictures/your-favorite-screen-actors-go-through-the-change.aspx (ac- cessed March 20, 2012).

Orenstein, Peggy. *Flux: Women on Sex, Work, Love, Kids, & Life in a Half-Changed World*. New York: Anchor Books, 2000.

———. "Mourning My Miscarriage." *New York Times*, April 21, 2012. http://www.nytimes .com/2002/04/21/magazine/mourning-my-miscarriage.html (accessed April 22, 2012).

———. *Waiting for Daisy: A Tale of Two Continents, Three Religions, Five Infertility Doctors, An Oscar®, an Atomic Bomb, a Romantic Night, and One Woman's Quest to Become a Mother*. New York: Bloomsbury, 2007.

"Over 1,000 Babies Born through Assisted Reproductive Treatment in 10 Years." *Nige-*

rian Tribune, November 6, 2012. http://tribune.com.ng/index.php/community
-news/50354-over-1000-babies-born-through-assisted-reproductive-treatment-in-10
-years (accessed December 5, 2012).

Overall, Christine. "Think Before You Breed." *New York Times*, June 17, 2012. http://opinionator
.blogs.nytimes.com/2012/06/17/think-before-you-breed/ (accessed June 23, 2012).

Parker, Andrew. "We Designed Our Baby to Be Safe from Cancer." *Sun*, October 7, 2012.
http://www.thesun.co.uk/sol/homepage/news/4576137/Nicky-Halford-gives-birth
-to-IVF-baby-designed-to-be-safe-from-cancer.html (accessed March 2, 2013).

Parker-Pope, Tara. "Can a 'Fertility Diet' Get You Pregnant?" *New York Times*, December
18, 2007. http://www.nytimes.com/2007/12/18/health/nutrition/18well.html (accessed March 2, 2012).

"Paropakar to Launch IVF Service Today." *Himalayan Times*, April 29, 2012. http://www
.thehimalayantimes.com/rssReference.php?headline=Paropakar+to+launch+IVF
+service+today&NewsID=330137 (accessed May 8, 2012).

Patrizio, Pasquale, MD. In interview with the author, May 1, 2012.

PBS NewsHour, October 19, 2012.

Peacock, Louise. "What's Wrong with Offering IVF Treatment as a Prize?" *Telegraph*, October
25, 2012. http://www.telegraph.co.uk/women/womens-life/9631684/Whats-wrong
-with-offering-IVF-treatment-as-a-prize.html (accessed December 3, 2012).

Pear, Robert. "Gender Gap Persists in Cost of Health Insurance." *New York Times*, March
19, 2012. http://www.nytimes.com/2012/03/19/health/policy/women-still-pay
-more-for-health-insurance-data-shows.html (accessed April 2, 2012).

Pearson, Catherine. "IVF and Birth Defects Could Be Linked, New Study Finds." *Huffington Post*, October 20, 2012. http://www.huffingtonpost.com/2012/10/20/ivf-birth
-defects_n_1989302.html (accessed November 3, 2012).

Peart, Karen N. "A New Method for Picking the 'Right' Egg in IVF." *Yale News*, May 31,
2012. http://news.yale.edu/2012/05/31/new-method-picking-right-egg-ivf (accessed June 24, 2012).

Peikoff, Kira. "Personhood vs. Stem Cell Research." *Atlanta Journal-Constitution*, May 25,
2012. http://www.ajc.com/news/news/opinion/personhood-vs-stem-cell-research/
nQT65/ (accessed October 13, 2012).

Peralta, Eyder. "Yahoo's Marissa Mayer Expands Parental Leave." NPR, April 30, 2013.
http://www.npr.org/blogs/thetwo-way/2013/04/30/180150731/yahoos-marissa
-mayer-expands-parental-leave (accessed May 2, 2013).

Perkowski, Jack. "China's One-Child Policy's Unexpected Issue: Infertility." *Forbes*, May 25,
2012. http://www.forbes.com/sites/jackperkowski/2012/05/25/chinas-one-child
-policys-unexpected-issue-infertility/ (accessed October 2, 2012).

Picardie, Justine. "The Real Gwyneth." *Harper's Bazaar*, March 2012.

Pirkle, Sunday, PhD. In interview with the author, January 8, 2013.

Plotz, David. "The 'Genius Babies,' and How They Grew." *Slate*, February 8, 2001. http://
www.slate.com/articles/life/seed/2001/02/the_genius_babies_and_how_they_grew
.html (accessed February 15, 2012).

Pogrebin, Abigail. "How Do You Spell Ms." *New York*, October 30, 2011. http://nymag
.com/news/features/ms-magazine-2011-11/ (accessed March 4, 2012).

Poma Traynor, Gabriela. In interview with the author, March 23, 2013.

Prentice, Alessandra. "Two U.S. Mothers Speak of Russian Adoption Joy." Reuters,
February 11, 2013. http://www.reuters.com/article/2013/02/11/us-russia-usa
-adoption-idUSBRE91A0YL20130211 (accessed February 24, 2012).

Press, Viva Sarah. "IVF Baby Boom in Israel." ISRAEL21c, May 13, 2012. http://
israel21c.org/news/ivf-baby-boom-in-israel/ (accessed May 16, 2012).

Profis, Michelle. "Lady Gaga Tells Oprah She Wants a 'Soccer Team' of Kids." PopWatch,
Entertainment Weekly, March 19, 2012. http://popwatch.ew.com/2012/03/19/lady
-gaga-on-oprah/ (accessed March 20, 2012).

"The Psychological Impact of Infertility and Its Treatment." *Harvard Mental Health
Letter*, May 2009. http://www.health.harvard.edu/newsletters/Harvard_Mental
_Health_Letter/2009/May/The-psychological-impact-of-infertility-and-its-treatment
(accessed May 3, 2013).

"Push for Insurance to Cover Egg Freezing." WCAX, October 26, 2012. http://www.wcax
.com/story/19926286/push-for-insurance-to-cover-fertilotiy-treatment (accessed
December 7, 2012).

Quenqua, Douglas. "Clinic Raffles Could Make You a Winner, and Maybe a Mother." *New
York Times*, October 20, 2012. http://www.nytimes.com/2012/10/21/health/ethical
-questions-raised-by-in-vitro-raffle.html (accessed December 2, 2012).

Queram, Kate Elizabeth. "Twin Births Rise Brings Concerns." *StarNews Online*, January 19,
2012. http://www.starnewsonline.com/article/20120119/ARTICLES/120119641
(accessed February 18, 2012).

Rabin, Roni Caryn. "Nearly 1 in 5 Women in U.S. Survey Say They Have Been Sexually Assaulted." Health, *New York Times*, December 14, 2011. http://www.nytimes
.com/2011/12/15/health/nearly-1-in-5-women-in-us-survey-report-sexual-assault
.html (accessed February 9, 2012).

Rahman, Rema. "The World at Seven Billion." BBC News, October 30, 2011. http://
www.bbc.co.uk/news/magazine-15494349 (accessed February 7, 2012).

Rasheed, PMA. "Monetary Aid Eases IVF Woes." *Gulf Today*, November 23, 2012. www
.gulftoday.ae/portal/cd204c96-f960-47bf-8aba-f147c2646a84.aspx (accessed December 11, 2012).

"Recurrent Pregnancy Loss." Patient Fact Sheet. American Society for Reproductive Medicine, August 2008. http://www.asrm.org/Recurrent_Pregnancy_Loss/ (accessed February 5, 2012).

Reese, Hope. "'Anger Boiled Up, and Betty Friedan Was There': 'Feminine Mystique' at 50." *Atlantic*, January 28, 2013. http://www.theatlantic.com/sexes/archive/2013/01/anger-boiled-up-and-betty-friedan-was-there-feminine-mystique-at-50/272575 (accessed February 2, 2013).

Reeves, Caroline. In interview with the author, April 23, 2013.

"Research and Markets: India IVF Treatment Market Analysis—Infertility in India Is Increasing due to Factors such as Urbanisation, Pollution and Chemical Exposure." *Business Wire*, May 2, 2012. http://www.businesswire.com/news/home/20120502005671/en (accessed May 12, 2012).

"Research with Worms May Shed Light on Women's Fertility." Health, *US News & World Report*, December 6, 2011. http://health.usnews.com/health-news/family-health/womens-health/articles/2011/12/06/research-with-worms-may-shed-light-on-womens-fertility (accessed February 20, 2012).

Rich, Adrienne. *Later Poems: Selected and New, 1971–2012*. New York: W. W. Norton, 2013.

Richards, Amy. *Opting In: Having a Child without Losing Yourself*. New York: Farrar, Straus and Giroux, 2008.

———. In interview with the author, April 30, 2013.

Richards, Sarah Elizabeth. "Alimony for Your Eggs." *New York Times*, September 6, 2013. http://www.nytimes.com/2013/09/07/opinion/alimony-for-your-eggs.html (accessed September 16, 2013).

———. "Coming Out of the Fertility Closet." *Time*, August 11, 2013. http://ideas.time.com/2013/08/11/coming-out-of-the-fertility-closet/ (accessed September 4, 2013).

———. *Motherhood, Rescheduled: The New Frontier of Egg Freezing and the Women Who Tried It*. New York: Simon & Schuster, 2013.

———. "We Need to Talk about Our Eggs." *New York Times*, October 22, 2012. http://www.nytimes.com/2012/10/23/opinion/we-need-to-talk-about-our-eggs.html (accessed October 28, 2012).

Richardson-Lyne, Tracy. "Why Do GPs Show So Little Sympathy for Women's Fertility Problems?" *Guardian*, August 29, 2012. http://www.guardian.co.uk/comment isfree/2012/aug/29/gps-no-understanding-womens-fertility (accessed August 30, 2012).

Richtel, Matt. "Housecleaning, Then Dinner? Silicon Valley Perks Come Home." *New York Times*, October 19, 2012. http://www.nytimes.com/2012/10/20/us/in-silicon-valley-perks-now-begin-at-home.html (accessed April 8, 2013).

Ritter, Malcolm. "3-Person IVF? Embryos from 2 Women, 1 Man Created in Lab." *Huffington Post*, October 24, 2012. http://www.huffingtonpost.com/2012/10/24/3-person-ivf-embryos-women-man_n_2011546.html (accessed October 30, 2012).

Roberts, Michelle. "Children with Older Fathers and Grandfathers 'Live Longer.'" BBC News, June 11, 2012. http://www.bbc.co.uk/news/health-18392873 (accessed August 9, 2012).

———. "Three-Person IVF Trial 'Success.'" BBC News, October 24, 2012. http://www
.bbc.co.uk/news/health-20032216 (accessed October 30, 2012).

Roberts, Soraya. "Hollywood's IVF Stigma's Strong." *Star*, April 29, 2013. http://www
.thestar.com/life/parent/2013/04/29/hollywoods_ivf_stigmas_strong.html (accessed
April 30, 2013).

Rochman, Bonnie. "Baby Contest: Couples Compete for Free IVF—Is This Exploitation of
Generosity?" *Time*, June 20, 2012. http://ideas.time.com/2012/06/20/baby-contest
-couples-compete-for-free-ivf-is-this-exploitation-or-generosity/ (accessed July 8, 2012).

———. "The Motherhood Penalty: We're in the Midst of a 'Mom-Cession.'" *Time*, August
17, 2012. http://healthland.time.com/2012/08/17/the-motherhood-penalty-were
-in-the-midst-of-a-mom-cession/ (accessed August 25, 2012).

Rodriguez, Diana. "10 Health Screenings All Women Should Have." *Everyday Health*,
April 20, 2012. http://www.everydayhealth.com/womens-health/10-screenings-all
-women-should-have.aspx (accessed April 24, 2012).

Rosenberg, Alyssa. "*New Girl*'s Fertility Episode Wants You to Panic about Your Eggs. Don't."
Slate, November 29, 2012. http://www.slate.com/blogs/xx_factor/2012/11/29/
new_girl_latest_episode_may_induce_unnecessary_fertility_panic.html (accessed
December 18, 2012).

Rosenhaus, Nancy. In interview with the author, April 26, 2012.

Rosin, Hanna. "The Gender Wage Gap Lie." *Slate*, August 30, 2013. http://www.slate
.com/articles/double_x/doublex/2013/08/gender_pay_gap_the_familiar_line
_that_women_make_77_cents_to_every_man_s.html (accessed September 5, 2013).

Rothenberg Gritz, Jenni. "Stephen Colbert Solves the 'Having It All' Dilemma in 5 Words."
Atlantic, July 17, 2012. http://www.theatlantic.com/business/archive/2012/07/stephen
-colbert-solves-the-having-it-all-dilemma-in-5-words/259936/ (accessed July 19, 2012).

Rowan, Karen. "Best Age to Raise Kids? Older Parents Say 30s." FoxNews.com, March
9, 2012. http://www.foxnews.com/health/2012/03/09/best-age-to-raise-kids-older
-parents-say-30s/ (accessed March 10, 2012).

———. "Fertility Decline Surprises Women over 40, Study Finds." Women, *Huffington Post*,
December 10, 2012. http://www.huffingtonpost.com/2012/12/10/fertility-decline
-women-surprised-over-40-ivf_n_2273122.html (accessed December 15, 2012).

"Royal College Warns Women Not to Leave Pregnancy Too Late in Life," 2009. http://
www.vitalab.com/infertility-news/royal-college-warns-about-late-pregnancy/ (accessed December 7, 2012).

Ruiz, Michelle. "Report: More US Women in Their 40s Never Have Kids." AOL News,
June 25, 2010. http://www.aolnews.com/2010/06/25/report-more-us-women-in
-their-40s-never-have-kids/ (accessed April 13, 2012).

Russell, Chrissie. "Why It's Time Men Opened Up about Infertility." *Irish Independent*, May
28, 2012. http://www.independent.ie/lifestyle/parenting/why-its-time-men-opened
-up-about-infertility-3120014.html (accessed June 2, 2012).

Sample, Ian. "IVF Could be Revolutionised by New Technique, Says Clinic." *Guardian*, May 16, 2013. http://www.guardian.co.uk/society/2013/may/17/ivf-revolutionised -new-technique-clinic (accessed May 19, 2013).

Sandberg, Sheryl. *Lean In: Women, Work, and the Will to Lead*. New York: Alfred A. Knopf, 2013.

Sandberg, Sheryl. "Why We Have Too Few Women Leaders." *TEDWomen*, December 2010. http://www.ted.com/talks/sheryl_sandberg_why_we_have_too_few_women _leaders.html (accessed June 28, 2012).

Schafer, Jenny. "Hugh Jackman on Wife's Miscarriages, The Joys of Adoption." *Celebrity Baby Scoop*, December 18, 2012. http://www.celebritybabyscoop.com/2012/12/18/ hugh-jackman-on-wifes-miscarriages-the-joys-of-adoption (accessed December 23, 2012).

Schapiro, Lillian. *Tick Tock*. Lincoln, NE: iUniverse, Inc., 2005.

Schilling, Mary Kaye. In interview with the author, May 2, 2012.

"Scientists Warn of Dangers in Delaying Motherhood." *Express Tribune*, April 10, 2012. http://tribune.com.pk/story/362393/scientists-warn-of-dangers-in-delaying -motherhood/ (accessed May 19, 2012).

Seligson, Hannah. "When the Work-Life Scales Are Unequal." *New York Times*, September 1, 2012. http://www.nytimes.com/2012/09/02/business/straightening-out-the-work -life-balance.html (accessed December 4, 2012).

Senior, Jennifer. "All Joy and No Fun: Why Parents Hate Parenting." *New York*, July 4, 2010. http://nymag.com/news/features/67024/ (accessed March 14, 2013).

Sharma, Gopal. "Japanese Octogenarian Becomes Oldest to Reach Everest summit." Reuters, May 23, 2013. http://www.reuters.com/article/2013/05/23/us-nepal -everest-oldest-idUSBRE94M05420130523 (accessed May 25, 2013).

Sheehy, Gail. *Passages: Predictable Crises of Adult Life*. New York: Random House, 2006.

———. *The Silent Passage*. New York: Pocket Books, 1998.

Shenfield, F., J. de Mouzon, G. Pennings, A. P. Ferraretti, A. Nyboe Anderson, G. de Wert, and V. Goossens. "Cross Border Reproductive Care in Six European Countries." *Human Reproduction* 25, no. 6 (2010): 1361–68.

Shlain, Leonard. *Sex, Time and Power*. New York: Penguin Books, 2004.

Shreffler, Karina, PhD. In interview with the author, May 21, 2012.

Shulevitz, Judith. "How Older Parenthood Will Upend American Society: The Scary Consequences of the Grayest Generation." *New Republic*, December 6, 2012. http:// www.newrepublic.com/article/politics/magazine/110861/how-older-parenthood -will-upend-american-society (accessed December 12, 2012).

Sidhu, Jasmeet. "How to Buy a Daughter." *Slate*, September 14, 2012. http://www .pulse.me/s/dhvor#/www.slate.com/articles/health_and_science/medical_examiner/ 2012/09/sex_selection_in_babies_through_pgd_americans_are_paying_to_have _daughters_rather_than_sons_.html (accessed September 23, 2012).

Silver-Greenberg, Jessica. "In Vitro a Fertile Niche for Lenders." *Wall Street Journal*, February 24, 2012. http://online.wsj.com/article/SB10001424052970203960804577241270123249832.html (accessed February 28, 2012).

Slack, Megan. "President Obama Speaks on the Shooting in Connecticut." *White House Blog*, December 14, 2012. http://www.whitehouse.gov/blog/2012/12/14/president-obama-speaks-shooting-connecticut (accessed December 17, 2012).

Slaughter, Anne-Marie. "There Are Lots of Ways to Help Make Men and Women Truly Equal." *Atlantic*, March 18, 2013. http://www.theatlantic.com/sexes/archive/2013/03/there-are-lots-of-ways-to-help-make-men-and-women-truly-equal/274084/ (accessed March 22, 2013).

Smith, Lizzie. "'I Chased My Career Instead of Chasing Guys': Giuliana Rancic Reveals How Her Infertility 'Blindsided' Her at 35." *Daily Mail*, October 30, 2012. http://www.dailymail.co.uk/tvshowbiz/article-2225299/I-chase-career-instead-chasing-guys-Giuliana-Rancic-reveals-infertility-blindsided-her.html (accessed November 2, 2012).

Smith, Rebecca. "British Man 'Fathered 600 Children' at Own Fertility Clinic." *Telegraph*, April 8, 2012. http://www.telegraph.co.uk/news/9193014/British-man-fathered-600-children-at-own-fertility-clinic.html (accessed April 23, 2012).

———. "Children with 'Three Parents' Could Become Reality." *Telegraph*, June 4, 2012. http://www.telegraph.co.uk/health/healthnews/9309023/Children-with-three-parents-could-become-reality.html (accessed July 3, 2012).

"Social Egg Freezing: The Reasons Some Women Freeze Their Eggs." My Fertility Choices, January 22, 2013. http://myfertilitychoices.com/2013/01/social-egg-freezing-the-reasons-some-women-freeze-their-eggs/ (accessed February 9, 2013).

Solomon, Andrew. *Far from the Tree: Parents, Children, and the Search for Identity*. New York: Scribner, 2012.

Sotomayor, Sonia. *My Beloved World*. New York: Alfred A. Knopf, 2013.

"Sotomayor's Life in Pictures." CNN, May 26, 2009. http://www.cnn.com/2009/POLITICS/05/26/gallery.sotomayor.life/index.html (accessed February 17, 2013).

Souter, Irene, MD. In interview with the author, April 24, 2012.

Spar, Debora L. "Why Women Should Stop Trying to Be Perfect." *Daily Beast*, September 24, 2012. http://www.thedailybeast.com/newsweek/2012/09/23/why-women-should-stop-trying-to-be-perfect.html (accessed October 2, 2012).

Springen, Karen. "The Mysteries of Miscarriage." *Daily Beast*, January 27, 2008. http://www.thedailybeast.com/newsweek/2008/01/27/the-mysteries-of-miscarriage.html (accessed February 15, 2012).

Stanley, Alessandra. "Mother of All Comedy Topics." *New York Times*, March 15, 2013. http://www.nytimes.com/2013/03/17/movies/tina-feys-admission-and-other-comedies-eye-maternity.html (accessed March 18, 2013).

"State Laws Related to Insurance Coverage for Infertility Treatment." National Confer-

ence of State Legislature. http://www.ncsl.org/issues-research/health/insurance
-coverage-for-infertility-laws.aspx (accessed February 13, 2012).

"The State of World Population 2011." United Nations Population Fund. http://www
.unfpa.org/webdav/site/global/shared/documents/publications/2011/EN-SWOP
2011-FINAL.pdf (accessed March 23, 2012).

Steenhuysen, Julie. "Gene Studies Begin to Unravel Autism Puzzle." Reuters, April 4, 2012.
http://www.reuters.com/article/2012/04/04/us-autism-usa-genes-idUSBRE83312
820120404 (accessed April 20, 2012).

Stein, Rob. "Chance to Pause Biological Clock with Ovarian Transplant Stirs Debate." NPR,
December 24, 2012. http://www.npr.org/blogs/health/2012/12/24/167705397/
chance-to-pause-biological-clock-with-ovarian-transplant-stirs-debate (accessed January 8, 2013).

———. "In Vitro Fertilization Can't Reverse Aging's Effects." *Washington Post*, January
15, 2009. http://articles.washingtonpost.com/2009-01-15/news/36883365_1_ivf
-infertile-women-treatment-cycles (accessed February 8, 2012).

Strachan, Julieanne. "Frozen Egg Birth Rate Remains Low." *Sydney Morning Herald*, July
1, 2012. http://www.smh.com.au/national/frozen-egg-birth-rate-remains-low-2012
0630-219d1.html (accessed July 17, 2012).

Strayed, Cheryl. *Wild*. New York: Vintage Books, 2013.

Sunderam, Saswati, PhD, Dmitry M. Kissin, MD, Lisa Flowers, MPA, John E. Anderson,
PhD, Suzanne G. Folger, PhD, Denise J. Jamieson, MD, and Wanda D. Barfield, MD.
"Assisted Reproductive Technology Surveillance—United States, 2009." Centers for
Disease Control and Prevention, November 2, 2012. http://www.cdc.gov/mmwr/
preview/mmwrhtml/ss6107a1.htm (accessed December 4, 2012).

Sullivan, Michele G. "ASRM: Egg Freezing No Longer 'Experimental.'" Ob.Gyn. News,
October 19, 2012. http://www.obgynnews.com/index.php?id=11146&cHash
=071010&tx_ttnews[tt_news]=137771 (accessed October 23, 2012).

"Supplement Touted as Way to Extend Fertility." CTV News, December 26, 2012.
http://www.ctv.ca/CTVNews/Health/20111223/coenzyme-q10-fertility-111226/
(accessed February 12, 2012).

"Supreme Court Justice Sonia Sotomayor Regrets Not Having Borne or Adopted Children in Memoir, 'My Beloved World.'" *NY Daily News*, Associated Press, December
10, 2012. http://www.nydailynews.com/news/national/sotomayor-regrets-borne
-adopted-children-memoir-article-1.1217303 (accessed January 4, 2012).

Summers, Lawrence H. "Remarks at NBER Conference on Diversifying the Science &
Engineering Workforce," January 14, 2005. http://www.harvard.edu/president/
speeches/summers_2005/nber.php (accessed March 15, 2013).

Szalavitz, Maia. "The Link between Infertility Treatments and Birth Defects." Health
& Family, *Time*, May 7, 2012. http://healthland.time.com/2012/05/07/the-link
-between-infertility-treatments-and-birth-defects/ (accessed August 3, 2012).

Tavernise, Sabrina. "Fertility Rate Stabilizes as the Economy Grows." *New York Times*, September 6, 2013. http://www.nytimes.com/2013/09/06/health/fertility-rate-stabilizes-as-the-economy-grows.html (accessed September 13, 2013).

Tewari, Mansi. "Vicky Donor Affect: Infertility Specialists in Meerut Get a Boost." *Economic Times*, May 30, 2012. http://articles.economictimes.indiatimes.com/2012-05-30/news/31900430_1_sperm-donation-sperm-banking-meerut (accessed June 3, 2012).

"Thirty-Seven Percent of Working Dads Would Leave Their Jobs If Their Family Could Afford It, CareerBuilder.com's Annual Father's Day Survey Finds." CareerBuilder .com, June 11, 2007. http://msn.careerbuilder.com/share/aboutus/pressreleases detail.aspx?id=pr375&sd=6%2F11%2F2007&ed=12%2F31%2F2007 (accessed March 8, 2013).

Thomas, Marlo. "Mom's Stifled Dreams." *Makers*. http://www.makers.com/marlo -thomas/moments/moms-stifled-dreams/ (accessed March 17, 2012).

Thompson, Derek. "Bye-Bye, Boomers: This Is the Age of the Baby Bust-ers." *Atlantic*, August 22, 2012. http://www.theatlantic.com/business/archive/2012/08/bye-bye -boomers-this-is-the-age-of-the-baby-bust-ers/261424/ (accessed August 30, 2012).

———. "Your Day in a Chart: 10 Cool Facts about How Americans Spend Our Time." *Atlantic*, June 25, 2012. http://www.theatlantic.com/business/archive/2012/06/ your-day-in-a-chart-10-cool-facts-about-how-americans-spend-our-time/258967/ (accessed July 7, 2012).

———. "The 4 Rich Countries Where Women Out-Earn Men (With 1 Huge Caveat)." *Atlantic*, December 17, 2012. http://www.theatlantic.com/business/archive/2012/12/ the-4-rich-countries-where-women-out-earn-men-with-1-huge-caveat/266343/ (accessed December 20, 2012).

Tomlinson, Simon. "'Women Will Have So Much Choice about When to Have Children': Scientists Can Stop Menopause with Ovary Transplants." *Daily Mail*, March 25, 2012. http://www.dailymail.co.uk/health/article2120102/Fertility-breakthrough-Scientists -halt-menopause-ovary-transplants.html (accessed March 29, 2012).

"Townterview Hosted by Bahrain TV." U.S. Department of State, December 3, 2010. http:// www.state.gov/secretary/rm/2010/12/152355.htm (accessed October 19, 2012).

Triggs, Charlotte. "Mariska Hargitay: My Double Adoption Blessing." *People*, October 31, 2011. http://www.people.com/people/archive/article/0,,20538446,00.html (accessed February 3, 2012).

Twenge, Jean. "How Long Can You Wait to Have a Baby?" *Atlantic*, June 19, 2013. http:// www.theatlantic.com/magazine/archive/2013/07/how-long-can-you-wait-to-have -a-baby/309374/ (accessed August 8, 2013).

"2009 Assisted Reproductive Technology Success Rates: National Summary and Fertility Clinic Reports." Centers for Disease Control and Prevention, American Society for Reproductive Medicine, and Society for Assisted Reproductive Technology, 2011.

"Ukrainian Women Increasingly Delay Motherhood for Future." forUm, October 25, 2012. http://en.for-ua.com/news/2012/10/25/153839.html (accessed October 28, 2012).

"Understanding Fertility." *Women in Business*, 2012.

"Understanding the Hague Convention." Intercountry Adoption. http://adoption.state.gov/hague_convention/overview.php (accessed March 8, 2012).

"A United Front: Dr. Dan Gehlbach Offers Support for Family Act of 2011 and Families Facing Infertility." PRWeb, August 7, 2012. http://www.prweb.com/releases/mrc familyact/08/prweb9766588.htm (accessed August 18, 2012).

Vaidyanathan, Rajini. "The Rise and Rise of New Bollywood." BBC News, June 7, 2012. http://www.bbc.co.uk/news/world-asia-india-18327901 (accessed September 15, 2012).

Valk, Kate. In interview with the author, April 27, 2012.

Vallejo, Victoria, Joseph A. Lee, Lisa Schuman, Georgia Witkin, Enrique Cervantes, Benjamin Sandler, and Alan B. Copperman. "Social and Psychological Assessment of Women Undergoing Elective Oocyte Cryopreservation: A 7-Year Analysis." *Open Journal of Obstetrics and Gynecology* 3 (January 2013). http://www.scirp.org/journal/ojog (accessed March 15, 2013).

Vinciguerra, Thomas. "He's Not My Grandpa. He's My Dad." *New York Times*, April 12, 2007. http://www.nytimes.com/2007/04/12/fashion/12dads.html (accessed March 19, 2012).

Waldman, Ayelet. "Is This Really Goodbye?" *Marie Claire*, October 18, 2012. http://www.marieclaire.com/world-reports/inspirational-women/hillary-clinton-farewell-3 (accessed October 24, 2012).

Walker, Ruth. "IVF Treatment: Shopping Abroad." *Scotsman*, November 11, 2012. http://www.scotsman.com/scotland-on-sunday/scotland/ivf-treatment-shopping -abroad-1-2628043 (accessed January 15, 2013).

Wallace, Benjamin. "The Virgin Father." *New York*, February 5, 2012. http://nymag.com/news/features/trent-arsenault-2012-2/ (accessed February 7, 2012).

Walton, Alice G. "Okay, We Get It: There's No Turning Back the Biological Clock." *Atlantic*, May 1, 2012. http://www.theatlantic.com/health/archive/2012/05/okay-we-get-it -theres-no-turning-back-the-biological-clock/256571/ (accessed May 18, 2012).

Warner, Judith. "The Opt-Out Generation Wants Back In." *New York Times Magazine*, August 7, 2013. http://www.nytimes.com/2013/08/11/magazine/the-opt-out -generation-wants-back-in.html (accessed August 8, 2013).

Waters, Abbie. "IVF Use in America: State IVF Rates and Rankings." http://www.fertility nation.com/united-states-of-ivf-state-ivf-rates-rankings-map-infographic/ (accessed May 3, 2012).

Weems, Marianne. In interview with the author, May 11, 2012.

Weidman Sterling, Evelina, and Angie Best-Boss. *Budgeting for Infertility*. New York: Fireside, 2009.

Weil, Elizabeth. "Puberty Before Age 10: A New 'Normal'?" *New York Times*, March 30, 2012. http://www.nytimes.com/2012/04/01/magazine/puberty-before-age-10-a-new -normal.html (accessed April 2, 2012).

Weisman, Jonathan. "Senate Votes Overwhelmingly to Expand Domestic Violence Act." *New York Times*, February 12, 2013. http://www.nytimes.com/2013/02/13/us/politics/ senate-votes-to-expand-domestic-violence-act.html (accessed February 15, 2013).

Weissmann, Jordan. "The Overhyped Rise of Stay-at-Home Dads." *Atlantic*, September 3, 2013. http://www.theatlantic.com/business/archive/2013/09/the-overhyped-rise -of-stay-at-home-dads/279279/ (accessed September 16, 2013).

———. "Why Are Women Paid Less?" *Atlantic*, October 17, 2012. http://www.theatlantic .com/business/archive/2012/10/why-are-women-paid-less/263776/ (accessed October 28, 2012).

Weller, Sheila. "'My Faith Pulled Me Through.'" *Good Housekeeping*, April 4, 2012. http:// www.goodhousekeeping.com/family/celebrity-interviews/mariska-hargitay-adoption (accessed April 15, 2012).

Westthorp, Tanya. "Couples Go to Asia to Select Baby Gender." Lifestyle, PerthNow, April 2, 2013. http://www.perthnow.com.au/lifestyle/parenting/couples-go-to-asia-to-select -baby-gender/story-fnhqgv0m-1226610697956 (accessed April 14, 2013).

"When There's a Baby between You and the Glass Ceiling." NPR, December 2, 2012. http:// www.npr.org/2012/12/23/167923727/when-the-glass-ceiling-is-a-baby-working -through-motherhood (accessed January 15, 2012).

White, Hilary. "Eugenics Threat Growing in IVF Industry: British Fertility Expert." LifeSiteNews.com, April 8, 2013. http://www.lifesitenews.com/news/eugenics -threat-growing-in-ivf-industry-british-fertility-expert/ (accessed April 20, 2013).

Williams, Alex. "Just Wait until Your Mother Gets Home." *New York Times*, August 10, 2012. http://www.nytimes.com/2012/08/12/fashion/dads-are-taking-over-as-full-time -parents.html (accessed August 12, 2012).

Williams, Mary Elizabeth. "Motherhood Is Not a Job." *Salon*, April 27, 2012. http://www .salon.com/2012/04/27/motherhood_is_not_a_job (accessed May 3, 2012).

Williams, Wendy M., and Stephen J. Ceci. "When Scientists Choose Motherhood." *American Scientist* 100, no. 2 (March–April 2012): 138. http://www.americanscientist.org/ issues/pub/when-scientists-choose-motherhood (accessed May 18, 2012).

Wilmhoff, Crystal. In interview with the author, May 29, 2012.

Wilson, Jacque. "Boys—Like Girls—Hitting Puberty Earlier." CNN, October 23, 2012. http://www.cnn.com/2012/10/20/health/boys-early-puberty/index.html (accessed October 28, 2012).

Winston, Robert. "The Bravery of Lesley Brown, Mother of the First IVF Baby." *Guardian*, June 21, 2012. http://www.guardian.co.uk/commentisfree/2012/jun/21/lesley -brown-mother-ivf-baby (accessed June 30, 2012).

Wise, Jeff. "About That Overpopulation Problem." *Slate*, January 9, 2013. http://www
.slate.com/articles/technology/future_tense/2013/01/world_population_may
_actually_start_declining_not_exploding.html (accessed March 12, 2013).

Wolff Perrine, Jennifer. "This Woman Has a Secret." *SELF.* http://www.self.com/
health/2010/08/breaking-the-silence-on-infertility/ (accessed February 13, 2012).

"Woman Who Underwent 2011 Womb Transplant 6 Weeks Pregnant." CBS/AP, April 29,
2013. http://www.cbsnews.com/8301-204_162-57581959/woman-who-underwent
-2011-womb-transplant-6-weeks-pregnant/ (accessed April 30, 2013).

"Women in Elective Office 2013." Center for American Women and Politics fact sheet.
Eagleton Institute of Politics. Rutgers, the State University of New Jersey. http://
www.cawp.rutgers.edu/fast_facts/levels_of_office/documents/elective.pdf (accessed
September 9, 2013).

"Women Graduates Wait until They Hit 35 before Having Their First Child." *Daily Mail*,
October 21, 2012. http://www.dailymail.co.uk/news/article-2220918/Women
-graduates-wait-hit-35-having-child.html (accessed October 21, 2012).

"Women and Science: A Look at Harvard Pres. Larry Summers," January 25, 2005. http://
www.democracynow.org/2005/1/25/women_and_science_a_look_at (accessed May
4, 2012).

"Women Still Confront Yawning Wage Gap—Study." Reuters, April 17, 2012. http://www
.reuters.com/article/2012/04/17/wages-gender-gap-idUSL2E8FH9IC20120417
(accessed April 20, 2012).

"Women University Grads Waiting Longer to Have Children." My Fertility Choices,
November 5, 2012. http://myfertilitychoices.com/2012/11/women-university
-grads-waiting -longer-to-have-children/ (accessed December 10, 2012).

"Women Warned of Infertility Trap." *CNN Health*, April 11, 2002. http://archives.cnn
.com/2002/HEALTH/04/11/women.infertility/index.html (accessed March 7, 2012).

Wong, Edward. "Reports of Forced Abortions Fuel Push to End Chinese Law." *New York
Times*, July 22, 2012. http://www.nytimes.com/2012/07/23/world/asia/pressure-to
-repeal-chinas-one-child-law-is-growing.html (accessed July 29, 2012).

Woodruff, Leigh Ann. "Genetic Test to Predict IVF Egg Production in Older Women."
Fertility Authority, March 19, 2012. http://www.fertilityauthority.com/articles/genetic
-test-predict-ivf-egg-production-older-women (accessed April 3, 2012).

Woods, Vicki. "Sofia Vergara: Dangerous Curves." *Vogue*, March 2013. http://www.vogue
.com/magazine/article/sofia-vergara-dangerous-curves/ (accessed March 20, 2013).

"The World's Number of IVF and ICSI Babies Has Now Reached a Calculated Total
of 5 Million." ESHRE, July 2, 2012. http://www.eshre.eu/ESHRE/English/
Press-Room/Press-Releases/Press-releases-2012/5-million-babies/page.aspx/1606
(accessed July 13, 2012).

"World's Oldest Person Celebrates his 116th Birthday in Japan. Reuters, April 19, 2013.

http://www.reuters.com/article/2013/04/19/us-japan-oldest-idUSBRE93I0KB20 130419 (accessed May 8, 2013).

Wurtzel, Elizabeth. "1% Wives Are Helping Kill Feminism and Make the War on Women Possible." *Atlantic*, June 15, 2012. http://www.theatlantic.com/politics/ archive/2012/06/1-wives-are-helping-kill-feminism-and-make-the-war-on-women -possible/258431/ (accessed June 22, 2012).

Yang, Calvin. "Using Books to Build a Ladder Out of Poverty." *New York Times*, April 29, 2013. http://www.nytimes.com/2013/04/29/world/asia/using-books-to-build-a-ladder -out-of-poverty.html (accessed May 8, 2013).

Yoon, Soon-Young. In interview with the author, May 11, 2012.

Young, Craig. "Funding Cut Threatens Loveland-Based Program That Encourages Adoption of Frozen Embryos; Women Tell Adoption Stories." March 10, 2012. http:// www.reporterherald.com/news/loveland-local-news/ci_20149489/funding-cut -threatens-loveland-based-program-that-encourages (accessed February 6, 2013).

Zarembo, Alan. "An Ethics Debate over Embryos on the Cheap." *Los Angeles Times*, November 19, 2012. http://articles.latimes.com/2012/nov/19/local/la-me-embryo-20121120 (accessed December 7, 2012).

Zoll, Miriam. "Know What You're Doing If You Decide to Wait." *New York Times*, July 10, 2013. http://www.nytimes.com/roomfordebate/2013/07/08/should-women-delay -motherhood/know-what-youre-doing-if-you-decide-to-delay-childbirth (accessed July 12, 2013).

Zoll, Miriam, and Pamela Tsigdinos. "Selling the Fantasy of Fertility." *New York Times*, September 11, 2013. http://www.nytimes.com/2013/09/12/opinion/selling-the -fantasy-of-fertility.html?emc=eta1&_r=0 (accessed September 14, 2013).

INDEX

ABOUT THE AUTHOR

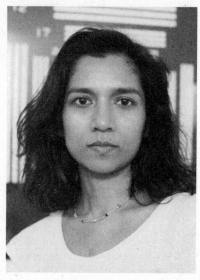

Tanya Selvaratnam is a writer, producer, actor, and activist. She has produced films by many directors and artists, including Gabri Christa, Chiara Clemente, Catherine Gund, Mickalene Thomas, Carrie Mae Weems, and Jed Weintrob; and has performed in shows by The Wooster Group and The Builders Association, among others. Tanya is also the Communications and Special Projects Officer for the Rubell Family Collection. As an activist, she has worked with the NGO Forum on Women, Ms. Foundation for Women, Third Wave Foundation, and World Health Organization. She received a BA in East Asian Languages and Civilizations, and an MA in Regional Studies–East Asia from Harvard University. Her master's thesis on the interplay of law and practice with regard to women's rights in China was published in the *Journal of Law and Politics*. She has been a fellow at Yaddo and Blue Mountain Center. Born in Sri Lanka and raised in Long Beach, California, Tanya now lives in New York City and Cambridge, MA. You can visit her personal site at http://tanyaturnsup.com and the book's website at http://www.thebigliebook.com.